OXFORD MEDICAL PUBLICATIONS

Women's Problems in General Practice

OXFORD GENERAL PRACTICE SERIES

Editorial Board

G. H. FOWLER, J. C. HASLER, J. HAYDEN, A.-L. KINMONTH, G. N. MARSH, M. ROLAND

Women's Problems in General Practice

THIRD EDITION

Oxford General Practice Series • 24

Edited by

ANN McPHERSON
General Practitioner, Oxford

Oxford   New York   Tokyo
OXFORD UNIVERSITY PRESS
1993

Oxford University Press, Walton Street, Oxford OX2 6DP
Oxford New York Toronto
Delhi Bombay Calcutta Madras Karachi
Kuala Lumpur Singapore Hong Kong Tokyo
Nairobi Dar es Salaam Cape Town
Melbourne Auckland Madrid
and associated companies in
Berlin Ibadan

Oxford is a trade mark of Oxford University Press

Published in the United States
by Oxford University Press Inc., New York

First edition © Ann McPherson and Anne Anderson, 1983
Second and third editions © Ann McPherson, 1987, 1993

First edition published 1983
Second edition published 1987
Third edition published 1993

A catalogue record for this book is available from the British Library

Library of Congress Cataloging in Publication Data
(Data available on request)
ISBN 0–19–262065–7

Typeset by Footnote Graphics, Warminster, Wilts
Printed and bound in Great Britain on acid-free paper by
Bookcraft Ltd, Midsomer Norton, Avon

Preface to the third edition

Interest in women's health problems has matured over the decade since the first edition of this book was published, and changing attitudes of society have forced the medical profession to pay more attention to this area. It can no longer be dismissed as a feminists' issue. Yes, we all have health problems, but, yes also, some of them are unique to women and need separate examination and explanation.

A rise of interest in women's health has also had a snowball effect of increasing awareness in those health problems that are unique to men, and a further book in this series is to be entitled *Men's problems in general practice*.

This, the third edition of *Women's problems in general practice*, continues to provide an up-to-date critical review of the management and treatment of the problems that women consult for at the primary care level. The book covers the major areas of women's health without trying to be rigidly comprehensive. Most of pregnancy, childbirth, and puerperal problems are dealt with in another book, as is the fast-changing subject of AIDS.

All the chapters have been updated or completely rewritten, and a new chapter on urinary incontinence has been included. I have once again avoided being rigid in the choice of authors and rather than choosing from a single group such as all GPs or all women, have instead sought those most appropriate both for their expertise in the subject and positive attitudes towards primary care. The preparation of this edition has raised further questions and revealed omissions which need to be addressed in the next edition: the involvement and views of practice nurses, and patients themselves, to highlight two. A section on controversies is included in the chapter on cervical screening. This has been well received by the reviewers of this edition. I hope that it will be possible to incorporate such a section in all chapters of the next edition.

I am indebted to the following people who have helped me enormously by their suggestions and general support: Angela Coulter, Jini Hetherington, Aidan Macfarlane, Alison Macfarlane, Klim McPherson, and Richard Peto.

The original volume was written and edited in conjunction with Anne Anderson. She died ten years ago, just as the first edition was published. I continue to miss her amusing and questioning cynicism about accepted medical practice, and this third edition still retains some of her thinking and deliberations.

Oxford   A.M.
November 1992

Contents

Contributors

Joan Austoker is the Director of the CRC Primary Care Education Group, University of Oxford Department of Public Health and Primary Care. She conducts research about breast and cervical screening, particularly relating to the role of primary care teams and the acceptability of screening programmes. She has published books for primary care on both breast and cervical screening.

Jean Coope graduated at Manchester University, entered general practice, and trained in family planning and cervical cytology. In the early seventies she carried out research into HRT in general practice. She has published many articles in medical journals and also a book for patients. Her pioneering clinic for menopausal women opened in January 1988. She lectures widely on the menopause and is the author of *Hormone replacement therapy* published by the Royal College of General Practitioners.

Lis Davidson trained in Nottingham and took some time travelling the country doing her VTS and then a variety of interim jobs (including working at Dublin Well Woman Clinic) before finally settling as Katy Gardner's 'other half' in a job share arrangement in a seven-doctor practice in Liverpool. With some of her 'other' time she works at Merseyside Brook.

Chris Freeman is a Senior Lecturer in Psychiatry and Consultant Psychotherapist in the Department of Psychiatry at Edinburgh University and the Royal Edinburgh Hospital. He runs a community-based out-patient and day-patient centre for individuals with a wide variety of 'neurotic disorders'. The unit has close links with community self-help groups and general practitioners. His current research interests include depressive disorders in general practice, eating disorders, and obsessive compulsive disorder.

Katy Gardner is currently a GP in inner-city Liverpool. She set up the first GP Well Woman Clinic in Liverpool, and her special interests are women's health and premenstrual syndrome (the latter both as a sufferer and as a doctor). She also works in Brook Advisory Centres.

Susanna Graham-Jones qualified from St Mary's Hospital Medical School, Paddington, in 1975, and then trained in psychiatry and general practice in Oxford. She has been a GP and lecturer in general practice in Liverpool since 1985, and is a member of Women in Medicine and the Women's Health Care Research Unit.

Jenny Griffiths pursued her early career in Public Health Departments in London and was very interested in epidemiology and the interface between health and social policy. She has been a Community Health Council Secretary. She then worked in health promotion and general health services planning at regional health authorities in London and Oxford. She is currently General Manager for Oxfordshire Family Health Services Authority, which has good links with primary care at all levels. Her interests are firmly rooted in the community health side of the NHS.

John Guillebaud is Medical Director of the Margaret Pyke Centre for study and training in family planning, and for the promotion of women's health in all respects. He is also a practising gynaecologist. During his training he worked as a locum in general practices, which gave him insight into the constraints of general practice. He is the author of numerous publications for the medical profession and the general public on population, birth control, and women's health issues. Professor of Family Planning and Reproductive Health, University College and Middlesex School of Medicine.

Keith Hawton works in Oxford as a Consultant Psychiatrist at the Warneford Hospital and also Clinical Lecturer in the University Department of Psychiatry. In addition to working as a general psychiatrist he has extensive research and clinical experience in the fields of sexual medicine, suicidal behaviour, and general hospital psychiatry. He has taken a particular interest in women's sexual disorders and their treatment, and is also involved in research into the outcome of depression in women. He has extensive research publications and is the author, co-author, or editor of seven books including the two Oxford University Press publications, *Sex therapy: a practical guide* and *Cognitive behaviour therapy for psychiatric problems: a practice guide*.

Jacqueline Jolleys is a Lecturer in General Practice at the University of Nottingham, and Medical Director of the Nottinghamshire Family Health Services Authority. Formerly a general practitioner in rural Leicestershire for fourteen years, she has a particular interest in the diagnosis and management of female urinary incontinence in general practice. She is on the steering committees of the British Association of Continence Care and the Association of Continence Advice Resource Centres.

Stephen Kennedy is a Clinical Lecturer/Senior Registrar in the Nuffield Department of Obstetrics and Gynaecology at the John Radcliffe Hospital in Oxford. His research interest is endometriosis and he is actively involved with the Endometriosis Society, an organization which helps women to understand the nature of their condition.

Ann McPherson works with four other partners in general practice in Oxford. She has, for many years, had a special interest in the health of women and teenagers. Her previous publications on women's health include *Cervical screening: a practical guide*, *Miscarriage*, and the first two editions of *Women's health problems in general practice*. Her books for teenagers, which include *Diary of a teenage health freak*, *I am a health freak too* and *Me and my mates*, introduce medical information for teenagers in a new fiction form. She represents the Royal College of General Practitioners on the Co-ordinating Cervical Screening Network, and lectures widely to GPs and students on women's health problems.

Richard Newton is a Senior Research Fellow and Senior Registrar in Psychiatry at the Royal Edinburgh Hospital. He has worked in the Mental Health Unit there for six years. As well as having an interest in eating disorders, he is involved in studies on psychiatric morbidity in street dwellers and the homeless in Edinburgh. He has recently been appointed Psychiatrist to the Eating Disorders Programme, Royal Melbourne Hospital, Australia.

Tom O'Dowd is a general practitioner in Nottinghamshire and a Senior Lecturer at Nottingham University. He has researched and published on both the urinary tract and bacterial vaginosis in general practice, and is a founder member of the British Association for Continence Care.

Catherine Oppenheimer is a Consultant Psychiatrist at the Warneford Hospital in Oxford. She has taught psychosexual counselling to general practitioners and family doctors. She is interested in the ethical issues of counselling and sexuality in old age.

Penny Owen is a Lecturer in General Practice at the University of Wales College of Medicine. She works as a general practitioner in a practice which for many years has carried out research into lower genital tract infections in women from the primary care perspective.

Moira Plant is a researcher in alcohol, drugs, and AIDS with the Alcohol Research Group in Edinburgh. She is a temporary consultant on women and alcohol to the World Health Organization. She is a group psychotherapist in the Alcohol Problems Clinic in Edinburgh. She has recently written a guide for general practitioners on how to take a drinking history.

Margaret Rees is the Parke Davis Fellow in the Nuffield Department of Obstetrics and Gynaecology at the John Radcliffe Hospital in Oxford, as well as a Supernumerary Fellow at St Hilda's College, Oxford. She has undertaken research into menstrual disorders and the menopause for over twelve years. She is also actively involved with the GP-led Primary Care Group in Gynaecology launched in February 1991 which aims to improve the quality of gynaecological care in family practice.

Diana Sanders is a research psychologist in the Department of Psychiatry of the University of Oxford. She has done research on the causes and treatment of premenstrual syndrome, and has experience in health education in primary care, including smoking cessation. She has a continuing interest in women's health, and is currently working on stress management.

Deborah Sharp is Senior Lecturer in General Practice at UMDS of Guy's and St Thomas's, and Honorary Senior Lecturer at the Institute of Psychiatry in the Section of General Practice and Epidemiology. She has been a partner in inner-city general practice for the last nine years. Her main research interest is psychiatry in primary care, particularly women's mental health. Recent studies include the epidemiology of childbirth-related emotional disorders, factors affecting the uptake of breast cancer screening, and the use of a computerized psychiatric interview in general practice.

Patti White was formerly Deputy Director of ASH and was a consultant on public information on tobacco for the World Health Organization's Regional Office for Europe before joining the Health Education Authority. She has a special interest in women and smoking, and is Convenor of the ASH Working Group on Women and Smoking, and Co-Chairperson for Europe for the International Union Against Cancer Tobacco Control Project.

1. Why women's health?

Ann McPherson

Although women live longer than men, they suffer more morbidity, take more drugs, see their GPs more often, and are more frequently admitted to hospital. Surely reason enough to look at specific aspects of women's health?

If further justification were needed, you need look no further than *The health of the nation* (Secretary of State for Health 1992), which has identified women's health as a specific issue. The Department of Health has published a booklet, *Your health: a guide to services for women* (DoH 1991). Cervical and breast cancer screening programmes are now well established in the UK. The problems are not just wombs and breasts; it is often forgotten that cardiovascular disease and lung cancer are the major causes of premature death in women. The overall causes of mortality and the relative risks from different causes are shown in Table 1.1, while Fig. 1.1 shows the mortality in 1989 from the most common cancers in the UK in men and women. The future will see changes. AIDS in the Western world is much commoner in men, but it is now increasing in women at a faster rate than in men, as it becomes established in the heterosexual community. Figure 1.2 shows the comparative causes of mortality between men and women.

Women may live longer, but with the extra years available comes the question of how worthwhile these years are. Neither men nor women want extra years of suffering or a twilight existence. Although expectation of life is going up for men and women, when active life between the sexes is analysed in greater detail, the 'gain' for women disappears. The expectation of life without disability for both men and women is increasing far

Table 1.1 *Approximate number of women in England and Wales who will die from the various causes listed (Beral, V., personal communication).*

	Before age 25	Before age 50	Before age 75
Breast cancer	1 in 100000	1 in 125	1 in 30
Lung cancer	1 in 100000	1 in 500	1 in 40
Heart attack	1 in 100000	1 in 250	1 in 12
Stroke	1 in 30000	1 in 300	1 in 30
Accidental death	1 in 500	1 in 200	1 in 100

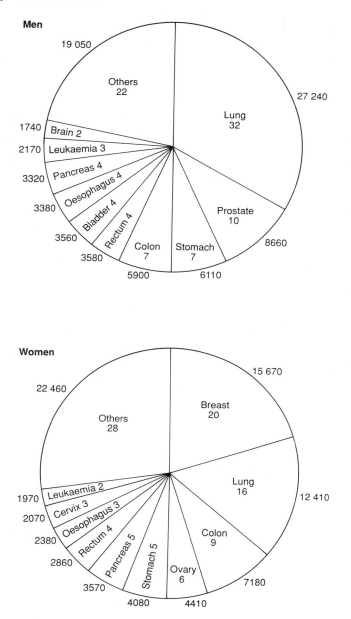

Fig. 1.1   Per cent mortality from the most common cancers in the UK in 1989. [From CRC 1991. Sources: Mortality statistics: cause, England and Wales 1989, HMSO (1991). Registrar General for Scotland, Annual Report 1989, Edinburgh (1990). Unpublished data, reproduced by kind permission of the General Register Office for Northern Ireland.]

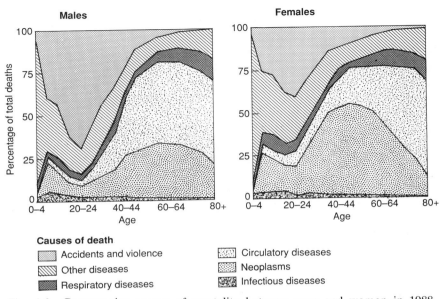

Fig. 1.2 Comparative causes of mortality between men and women in 1988. (From OPCS Mortality Statistics 1988.)

more slowly than is life expectancy, with 60 per cent of women over the age of 80 living alone. Because of this, some of the new agendas concern euthanasia and 'care of the elderly'. Both obviously will be of great concern to women.

HISTORY

The development of contemporary medical attitudes to women's health can be best understood within a historical and social context.

There have always been differences between the health problems of men and those of women, and even in primitive hunter–gatherer societies it is not difficult to imagine that the major causes of death would have been different for the different sexes. In more recent history much of the emphasis on women's health has concentrated on childbearing, but, with the advent of more effective contraception and the conquest of infection, the broader and more subtle aspects of women's, as against men's, health became apparent.

The last 150 years

The general health of both women and men has improved dramatically since the 1800s. The expectation of life at birth in 1841 for men was 40, and in 1987–89 it was 72; whereas for women in 1840 it was 42 and in 1988 it was 78.

The main cause of death in the 1800s, and even in the early part of this century, in both sexes, was infectious diseases. The heroines of novels and opera wasted away with consumption or tragically died in childbirth. Even as late as between 1921 and 1930, records show that tuberculosis accounted for 26 per cent of deaths in women under the age of 45 and that maternal mortality (mainly puerperal fever) over the same period and in the same age group accounted for 17 per cent of deaths. Many factors, both specific to women and general to both sexes, played a part in the eradication of these causes of death, particularly improvements in the general standards of living including better nutrition, improved housing, public health measures, more effective contraception, safer childbirth, the introduction of antibiotics, the treatment of anaemia, and various other medical advances.

From 1911 the Health Insurance Act entitled specific groups of working men and working women, depending on income, to the services of a panel doctor and free medicine. This, however, did not cover hospital treatment or give help to a dependant—other than a maternity grant to the working man's wife. For example, according to the 1911 census only 10 per cent of married women were working outside the home, so that health care facilities were not available to 90 per cent of married women unless they were paid for. It would be untrue to say that there were no free health care facilities for women working at home, as provision was made for advice to be given in the local authority or voluntary infant welfare clinics and municipal antenatal clinics which were being developed at this time. These were available to those who were pregnant or who had just had a baby. Women used these clinics, many not till later on in the pregnancy, for antenatal advice, but very few were seen for postnatal check-ups.

Further evidence concerning women's illnesses was provided by the Women's Health Enquiry Committee which in 1939 received over a thousand replies from working-class married women to a questionnaire sent out via health visitors. It was found that the ailments most mentioned were anaemia, headaches, constipation, rheumatism, gynaecological trouble, dental problems, varicose veins, and ulcerated legs. From the results, the Committee felt that only a third of women were in good health and that another third were actually in poor health. Although many women who replied had consulted a doctor, only a very small number (5 per cent) felt that they had received any 'health' teaching. A study looking at illness, incapacity, and medical attention among adults in 1947–49 (Logan 1950) reflected the official figures of the changing morbidity patterns immediately before and after the introduction of the National Health Service. The main difference between the years 1947–48 and 1948–49 was that medical consultation rates increased over the whole country.

The increase was 6 per cent for men under the age of 65 and 9 per cent for those over that age. For women the increases were much greater, 18 per cent for the younger age group and 22 per cent for the older women. Therefore there can be little doubt that before the start of the NHS many women failed to seek medical advice for economic reasons, but once the financial disincentive was removed they consulted their doctors more for the same relative amount of sickness. The NHS theoretically provides free health care for all, and although women are no longer discriminated against in the same direct economic way as prior to 1948, the continuing differences in the use of the health service facilities by different social classes give some indication of the complexities involved.

THE INFLUENCES OF FASHION AND FINANCES ON HEALTH

The classification of ailments raises the question of how society, and the individual within society, defines disease. Changing patterns of what has classically been considered pathological disease and the increasing medicalization of areas such as childbirth, sex, prevention, relationship problems, etc., are in part responsible for the relatively high rate at which women now attend the surgeries of general practitioners (see below). These changes have led to an increasing awareness of 'health fashions' which are based to a variable degree on new scientific evidence. Changes in fashion are particularly abundant in the area of women's health, and one example is the changing attitudes towards the menopause and premenstrual tension.

Although there is naturally little direct reference to such *risqué* areas in Victorian literature, it is possible that some characters, Mrs Nickleby, for instance were in fact menopausal. However, the lack of references to the menopause in literature may not only have been due to prudery but also to the fact that far fewer women succeeded in surviving long enough to experience it! Doctors were slow to accept menopausal symptoms as a problem to which they could offer any contribution until patients and the media forced them to take notice. In this atmosphere of increased awareness, the drug companies devoted themselves to producing and marketing suitable hormone therapy. Thus the interdependency of medical, pharmaceutical, and lay interests has encouraged the view that symptoms of the menopause are pathological. Nevertheless, permanent cessation of menstruation is something that happens to all women and cannot therefore in itself be classified as disease, though it is likely that some women will have symptoms which do need treatment. The symptoms themselves are not the only determining factor of therapy. As always in medicine they have to be balanced against the side-effects of the therapy used. Prevention of osteoporosis and heart disease, and prolongation of an active sexual life, by the use of hormone replacement therapy (HRT) is being presented by the drug companies as the only way forward for women in their middle years; an attitude challenged by others who have anxieties about increased risks of breast cancer, and cannot believe that it is the norm for all women to need hormone replacement. Unfortunately, the arguments are becoming polarized, with the ever printworthy Germaine Greer almost labelling some women as HRT wimps, while some doctors compare the use of HRT with 'needing to wear glasses' for age-onset presbyopia. Some women will undoubtedly benefit from hormone replacement, while others will suffer more than they gain. What is certain is the uncertainty that still remains.

SELF-HELP

In a perverse kind of way the knowledge of the side-effects of drugs used, for example in the treatment of the menopause, has led to the use of untried natural remedies for many disorders. There is a general misconception that the word 'natural', as in natural remedies, automatically means safe. However, this is clearly not so, for example it is possible to take an overdose of vitamin A, and some so-called natural diets are in fact deficient in some basic elements. Ginseng, vitamins, diets, herbs, homeopathy, and so on, though fashionable as natural remedies at the moment, have never been properly assessed either for their efficacy or for their side-effects. Nevertheless, it is likely that there are far more benefits than disadvantages in the movement towards self-help.

Self-help for women has always been an alternative to professional care but has recently become something of a growth industry. It is by no means new, and in the past it may have come from a similar impetus to the contemporary movement. There is a manuscript dating from 1500 published in 1981 under the title *Medieval woman's guide to health*. This was produced, as the editor comments, 'because women were dissatisfied with their treatment at the hands of male physicians and were endeavouring to instruct one another as to how to help women with their gynaecological problems'.

The publication of *Our bodies, ourselves* as a modern counterpart by a group of non-medical women in Boston in 1971 produced a focus for women on the possibilities and increased self-respect that self-help in health might offer them. The book challenged the idea that help was only the medical profession's prerogative—the authors all having experienced 'frustration and anger towards specific doctors and the medical maze in general'; and the basic aim was 'learning to understand, accept and be responsible for our physical selves'. In the United States the book rapidly became a bestseller but when the first English edition was published in the late 1970s it went unheralded. The difference in the reactions to the text and its philosophy in the two countries may in part have been because in the early 1970s American medicine, including family planning and child health, was almost entirely male-dominated (only 7 per cent of doctors were female), whereas in England there were relatively more women doctors (though they were still in the minority) and certainly in the areas of family planning and child health it was very likely that women patients would come into contact with female doctors.

This apparent predominance of interest by women in self-help in health is perhaps because in their role as carers and nurturers women have to be more sensitive to the emotional side of well-being—something that they obviously felt was sadly lacking in many of the medical services provided. The health areas in which women are able to support each other are many—as represented by such organizations as the Mastectomy Association, The National Childbirth Trust, The Postnatal Support Group, the UTI (Urinary Tract Infection) Club, etc. For a complex variety of reasons women predominate, both as users and as providers, whichever way health in the community is considered. With the continuing shortfall in NHS financing, self-help has now achieved official status, with the official title 'health practice and education'. Much of this is directed towards women who have the traditional role as the family carers.

CONSULTATION RATES

General practitioners see more women than men as patients and give them more medicine. Why is this? Who are these women? What illnesses do they have, and what medicines do they take?

There are, of course, more women than men in the community as a whole—the slightly larger number of males than females in the community up to the age of 45 being more than offset by the longevity of women. In England and Wales in 1990, of the 3.6 million individuals aged 75 or more, 63 per cent were women. Thus the diseases of ageing, for example dementia and cancer, will tend to be diseases affecting women.

Information on consultation rates comes from the General Household Survey (a continuous monitor of a random sample of the population), the Health and Lifestyle Survey, and the Third National Morbidity Survey done by a non-random set of general practitioners in 1980–81. Thus the consultation rates are collected in different ways and at different times and sometimes with different results. The National Morbidity Survey, now 10 years old, showed that 61 per cent of consultations with family doctors involve women. On average women visit their doctor six times per year, while for men it is four times per year, with 17 per cent of women and 12 per cent of men consulting in a two-week period prior to being questioned.

Although it may appear that women do consult their doctors more often than men, from the crude figures—and crude they are—it does also seem that women actually suffer more from disease and do not simply consult more often for each episode of illness. Much of the disease is 'gender related'. There was still a difference, but the differences between men and women were much smaller once consultations which were not for illness were removed; and virtually disappeared after consultations for pregnancy and childbirth and diseases of the male and female genito-urinary systems were excluded.

The reasons for which women and men consult their doctors also show differences. For instance, women consult more for endocrine/nutritional/ metabolic diseases, diseases of the blood and reproductive organs, mental disorders, diseases of the circulatory system, genito-urinary disorders, and muscular and connective tissue disorders. A further category of complaints entitled 'symptoms and ill-defined conditions' is twice as common in women. The only category for which consultation rates are commoner in males is accidents, poisoning, and violence. Consultation rates are roughly the same in both sexes for infectious and parasitic diseases, neoplasms, diseases of the nervous system (excluding mental disorders), diseases of the respiratory system, and disorders of the digestive system and of the skin, though in nearly all these female/male ratio slightly favours the females.

A further difficulty lies in interpretation of the consultation statistics because of the question of who deals with what problems where. For instance, the figures for consultation rates with general practitioners show that there are 139 consultations per 1000 women for genito-urinary problems compared with 29 per 1000 for men. The reasons for these consultations in women cover a wide range of problems such as menstrual irregularities, abortion, menopausal problems, vaginal discharge, etc. The equivalent problems in men, such as urethral discharge, are most likely to be dealt with in hospital venereal disease or genito-urinary clinics where female/ male ratio of attenders is 1:3, but obviously one is not comparing like with like.

Likewise, although, as already mentioned, many men will consult their GP for injuries, they are also more likely to go directly for treatment to hospital. Parents (usually women) have other sources of medical advice, such as child health clinics, which will not be documented as their own consultation. Those who run child health clinics well recognize that the problems they most frequently encounter, such as feeding problems, sleep problems, etc., have as much to do with the stresses and strains on women and parents in our present society as any actual illness in the child.

Consultation rates are, therefore, hardly an accurate reflection of illness. The GP is consulted for only one in 18 illness episodes, the rest being 'coped with' without formal medical consultation; while there is an average of 11 lay consultations for every medical consultation. This rate is a reflection of what patients and doctors consider as appropriate to be dealt with by the GP, and goes some way towards demonstrating the actual workload he or she has to deal with.

MEDICATIONS

If women appear to like their doctors' company then it is also clear that they consume a diet rich in pills, both prescribed and non-prescribed. The General Household Survey, for instance, showed that in a fortnight previous to the survey, half the women and a third of the men reported that they had taken prescribed medicine, and another study showed that twice as many women as men had treated themselves (17 per cent versus 8 per cent). This pattern did not apply to girls under the age of 15, where the reverse was true, so that one cannot conclude that early experience plays a significant role, although girls may see their mothers taking tablets as being a part of female adult life. However, a study in Oxfordshire in 1985 of 14-year-olds showed that 77 per cent of girls had taken medicines in the previous four weeks compared to 63 per cent of boys.

The prescribing practices of GPs can provide valuable information. A general practitioner-based study over three years (Jones *et al.* 1984) showed that twice as many women as men received psychotropic drug prescriptions, and women were three times as likely to have had a psychotropic drug as men, and other studies have shown similar patterns.

Thus women were not only prescribed drugs more often, the drugs were also prescribed for longer periods of time. It does seem that women are prescribed more medicine by their GPs but it is difficult to compare consultation rates and prescriptions as few studies relate symptoms to prescriptions for specific drugs.

Whether consultation rates and prescribing rates are linked or not, it does seem that women take more pills and it is difficult to find the reason, though obviously both patients and doctors are involved. Regular contact with services such as family planning, antenatal care, and child health clinics might encourage women to think of drug taking as acceptable. Further, women as shopper-consumers—at whom most advertisements are directed—have, in shops and elsewhere, more easy access to medicines, and women's magazines with their widespread circulation give further credence to the idea of taking medicines to cure certain ills. These ideas must remain speculative and do not give the full explanation. If they did, one would expect to see a more significant difference between the sexes in the self-medication rates compared with the prescribed rates, and the studies done in this area are conflicting. It may be that historically women have tended to take medicines and pills whereas men have taken alcohol. Laudanum and various other tonics containing psychotropic components might have been the mother's little helper of Victorian times, replaced now by diazepam and other such drugs: throughout this time beer drinking and the group psychotherapy camaraderie in the pubs and other leisure centres has probably been the equivalent medication available to men!

Perhaps doctors have a preconceived idea that the male patient should be able to cope without help and that the female 'being the weaker sex' needs the support of drugs. A quick glance through the drug advertising in medical journals still reinforces the picture of the downtrodden woman patient as a headachy, premenstrual, depressed person with chronic back-ache and lines of worldly care across her face, in obvious need of immediate help from her GP, probably in the form of a prescription.

ENVIRONMENT, SOCIAL CLASS, AND DISEASE

Women may be represented in advertisements in this way for good reason, and sociological studies have helped to give general practitioners insight into some of the environmental influences on the health of women. Brown and Harris (1978), for instance, looked at depression in a random sample of women in south London (there was no similar study for men), and their findings confirmed what had been for many GPs a clinical impression. They found that the incidence of depression was significantly greater in the lower social classes and identified certain vulnerability factors that preceded the depression. These included loss of mother in childhood, three or more children aged less than 14 living at home, lack of a confiding or intimate relationship with a husband or boyfriend, and lack of full- or part-time work. The effect of employment was especially interesting, as even when all the other factors were present, many more women developed depression if they did not have paid employment. This is a finding that is in line with more recent research and with the rising levels of unemployment has important implications for medical practice. Other important findings were that less than half the women with clinical symptoms of depression had seen their general practitioner, and very few of those who had were referred to a psychiatrist.

The differing standard mortality ratios in men by occupation and social class are well documented (for example, the Black Report 1980), but the implications of the differences for women have received less attention. For instance, why is cervical cancer in coalminers' wives so much higher than expected, even allowing for social class, and why is suicide so much higher than expected in doctors' wives? And not only do women appear to suffer from the effects of their husband's occupation, but also more directly from their own occupations and their own social class.

Data are now available to look directly at the effect of women's occupation on various disease processes. Social class differences in mortality, however, are best seen when married women are tabulated according to their husband's occupation rather than their own, so it is important that social class differences are looked at in both ways—by the husband's occupation and the woman's. The effect of social class is different according to whether the man or the woman is the main earner in the household—generally according to which rates the higher social class.

Some evidence for this is the apparent increase of spontaneous abortion rates in female anaesthetists, and the fact that women working in the textile industry appear to have a higher incidence of vascular disease. In the United States such findings have led to claims that certain occupations are closed to women, unless they agree to be sterilized, because of risks to a potential fetus. Almost all ill health and mortality is increased in social classes IV and V, a fact present from birth with the doubling of perinatal mortality in babies born to women of this class and the tripling of infant mortality rates in the same social class. Of course, classifications of social class are traditionally likened to a temperature taken with a thermometer—they tell you something is wrong without being able to define what it is; but the effects of social class on health permeate almost every aspect of health care.

General environmental influences, such as the effects of exercise, weight, etc., on coronary artery disease and the effects of smoking on the incidence of lung cancer, have also been examined more thoroughly in men than in women. Nevertheless, coronary artery disease is the significant cause of death in women (albeit less so than in men) and the quit rate among female smokers is less than that in male smokers. In 1950 women in Britain smoked half as many cigarettes as their male contemporaries, while in 1980 they smoked nearly as many and by 1990, in younger age groups, women smoked more than men. Not surprisingly, therefore, the rates of lung cancer in women are soaring. Attempts have been made to aim some of the anti-smoking health education programme specifically at women (usually only during pregnancy) with notable lack of success. Little attention has been paid to why there are differences in the changing smoking patterns in men and women, but recent information on smoking habits emphasizes the need for the general practitioner to use different tactics when counselling women and different methods with different groups of women.

Diet and exercise are two further areas where men and women behave in different ways. Obesity is twice as common in women as in men. The Health and Lifestyle Survey showed that there was little difference between the consumption of red meat and butter between men and women, but that in the 18–39 age group, twice as many males as females ate fried foods. Women generally attributed more importance to diet as an influence on health than men, but alas, many of us still remain fat!

There are signs from the General Household Survey that more women are taking part in sports and other physical activities than in previous years, but this still remains less than men. For instance, when asked about participation in the four weeks prior to interview, 24 per cent of women compared with 39 per cent of men had been active in an outdoor sport.

WOMEN DOCTORS, WOMEN PATIENTS

Women are not only the main users of the health service but are also, as nurses, midwives, health visitors, hospital ancillary staff, radiographers, physiotherapists, to a large extent the providers. On the other hand, the majority of doctors are men, but in 1991, for the first time, over 50 per cent of the medical student intake throughout the country were women. Few regional health authorities have addressed the problem of part-time training, and many have not yet faced up to the fact that a large part of their potential workforce will not continue training, or be available in specialties where they are needed, unless part-time working facilities and crèches/nurseries are provided. The Department of Health, in its recent report on opportunities for women doctors, showed that at consultant level, in all hospital medical specialties, only 15 per cent were women, which is much lower than might be expected given the previous percentage of female medical graduates.

Even in general practice, at 23 per cent women are still very under-represented as partners, though 45 per cent of trainees are women. Prior to 1990 the number of women general practitioners was increasing. The full effect of the new GP contract on women's employment in general practice is still unknown, but there are anxieties that it will make things worse rather than as stated that it will improve the situation. It is a matter of concern that the new requirement for a doctor to give 26 hours per week of patient contact fully distributed across the working week will be a disincentive to taking on new partners who want to work part-time.

The Institute of Manpower Studies (1990) found that only 59 per cent of married women with certified GP training had principal posts, compared to 85 per cent of married male GPs. More women GPs than men were dissatisfied with their current employment status. However, women doctors are more likely than other professional women to continue working once they have children. It is children that interfere with career achievement. Even in the age of the 'new man', full-time working women have an average of 17 hours a week less leisure time than men. The data on the outcomes of the effect of different types of childcare arrangements are conflicting. But it seems strange that in a profession that is producing evidence to show that there may be some adverse outcomes if a child is in childcare for more than 20 hours a week in the first year of life, so little is being done to enable women doctors (or any other women in the health service) to fulfil their potential by appropriate part-time training schemes and career posts.

Some will argue against equal opportunities as a philosophy. But even if this line is taken, it is hard to argue against the wishes of patients who want to see a woman doctor. The Women's National Commission, an advisory committee to Her Majesty's Government, carried out a survey in 1984. Of 5850 respondents, 72 per cent felt that women should be offered the choice of seeing a female or male doctor for hospital treatment. This figure rose to 90.4 per cent in the 16–24 age group, and 74 per cent in the over-65 age group. However, at that time only three of the health authorities answering the questionnaire could offer such a choice. For preference of the sex of their general practitioner 18.3 per cent of the respondents chose a female doctor, rising to 35.6 per cent among the 16–24 age group. 74.2 per cent said they had no preference (with some explaining that they had never had a female doctor and therefore no experience from which to make a choice), while 7 per cent had a preference for a male doctor. 42 per cent expressed a preference for a female GP when needing advice on menstrual, gynaeco-logical or mammary problems, 36 per cent for family planning, and 25 per cent for maternity care. The main reasons given for wanting a woman GP were that: (a) as a woman she would have a better understanding of women's problems (82 per cent); and (b) a female doctor would be easier and less embarrassing to talk to (70.5 per cent).

A recent survey (1990) commissioned by the National Council of Women looked at womens views of doctors. 78 per cent of all the women surveyed expressed a preference to consult a woman doctor, but there was a difference according to age, with 87 per cent of 15–24 year-olds experiencing a preference. In 1990 Graffy found that more than half the women patients attending a south London practice preferred to see a woman GP for specific problems, and nearly four out of 10 wanted to see a woman doctor on every visit to the surgery. The majority of men did not feel the doctor's sex mattered. Figures for April 1991 reveal that in almost half the practices in England, that is, in 4386 partnerships, patients do not have access to a woman doctor (Newman 1992).

Women doctors see more female patients than male. Cartwright and Anderson (1981) found that, whereas in 1964 75 per cent of women doctors' patients were women, this had decreased to 60 per cent by 1977. There is so much written about women, be they doctors, patients, lawyers, or whatever, perhaps the most surprising finding in Ann Cartwright's study is that there was very little overall difference between the male and female general practitioners in their attitudes and behaviour towards women patients, although this may have something to do with the type of training doctors go through. A study in one group practice looked at consultation patterns of male and female partners (two male and two female). There was no truth in the myth that the woman doctor did not pull her weight with regard to the number of consultations carried out. The women partners had a slightly higher, or at least an equal, consultation rate than their male colleagues; doctor-initiated appointments were higher for women patients of women doctors than for their male patients; of the men consulting a woman doctor, younger rather than older men chose to consult; and patients chose to consult a doctor of their own sex not only for sex-specific disorders but also for conditions which were not sex linked.

CONCLUSION

I have, in this introduction, presented some ideas influencing women's health in general, but also more specifically in relation to general practice. It was obvious to me, when reviewing the facts available, that they are open to many interpretations. Nevertheless, I hope that the issues raised provide a background for the chapters of this book which deal in large part with the more specific problems for which women consult their general practitioners. Just as it has been traditionally necessary for a surgeon to be aware of the female/male differences in the anatomy, with the increasing specialist training, especially now for general practice, it has become essential that the more subtle female/male differences in behaviour and psychological attitudes towards disease should also be taught and learnt.

Many changes are taking place in the health service. It is an ideal opportunity to monitor what is the best and most sensitive way of giving care. Women are not asking for a separate health care system, but within a comprehensive system there needs to be evaluation of the outcomes of alternative ways of offering care within the primary health care system.

REFERENCES AND FURTHER READING

Black, D. (1980). *Inequalities in health*. Report of a Research Working Group. Department of Health and Social Security, London.

Brown, G. and Harris, T. (1978). *Social origins of depression*. Tavistock Publications, London.

Cartwright, A. and Anderson, R. (1981). *General practice revisited*. Tavistock Publications, London.

Cooke, M. and Ronalds, C. (1985). Women doctors in urban general practice: the patients. *British Medical Journal*, **290,** 753–4.

Department of Health (1991). *Your health: a guide to services for women*. O/N 13916 (HSSH) J1299NJ. DoH, London.

Dunnell, K. and Cartwright, A. (1972). *Medicine takers, prescribers and hoarders*. Routledge & Kegan Paul, London.

Fry, John (1979). *Common diseases* (2nd edn). MTP, Lancaster.

Gold, E. B. (1984). *The changing risk of disease in women. An epidemiological approach*. Collamore Press, Toronto.

HMSO (1980). *Social trends*. HMSO, London.

Jones, L., Simpson, D., Brown, A. C., *et al*. (1984). Prescribing psychotropic drugs in general practice: three year study. *British Medical Journal*, **289** 1045–8.

Leeson, J. and Gray, J. (1978). *Women and medicine*. Social Science Paperbacks. Tavistock Publications, London.

Logan, W. P. D. (1950). Illness, incapacity and medical attention among adults, 1947–49. *Lancet* **i**, 773–6.

Macfarlane, Alison (1990). Official statistics and women's health and illness. In *Women's health counts* (ed. Helen Roberts). Routledge, London.

Medial and dental staffing prospects in the NHS in England and Wales 1988. *Health Trends 1989* **21**, 99–106.

Morrell, D. C. and Wale, C. J. (1976). Symptoms perceived and recorded by patients. *Royal College of General Practitioners*, **26**, 398–403.

National Council of Women (1990). *Are we fit for the 90s?* National Council of Women, London.

Newman, L. (1992). Second among equals. *British Journal of General Practice*, **42**, 71–4.

Preston-Whyte, M. E., Fraser, R. C., and Beckett, J. L. (1983). Effect of a principal's gender on consultation patterns. *Journal of the Royal College of General Practitioners*, **255**, 654–8.

Report of a Women's National Commission Ad Hoc Working Group (1984). *Women and the health service*.

Rowland, Beryl (ed.) (1981). *Medieval woman's guide to health*. Croom Helm, London.

RCGP (Royal College of General Practitioners) (1979). *Trends in general practice*. Royal College of General Practitioners, London.

Secretary of State for Health (1991). *The health of the nation*. Cm. 1523. HMSO, London.

Silman, A. J. (1987). Why do women live longer and is it worth it? *British Medical Journal*, **May,** 1311.

Skegg, D. C. G., Doll, R., and Perry, J. (1977). Use of medicines in general practice. *British Medical Journal*, **1**, 1561–3.

Wells, M. (1987). *Women's health today*. Office of Health Economics, London.

2. Breast cancer and benign breast disease

Joan Austoker and Deborah Sharp

INTRODUCTION

Breast cancer is by far the most common type of cancer in women, accounting for 21 per cent of all new female cases. Overall in the UK it is estimated that about one in 12 women will develop the disease at some stage in their life. A diagnosis of breast cancer is likely to herald the onset of significant physical and psychological difficulties for the patient, as well as gloom and despair in her family and carers. Although our understanding of breast cancer has increased enormously over the last two decades and treatment has become more rational, progress is slow and improvement in case survival modest.

Breast diseases of all sorts account for a substantial number of consultations each year in general practice. The Third National Morbidity Survey (RCGP/OPCS/DHSS 1986) reported all ages consultation rates per thousand women at risk of 9.7 for breast cancer, 2.3 for benign neoplasms, 7.3 for fibroadenosis and other dysplasias, and 10.8 for other miscellaneous conditions of the breast—a total of 30.1. This compares with rates of 12.9 for dysmenorrhoea, 16.0 for premenstrual syndrome, and 22.6 for menopausal symptoms.

This chapter focuses equally on both breast cancer and the management of benign breast disease since the latter forms the majority of the consultations for breast symptoms in general practice and as such constitutes a large cost to the NHS in terms of medical, nursing, and administrative time. It is also a cause of a great deal of anxiety in the women who have these symptoms. We begin by considering the epidemiology of breast cancer and the strategies available to promote its early diagnosis. We then discuss the management of a woman who presents with symptoms of breast disease, including information on examining the breasts. The general management of benign breast disease is considered in some detail. This is followed by sections dealing with the diagnosis and treatment of both early and advanced breast cancer. We conclude with a consideration of the adverse effects of treatment and the psychological aspects of breast cancer.

EPIDEMIOLOGY

The size of the problem

Each year in the United Kingdom, 26 000 women are newly diagnosed with breast cancer and nearly 16 000 die from it (CRC Factsheet 6, 1991). Breast cancer is the leading cause of female cancer death in the UK. Moreover, it is the commonest single cause of death in women aged 35 to 54 years. The UK is in the unenviable position of having the highest breast cancer mortality rate world-wide. Between the late 1950s and early 1970s mortality in women aged 15 to 44 increased by 16 per cent, but since then it has shown a slight decrease. However, in older age groups it has continued to show a slight increase. Incidence rates have changed little in women aged under 55 over the past decade, but in older women there has been a slight increase.

The aetiology of breast cancer

Many studies of the aetiology of breast cancer have been reported and a vast literature exists on the subject. Only a very brief review will be given here. More comprehensive information can be found in Henderson *et al.* (1984), and Mant and Vessey (1991).

Family history

A woman with a first-degree relative (mother or sister) with breast cancer is herself at an increased risk. The relative risk among relatives of women with unilateral breast cancer is of the order of a two- to threefold increase. The risk is likely to be greater if the index case developed premenopausal breast cancer, and greatest in relatives of those with bilateral premenopausal breast cancer.

Medical history

The risk of developing a second primary breast cancer after a first is reported to be up to five times the general risk and is inversely related to age at presentation of the first primary cancer. Primary ovarian or endometrial cancer is also associated with an increase in risk, but the risk is probably less than twice that of the general population.

The cancer risk of benign breast disease is in general very low. Fibrocystic disease, commonly diagnosed in middle-aged women, is associated with about a twofold increase in the risk of breast cancer. The excess risk is particularly associated with epithelial hyperplasia lesions. Moderate or florid hyperplasia without atypia is thought to carry a slightly increased risk (1.5- to twofold) and lobular or ductal hyperplasia with atypia (which are rare) show a moderate increase in risk (four- to fivefold) (Dupont and Page

1991). In fibroadenoma, diagnosed most frequently in young women, any associated increase in breast cancer risk is less well established.

Particular mammographic patterns (Wolfe patterns) may also be interpreted as describing a type of benign breast disease associated with an increased risk of breast cancer. There is some evidence of a two- to threefold increase in risk in women whose mammograms show dysplasia or a greater than normal amount of prominent ducts.

Menstrual factors

An early onset of menarche is associated with a twofold or less increase in breast cancer risk. This effect decreases with age and is small after the menopause. A recent study has found that breast cancer cases established regular menstrual cycles more rapidly than controls, and that the combination of early menarche (age 12 years) and early establishment of regular cycles (within one year of menarche) was associated with a more than threefold increase in risk (Henderson *et al.* 1981).

For individual women, menopause before the age of 45 leads to a twofold reduction in risk compared with menopause occurring after age 55. Artificial menopause induced by medical treatment has a protective effect similar to that of natural menopause.

These findings all indicate a positive association between the number of menstrual cycles and the risk of breast cancer. The possible carcinogenic role of oestrogen has been widely explored. Other hormones have also been investigated but the precise relationship between endogenous hormones and breast cancer risk remains unclear.

Reproductive factors

An early full-term pregnancy has an important protective effect. Women who deliver their first child before age 20 have approximately half the risk of breast cancer of nulliparous women, or of women whose first child is born when they are aged 30 to 35 years. The risk is highest in women whose first full-term pregnancy occurs after the age of 35 years. Parity is associated with age at first birth, but there is some evidence that high parity may provide some additional protection.

The protection gained from an early first pregnancy only exists if the pregnancy continues to term. Two recent studies have suggested that first trimester abortion before first full-term pregnancy is associated with a substantial increased risk of breast cancer, but this finding has not been replicated in other studies. Abortions after the first full-term pregnancy do not carry any increased risk.

The independent effect of lactation on risk remains a subject of continuing debate. A protective effect of lactation has recently been reported in two studies (McTiernan and Thomas 1986; Byers *et al.* 1985).

Exogenous hormones

Recently, several case control studies have reported an association between oral contraceptive usage at a young age and breast cancer (e.g. UK National Case–Control Study Group 1990). These studies are by no means unanimous as several other studies seem to show no association. There is the possibility that there is an adverse effect when combined oral contraceptives are taken for long periods at a very early age or before the first full-term pregnancy. At older ages there is no evidence of an increased risk and recently there has been the suggestion of a slight reduction in risk. The subject remains controversial—we cannot say yet whether the Pill is or is not implicated in breast cancer causation (McPherson and Doll 1991). Among the problems to be confronted are the relatively recent widespread use of oral contraceptives, the possibility of a longer latent interval between oral contraceptive use and the onset of cancer, and the changing oestrogen and progestogen content of oral contraceptive preparations over the past two decades.

The relationship between HRT and breast cancer remains controversial. The majority of studies, especially the more recent, suggest some increase in risk of breast cancer with long-term use of oestrogens (a relative risk of approximately 1.5 after 15 years' use) (Vessey 1984; McPherson and Doll 1991). It is important to note that most of the information relates to oestrogen on its own. Unfortunately there is virtually no data on the effects of combined oestrogen/progestogen usage and, in view of the probable latent period of 10 to 20 years, it may be some time yet before conclusive data become available about the forms of HRT now in common use in the UK.

Weight, diet, and alcohol

Most studies indicate that breast cancer risk is directly proportional to relative weight, with obese women experiencing an increased risk of 1.5 to twofold. This increased risk is restricted to postmenopausal women.

The issue of diet as a cause of breast cancer has been dominated by fat. Some have judged the evidence convincing enough to warrant dietary recommendations, others find the evidence very weak (for a review, see Kinlen 1991). Population correlation studies have suggested that animal fat or meat consumption may be of primary importance in determining breast cancer risk. However, individual case controls studies have provided only very weak evidence confirming this finding and a large prospective study of nurses has failed to show any relationship between fat intake and subsequent breast cancer during the first four years of follow-up.

The relationship between alcohol consumption and breast cancer is still the subject of debate.

Ionizing radiation

There is direct evidence of the carcinogenic effect of radiation on breast cancer risk, both from Japanese atomic bomb survivors and from women exposed to high doses of ionizing radiation for the treatment of mastitis and TB. The extent of risk is directly proportional to the radiation dose and inversely proportional to the age of the woman at the time of exposure.

This relationship has raised anxieties about the use of mammographic screening. However, the probability of a middle-aged woman developing breast cancer as a result of a single mammographic examination is very low—one in 2 000 000. This risk is far outweighed by the potential benefits of screening (see below).

Non-risk factors

A number of factors have been considered as possible indicators of breast cancer risk but should now be considerd as 'non-risk factors'. These include exposure to diazepam and hair dyes, and the occurrence of cholecystectomy and thyroid disease. Importantly, cigarette smoking is a non-risk factor, but this does *not* imply that it is a protective factor.

EARLY DIAGNOSIS OF BREAST CANCER

Based on the present somewhat inadequate understanding of the aetiology of breast cancer, the scope for primary prevention is limited. At present strategies for early diagnosis are considerd more promising, based on the belief that these will improve the outlook for a woman with breast cancer. The inference is that, for the vast majority of women presenting with early stage disease, the cancer will be confined to the breast. Although this proposition is intuitively attractive, the belief that breast cancer spreads in a step-wise manner from a primary tumour to regional lymph nodes and then to distant sites is now out-moded. Even in women presenting with so-called 'early' stage disease, the cancer can either be confined to the breast or else already be disseminated via vascular and lymphatic channels more or less simultaneously.

Breast cancer is almost unique in that distant metastases may occur almost from the date of the inception of the cancer, yet remain occult for several decades before becoming clinically apparent. Lymph node involvement is a marker of a spreading tendency rather than the first step in a sequence of events. The probability of developing distant metastases is unaffected by treatment of lymphatic pathways.

Despite the biological complexity of breast cancer, there is a considerable body of evidence that early diagnosis *does* confer benefits. This is a matter of probabilities rather than certainties. Thus, while there may be a general benefit to the population, this cannot necessarily be taken to confer benefit to each individual, providing obvious difficulties for general practitioners in that the potential for benefit cannot be translated with certainty into individual terms.

The probability of haematogenous dissemination does correlate closely with tumour size. Invasive cancers detected when less than 2 cm are less likely to have metastasized to local lymph nodes or distant sites than larger tumours. Non-invasive or very small invasive tumours are generally regarded as constituting 'early stage' disease. The stage at which a woman has her breast cancer diagnosed greatly influences her survival chances. Generally speaking the earlier the breast cancer is diagnosed, the better are the survival rates (see Table 2.1). By identifying tumours earlier in their evolution, effective treatment is expected to be curative in a greater proportion of women. This is the basis of population-based screening discussed below.

Table 2.1   *Breast cancer stage and 5-year relative survival*

Stage	Description	% 5-year relative survival
I	Small mobile tumour less than 2 cm and confined to the breast. No lymph node involvement.	84
II	As I, but with some nodal involvement, or larger tumours (2 to 5 cm) with or without nodal involvement. No known distant metastases.	71
III	Locally advanced tumour possibly attached to the chest wall. Nodal involvement. No known distant metastases.	48
IV	Distant metastases present.	18
All stages		63

Source: CRC Factsheet 6 (1991).

Breast cancer screening

As has just been stated, there is considerable potential for reducing population mortality from breast cancer by a systematic approach to improving the stage at presentation by early detection. About 70 to 80 per cent of screen-detected cancers may have a good prognosis. At the initial screen up to 20 per cent of cancers may be *in situ*, a further 20 to 25 per cent are likely to be invasive lesions under 1 cm in diameter, and another 25 per cent will be between 1 and 2 cm.

Breast screening by mammography is the only cancer screening method for which the value has been demonstrated quantitatively by rigorous randomized trials (Day 1991). There have in addition been a number of non-randomized population-based breast screening trials. For women aged 50 years and over at entry into the trial, all trials show a reduction in breast cancer mortality although the results are not statistically significant in all cases. The randomized trials show a reduction in breast cancer mortality ranging from 20 to 40 per cent, and the design of these trials has been such as to avoid the problems of bias. The non-randomized geographic and case control studies, while not avoiding the problems of bias, support the concept that a significant benefit can be derived from mammographic screening. For women under the age of 50, no significant mortality reduction has yet been demonstrated.

For women aged 50 and over, the results are encouraging. However, central to any debate on the merits of breast screening is a consideration of the benefits versus the adverse effects. In all considerations of its efficacy, the most important factor to be taken into account is whether and by how much screening can reduce the very high mortality from breast cancer, and if so at what costs. If the costs are too high (human as well as economic), the benefits are marginalized. The acceptability of screening to women, the accuracy of diagnosis, the safety and frequency of the screening tests, the potential for 'over-diagnosis' and therefore over-investigation, anxiety and unnecessary morbidity in 'false positives', the availability of effective treatment, and the economics of the whole process, must be taken into account.

Since March 1988, health authorities in the UK have been phasing in the National Breast Screening Programme. A nationwide service was established by 1991 and by the end of 1994 all eligible women should have received an invitation to be screened. The aim of the programme is to reduce mortality from breast cancer through early diagnosis by mammography. Routine screening is being offered to all women aged 50 to 64 years. Women aged 65 and over may be screened on request but not more than once every three years. Women under 50 are not being offered routine screening as mammography has not been shown to be of benefit in this age group. Screening by single oblique view mammography is taking place at an initial frequency of three years. These guidelines are being kept under review and are the subject of national research trials which are now in progress.

Ideally, all eligible women from a whole general practice should be screened once every three years rather than screening a third of the women from a practice each year, or smaller groups on a continuous basis. Screening by whole practice allows publicity to be concentrated in a specific area, providing better information to primary care teams and women.

For the National Breast Screening Programme to be successful the contribution and co-operation of primary care teams is essential (Austoker

1990*a*; 1990*b*). Primary care teams can help to improve the quality of the programme, increase uptake, and provide information and counselling related to all aspects of the programme. Good communication between practices and the screening office will ensure that practices are well prepared in advance, understand the procedures, and know the time schedule for the entire screening process.

An abnormal result will create anxiety, and general practitioners can help in allaying fears, although most often in the breast screening programme these fears and anxieties are being dealt with by the staff at the assessment centre. Women may wish their GPs to provide further information about the implications of a result that requires further investigation. It is important for GPs to appreciate the complexity and limitations of mammography and the corresponding need to call back a number of women who will subsequently be found to be normal. It is equally important, however, not to provide false reassurance at this stage. GPs will need to be able to explain the range of diagnostic techniques that are available and what these may entail. Most women who have abnormal mammograms will be found to be normal on assessment and will rejoin the routine recall system. Some women will have cancer diagnosed by fine needle aspiration cytology and will not need a biopsy. A few may require a biopsy to allow a firm diagnosis or exclude the possibility of cancer. The GP should be notified as soon as the need for a biopsy is identified.

If a woman is found to have breast cancer her GP will be informed and asked to refer her for treatment. A woman may be referred to the surgeon from the specialist team, or the GP in consultation with the woman may wish to arrange alternative referral.

GPs, practice nurses, and health visitors are in an ideal position to discuss breast screening with non-attenders, either when the woman next consults or directly by contacting non-attenders to offer further information and advice. If the woman has fears and anxieties these need to be carefully explored. Ultimately women have the right to choose not to participate in the screening programme. They should have access to accurate information to enable them to arrive at an informed decision. It is important not to create feelings of guilt or inadequacy by this process.

The National Breast Screening Programme has, to date, exceeded the short-term quality standards which have been set for the programme as a whole. The ultimate aim of the programme is clear and unambiguous—to reduce mortality from breast cancer. It will be some years before the success of the programme in meeting this aim can be determined. Current estimates suggest that by the year 2000 the screening programme can be expected to reduce death from breast cancer by approximately 25 per cent in the population of women invited for screening provided that 70 per cent of these women attend. This should result in a reduction of 1250 breast cancer deaths each year in the UK.

Breast self-examination (BSE)

The role of routine breast self-examination following a set technique is controversial. In the past BSE has been advocated as a means of promoting the early diagnosis of breast cancer, both as an adjunct to screening and as a technique in its own right. To date, 14 studies of BSE have been conducted. None of these has shown a reduction in breast cancer mortality in women carrying out BSE compared with controls. Eight of these studies showed somewhat more favourable tumour characteristics in BSE performers than controls, but as none of the studies was randomized, the results are subject to a number of biases. This means that any differences in stage observed in BSE performers does not guarantee a survival benefit.

The BSE studies show low positive predictive values for presented breast lumps. This means that only a small proportion of women with a 'positive' test result will on further investigation be shown to have breast cancer. All studies to date have experienced difficulty in achieving good acceptance rates. Evidence about the effectiveness of different approaches to BSE instruction is inadequate and conflicting. There is also considerable variation and inconsistency in suggested techniques, both between studies and, on occasion, within studies.

The 10-year update of the UK Trial of Early Detection of Breast Cancer shows no overall reduction in breast cancer mortality in the combined BSE districts compared with the comparison districts (Chamberlain 1991, personal communication). A USSR/WHO randomized study of BSE in over 120 000 women, currently under way in Leningrad, has shown no difference at five years in the cancer detection rate between BSE performers (3.15 cancers/1000 women) and controls (3.19 cancers/1000 women) (Semiglazov 1991). Comparison of women from both groups with regard to the size of the primary tumour and the incidence of metastatic lesions in the regional lymph nodes showed no difference. The BSE group showed a higher frequency of visits to doctors with breast complaints, a higher rate of referral for further investigation, and a higher number of excision biopsies due to a benign lesion.

The practice of routine BSE may cause a number of problems for women. It may raise anxiety in that women associate its practice with breast cancer, thereby stimulating rather than allaying fears. Many women may be reluctant to touch and examine their own breasts. If BSE is promoted in accordance with a formal procedure and a particular technique, women may worry that they are not doing it correctly, or that they have forgotten to do it on the 'right day'. If they are unfamiliar with the changes in their normal breast tissue, they may be alarmed by the lumpy nature of normal premenopausal breasts. BSE practice may also lead to a high number of unnecessary investigations and biopsies.

BSE is therefore a procedure for which there is only fragmentary evidence of benefit and, furthermore, which only a small minority of women practice despite a high awareness of its existence. There is currently no evidence to support the view that BSE should be regarded as a primary screening technique, nor that it should be conducted on a routine basis following a set technique which requires formal instruction. However, most breast cancers are found by women themselves, and we need to optimize the chances of them doing so. Accordingly, in the UK a more general breast awareness is being encouraged, based on knowing what is normal, knowing what changes to look out for, and, above all, encouraging the prompt reporting of any such changes. A new leaflet, *Be breast aware*, has been produced. GPs and practice nurses will play an important role in facilitating the raising of breast awareness. The four major symptoms with which women present are discussed in detail on pp. 28–34.

Reducing the delay in obtaining diagnosis and treatment

Reducing the delay between the onset of symptoms of breast cancer and definitive treatment is likely to have important consequences in terms of lowering the overall mortality from breast cancer. It has been estimated that approximately 20 per cent of women with symptoms of breast cancer delay seeking advice for three months or more (Williams *et al*. 1976). It has been suggested that delay among British women in consulting about breast symptoms may well be contributing to the very high mortality rate in Britain (Ellman 1989). In Sweden where women report promptly with symptoms, and where screening trials have had a very high uptake, the ratio between breast cancer mortality and incidence is reported to have decreased from 60 per cent in 1960 to 36 per cent in 1982–4. Unfortunately the corresponding figure for Britain at present is 63 per cent. In Norway it is reported that only 9 per cent of women have locally advanced disease when breast cancer is first diagnosed, in the USA 11 per cent. By contrast in 1990 in Edinburgh in the control population for the UK Trial of the Early Detection of Breast Cancer this was 35 per cent, little different from a decade previously.

The delay in presentation of breast symptoms for consultant investigation has been described in several series of patients (Adam *et al*. 1980; Nichols *et al*. 1981). The characteristics of these patients is not well understood, but denial is a common strategy employed by women. Most often this takes the form of suppression rather than frank denial. While some women are genuinely ignorant of the sinister implications of their symptoms, the majority understand their symptoms, but are characterized by a diversity of beliefs and behaviour including an overwhelming fear of doctors, hospitals, illness in general, and cancer in particular (Fallowfield 1991). Several studies report that delayers are generally older women of lower socio-economic class, less well educated than non-delayers, more depressed or anxious, and more pessimistic about the treatment or fearful of the consequences of surgery (Greer 1974; Williams *et al.* 1976). Whatever the case, the underlying reasons for delay are likely to be complex and by no means entirely due to the woman. Delay also occurs after the general practitioner consultation. This may be for a variety of reasons including delay in referral, delay in reaching a diagnosis, and delays due to waiting times for hospital admission for treatment. Delay at any stage is also likely to occur when the presenting symptoms differ from the 'painless lump', despite the fact that a significant proportion of breast cancers may not present in this stereotyped way. This reinforces the need to raise a better awareness of what changes to look out for and what to do if such changes are found.

CONSULTATION WITH A WOMAN WITH BREAST SYMPTOMS

The most important aspect of management for any patient presenting with a problem related to the breast is to exclude cancer through accurate diagnosis and in so doing provide effective reassurance to the patient. It is not only women presenting with a lump who are anxious about the possibility of breast cancer. Other symptoms such as pain, nipple discharge, nipple retraction, or other skin changes may be equally potent in causing anxiety with respect to the possibility of malignant disease being the underlying cause. Furthermore, the level of anxiety induced by breast symptoms may in some women be of such magnitude as to impede their ability to seek medical help. These women may present to their general practitioner with a hidden agenda offering some totally unrelated reasons for consultation. Alternatively, denial may take over and women with a symptom that does eventually turn out to be due to cancer, delay so long that their prognosis is adversely affected (Phelan *et al.* 1991).

Thus all women who present to their GP with a lump or other symptom related to their breasts should be seen without delay in order to exclude cancer where possible and thus alleviate anxiety. If there is any doubt in the GP's mind as to the cause of the problem, prompt diagnostic procedures or referral can then be instituted.

The consultation process for a women with breast symptoms

As with all presenting complaints, the first essential is for the doctor to take an appropriate history. The age and menstrual status of the patient should be noted together with an accurate account of the symptoms including when the woman first noticed them. A family history of breast disease should be ascertained, as should information about whether the patient is taking any hormonal preparation (oral contraceptive or HRT) as well as other drugs such as antidepressants, antihypertensives, H2 receptor antagonists, or opiates. Any fluctuation in the size of lumps and associated pain during the menstrual cycle should be discovered. If there is a nipple discharge, questions as to its nature should be asked. A carefully taken history will begin to shape one's 'index' of suspicion. Age plays an important part in this, as breast lumps are increasingly likely to be malignant as the age of the patient increases, but stereotypes can be misleading. Breast cancer may be present in women who present with a symptom other than the typical painless lump. A woman in her twenties with a lump, with or without pain, may indeed have cancer. And a woman may present for the first time with symptoms due to metastatic breast cancer—such as anaemia, unexplained backache, or other generalized symptoms.

Examination of the breasts

As far as clinical examination is concerned, the main objective is to determine whether or not a mass is in fact present. To this end, the breasts should always be examined systematically. Inspection of the breasts, with the woman sitting facing the doctor, may reveal a change in outline, size or shape of the breast and puckering or dimpling of the skin or nipple. These changes are accentuated if the patient presses her hands on her hips. Any pain or discomfort associated with a lump should be ascertained.

Palpation of the breasts should be carried out with the flat of the fingers in a systematic fashion so that each part of the breast is examined. Some people prefer to do this in a spiral fashion working from the nipple outwards, others quadrant by quadrant. The periphery and axillary tail must not be forgotten—the latter being best examined with the patient's arm by her side. If the lump that the patient is complaining of cannot be found, she should then be asked to palpate the breast herself to locate it for the doctor. Finally, the axillae and supra- and infraclavicular fossae should be examined and the neck palpated for cervical nodes.

BENIGN BREAST DISEASE

About 50 per cent of women in the UK will experience symptoms of benign breast disease during their reproductive years (Hughes *et al.* 1989). Benign conditions of the breast have always been neglected in comparison to cancer, despite the fact that only about 1:10 patients attending breast clinics will turn out to have cancer, and this ratio is increasing with the advent of the National Health Service Breast Screening Programme (1:14). Compared with breast cancer there has been relatively little work on the epidemiology of benign breast disease. However, a 23-year prospective study of 726 nurses in Canada found that 30 per cent had reported breast symptoms requiring medical advice and 14 per cent had had a biopsy with a benign result (Hislop and Elwood 1981). These figures are somewhat greater than those from a study in Edinburgh (Roberts *et al.* 1987) which found that GPs were seeing an average of 13 patients with breast problems each year. Similar results were reported from a study in Southampton (Nichols *et al.* 1980).

Classification of benign breast disease

The management of benign breast conditions is critically dependent on an understanding of the normal and histological processes within the breast and the aberrations which lead to clinical presentation. Terminology in benign breast conditions has been confused by a multiplicity of terms which do not relate accurately to clinical or histological patterns and which are not based on sound concepts of pathogenesis. The ANDI Classification (Aberrations of Normal Development and Involution) (Hughes *et al.* 1987) has been put forward as a nomenclature based on pathogenesis to replace the division of benign breast disorders into normal and disease (see Table 2.2). It recognizes that a spectrum exists for most conditions which extends from normal through mild abnormality to aberrations and finally disease.

An important point in the classification is the replacement of the term 'disease' by 'disorder'. It recognizes that most breast complaints are due to disorders based on the normal processes of development, cyclical changes, and involution. Such disorders occasionally become frankly abnormal and then can be considered as disease. The main benign breast disorders which will be considered in this section are fibroadenomas, cysts, breast pain, and nipple discharge.

The four major symptoms

The four major symptoms which women present with are lumps, nipple discharge, nipple retraction, and pain. Faced with a lump, the general practitioner needs answers to the following questions: who found the lump (patient, partner, or physician, or nurse), was its onset sudden or gradual, is it single or multiple, is it diffuse, is it smooth or are the margins irregular, and is it mobile or tethered? If nipple discharge is being complained of the GP should note whether it is spontaneous or present only on expression, if it is scanty or profuse, unilateral or bilateral, from single or multiple ducts, and what colour, i.e. milky (galactorrhoea), green, watery (serous), or bloody. With regard to nipple retraction, there are several features which will help in diagnosis—the length of the history, whether it is unilateral or bilateral, transient or permanent, partial or complete, linear or circumferential, and real or apparent (e.g. eroded nipple). Similarly there are specific features of breast pain which will aid diagnosis—its cyclicity, whether it is diffuse or well localized, whether it is unilateral or bilateral, if it is confined to the breast, and whether it originates in the breast or elsewhere.

Table 2.2 *A broad classification of benign breast disorders*

---

1. ANDI (Aberration of Normal Development and Involution)

   (a) Development

      Lobular   Fibroadenoma

      Stromal   Adolescent hypertrophy

   (b) Cyclical change

      Hormonal activity   Mastalgia

                             Nodularity—focal/diffuse

   (c) Involution

      Lobular   Cyst formation

                             Sclerosing adenosis

2. Duct ectasia/periductal mastitis

3. Epithelial hyperplasias

4. Conditions with well-defined aetiology, for example

    Lactational abscess

    Traumatic fat necrosis

Reproduced with kind permission of Professor L. Hughes.

General principles of management

Having taken a history and examined the patient, the general practitioner has to ask him or herself several questions. Is there a true lump present? Sometimes lumps can be confused with induration in the breasts after trauma or with a costochondral junction. Some women may experience a lump or lumps as part of the menstrual cycle or in association with pregnancy. If there is definitely no lump, and no other significant abnormality has been found in the history and examination, or the symptoms can be satisfactorily explained as being due to trauma or hormonal fluctuations, reassurance should suffice even if a specific diagnosis cannot be made. Care should be taken to ensure that the patient is not harbouring a particular fear of breast cancer (cancer phobia) which might necessitate further investigation and/or referral. The woman should always be advised about breast awareness and invited to re-consult should there be any further problems.

The finding of a discrete lump is in some ways easier to deal with. Even though most lumps are benign, all women should be referred to hospital, preferably to a specialist breast clinic (Yelland *et al.* 1991). However the very act of referral will undoubtedly induce anxiety. Thus the delay in the very act of referral will undoubtedly induce anxiety. Thus the delay in the outpatient appointment should be as short as possible and the GP should advise the woman as to what is likely to happen to her in the way of investigations when she attends the hospital: for example, aspiration cytology, needle biopsy, ultrasound, and mammogram. But in a substantial percentage of women complaining of breast symptoms, especially those in their thirties or forties with 'lumpy breasts', it may be more difficult for the GP to make a definite diagnosis. Sometimes it can be helpful to ask the woman to return at a different time in the menstrual cycle, especially after a period, for another examination. If, at the second examination, there is some abnormality, nodularity, or thickening, referral to a specialist is probably the safest course of action. Other symptoms such as galactorrhoea or breast pain may justify blood tests and X-rays by the GP before the decision to refer is made. The results of these investigations will help the GP to be sure whether the symptom is originating in the breast or elsewhere. For example, breast pain can be confused with pain from the chest wall (Tietze's syndrome) or from the cervical spine or pleura. Nipple discharge may be drug induced or arise from an exudate due to eczema of the nipple or areola.

Breast lumps—fibroadenomas and cysts

Consistency, surface characteristics, and mobility in relation to surrounding tissues are each important in diagnosing benign lesions. Fibroadenomas account for about 12 per cent of all palpable symptomatic breast lumps (Dent and Cant 1989). They are particularly common in the 15–30 age group. They have a rubbery consistency, a smooth surface, and are extraordinarily mobile. Palpation of a moderately tense cyst is equally characteristic, but clinical findings vary with the degree of intracystic tension. A cyst can be completely missed if it is soft and, on the other hand, diagnosed as cancer if it is very hard. The passage of a fine needle in every breast lump can be justified because in the event of finding fluid, the patient may be saved much distress and unnecessary surgery.

The relative frequency with which a fibroadenoma is the cause of a breast lump is shown in Fig. 2.1. A fibroadenoma may grow progressively, remain the same size, or regress, but since they are rare in older women it is likely that most regress. The best way to make a diagnosis is to use clinical examination, ultrasound, and aspiration cytology. Since they are benign and without a malignant potential they can be safely left *in situ*, but many women wish for them to be excised. This can be done under local anaesthesia.

Breast cysts are most common in the 40–50 years age group. In more than 50 per cent of patients they occur multiply and are most often in the upper outer quadrant. They are the commonest abnormality in patients

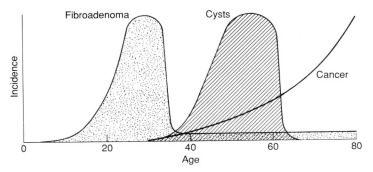

Fig. 2.1 Frequency distribution of breast lumps with age.

presenting to a breast clinic (Haagensen 1986). They are frequently asymptomatic and noted accidentally by the patient when touching the breast.
They can be accompanied by pain, probably due to leakage of fluid into
surrounding tissues. Pain is not usually related to the menstrual cycle, nor
is variation in the size of the cyst. Mammography is not very useful as it is
difficult to differentiate cysts and fibroadenomas. Ultrasound is useful but
hardly necessary when needle aspiration is readily available. Over the last
40 years, the trend in management has gone from mandatory excision
through selective aspiration with cytological examination to routine (and if
necessary repeated) aspiration alone. Cytological examination of the cyst
fluid is not useful unless the fluid is blood-stained. If the mass does not
disappear completely after aspiration it should be treated as any other
persistent mass as indicated by the individual circumstances. About 10 per
cent of cysts refill to become palpable and approximately 50 per cent of
women will develop another cyst elsewhere in the breast. Recurrence need
not be regarded as sinister but may be an indication for mammography.

Breast pain and nodularity

Breast pain (mastalgia) and nodularity form part of the ANDI Classification of benign breast disorders and as such are an excellent example of the
spectrum from abnormality through aberration to disease. Many women
develop mild premenstrual breast pain with or without associated nodularity
which lasts for a variable length of time but always resolves with menstruation. Severe pain and nodularity are aberrations of the normal cyclical
changes that occur in the breasts of all women during their reproductive
years. In a few women the severity and duration of the pain would be of a
degree such that the term disorder could be applied. Pain is a presenting
symptom in about 50 per cent of women attending a breast clinic (Hughes
et al. 1989) and is the most frequent reason for breast related consultations
in general practice (Roberts *et al.* 1987).

There are three main clinical syndromes of mastalgia. The commonest is cyclical mastalgia which shows a definite relationship to the menstrual cycle and is often associated with nodularity of varying degree, maximal in the outer upper quadrant and showing a similar cyclicity. It presents most commonly during the third decade of life and tends to be of a chronic relapsing nature with resolution of the symptoms around the time of the menopause. The second largest group, non-cyclical mastalgia, has no relationship to the menstrual cycle and tends to present a decade later with a shorter duration of symptoms that resolve spontaneously in about 50 per cent of cases. The pain tends to be well localized in the breast and nodularity is less prominent than in the cyclical group. The third group is Tietze's syndrome which is not true breast pain, but pain occurring in the costochondral junction. The pain is often felt in the region of the breast that overlies the costal cartilages. Typically the pain is felt within the medial quadrants of the breast and worsens when pressure is applied to the affected cartilage.

The aetiology of mastalgia is unclear. The long-held views about water retention and its prevalence in neurotic women have not been substantiated in well-controlled clinical trials and it is more likely that there are abnormalities in the control mechanisms of the pulsatile secretion of gonadotrophins and/or prolactin. The relationship of the Pill to mastalgia is unclear. There does not appear to be any clear correlation between the brand of pill, its hormonal content, and the occurrence of breast pain. If mastalgia is experienced by a woman on the Pill, then it is worth changing the type of pill assuming that she is already on a low-dose preparation. HRT in peri- and postmenopausal women is a well-known cause of mastalgia. It is treated by withdrawing the exogenous oestrogen completely or using a low-dose combined preparation for a short time only.

If clear pathological causes of pain can be excluded, such as abscess, periductal mastitis, sclerosing adenosis, and cancer, most patients can be managed by explanation of the likely physiological nature of the symptoms and reassurance that they do not have cancer. However, in about 15 per cent of women the pain is so severe that it affects their lifestyle and requires treatment. Bromocriptine, danazol, gamolenic acid, and tamoxifen have all been shown in placebo controlled trials to be useful in the treatment of breast pain. Diuretics, the most popular treatment in general practice, progestogens, and B_6 have not been shown to be any more efficacious than placebo.

Bromocriptine reduces the secretion of prolactin. At a dose of 2.5 mg twice daily it is helpful in women with cyclical mastalgia but not in those with non-cyclical mastalgia. However, many women experience side-effects such as nausea, vomiting, and dizziness sufficient for them to terminate treatment. Danazol, a gonadotrophin release inhibitor, is the most effective treatment for women with severe cyclical mastalgia. At a dose of 200 mg daily it can relieve symptoms in 70 per cent of women, and if the dose is lowered to 100 mg either daily or on alternative days after the first two months of treatment, troublesome side-effects can be kept to a minimum. Evening primrose oil, gamma-linolenic acid, has been shown to reduce pain, tenderness, and nodularity at a dose of 3 g daily. It is similar in efficacy to bromocriptine but less so than danazol. However, its very low incidence of side-effects makes it especially useful. Tamoxifen, an anti-oestrogen, has been found to improve mastalgia at doses of 10 to 20 mg daily. There are concerns about its use, particularly in premenopausal women, because it has some oestrogenic activity and thus it should not be prescribed unless all other treatment has failed. Early results from a placebo controlled trial with goserelin, an LHRH analogue, are encouraging, but it should only be used as a last resort in a specialist clinic.

Nipple discharge

Nipple discharge is a relatively uncommon presenting complaint. However, women may present because they fear the diagnostic implications, because it is socially embarrassing, or because it is in association with another breast symptom such as a lump. If it is the latter, then the lump will take precedence as far as investigation is concerned. Nipple discharge is potentially most significant when it occurs spontaneously and as the dominant symptom.

Three main groups of discharge are described: bloody, coloured opalescent, and milky. A serous, sero-sanguinous, or frankly blood-stained discharge all carry the same significance. They are usually due either to a hyperplastic epithelial lesion or duct ectasia (see below). The epithelial hyperplasia is usually benign, due to one or more duct papillomas, but the risk of malignancy increases with age, being much greater after the menopause. The discharge from a duct papilloma usually arises from a single duct and a nodule may be felt below the skin which upon pressure results in a small jet of discharge from the duct. Galactorrhoea is the term used to describe secretion of human milk from the breast unrelated to breast-feeding. Its cause is more often physiological than due to pathology in the breast and as such should be sought elsewhere. A raised prolactin level is often to blame. This is rarely due to a pituitary tumour and more often due to medication such as phenothiazines, butyrophenones, or metoclopramide.

Discharges other than sanguinous or milky can for most purposes be considered together and are not associated with an increased risk of cancer. They occur more commonly in the later years and can be very profuse. Multiple ducts of one or both breasts are involved and the underlying pathology is usually duct ectasia. The discharge can be nearly any colour and in about 50 per cent of cases contains blood. This disorder may also present with nipple inversion, inflammatory masses, abscess formation, and mammillary fistulae.

The management of nipple discharge depends on its nature and the age of the patient. The management of galactorrhoea is that of the underlying cause together with bromocriptine. In a young patient with a blood-stained discharge, the risk of malignancy is so low as to require simple observation after a full assessment has been made. However, in women over 45, the risk of malignancy is such that excision of the major duct system on the affected side is appropriate. The use of appropriate antibiotics, especially those effective against anaerobic organisms, can help resolve the inflammatory element of duct ectasia. A coloured opalescent discharge only requires treatment, by duct excision, if it is so copious as to require the use of pads. The laying open of a single mammary duct fistula is usually effective in allaying chronic recurrent abscesses.

Infection of the breast

Infection of the breast may occur as a localized phenomenon or as part of a systemic illness. The incidence of acute puerperal breast abscesses, the most common cause of breast abscess in general practice, is not known but appears to be decreasing (Benson 1982). Attention to care of the breast during pregnancy and after in breast-feeding mothers can do a great deal to lower the risk of mastitis and subsequent abscess formation. Although the vast majority of puerperal infections are caused by *Staphylococcus aureus*, there are a substantial number of cases of non-infective mastitis, where the early symptoms are identical. These symptoms of a painful, red, and swollen breast with some constitutional upset require in the first instance the same management regardless of the underlying pathology. Emptying the breast, either by suckling or expression, is of vital importance and these days it is *not* advised to stop feeding from the affected side. Hot soaks to the breast as frequently as possible with an anti-pyretic/anti-inflammatory drug are also recommended and in the case of non-infective mastitis should see the resolution of symptoms within twenty-four hours. Flucloxacillin, 500 mg four times a day, is the antibiotic of choice and in most cases will arrest infection with resolution at the cellulitic phase. However 5–10 per cent of women will go on to develop an abscess requiring surgical drainage with periductal mastitis/duct ectasia characterized by inverted nipples and a chronic nipple discharge (see above). In these cases, the causative organism is more likely to be an anaerobe and to give rise to recurrent infections which are best treated surgically.

DIAGNOSIS OF BREAST CANCER

Pre-operative diagnosis

In the past, pathological examination of breast disorders was carried out almost exclusively on tissue removed at surgical operation. In recent years, there has been an increasing tendency to obtain a tissue diagnosis before surgery. With a firm diagnosis of carcinoma, patients can be counselled and staged prior to surgery and the various treatment options can be discussed. The psychological trauma of intra-operative diagnosis by frozen section with open-ended consent for mastectomy should cancer be diagnosed is avoided. Furthermore, the patient can be reassured if the diagnosis is benign.

The two main methods of obtaining a pre-operative tissue diagnosis are fine needle aspiration cytology (FNAC) and wide bore needle (trucut) biopsy (Sloane 1991). The advantage of a trucut biopsy is that structural as well as cytological information can be obtained. This is especially important in distinguishing *in situ* from infiltrative carcinomas. However, FNAC offers distinct advantages over a trucut biopsy in that it is a much quicker and simpler technique which does not require the local anaesthetic needed for needle biopsy and causes less discomfort to the patient. Furthermore, small lesions are more easily located and the procedure does not result in significant distortion of mammographic appearances which may occur after trucut biopsy. FNAC is becoming the method of choice in most centres given the relative ease with which it can be undertaken.

Stereotactic FNAC is now an important means of diagnosing impalpable lesions. Various stereotactic devices are currently available. If a stereotactic pair of radiographs of an object are made then the exact position of a small target area within the object can be located by calculation. The immediate reporting which FNAC allows reduces the length of time the patient has to wait for a diagnosis and thereby reduces anxiety. Furthermore, it enables future management to be planned at the first visit, reducing clinic visits.

Pre-operative dignosis should not rely on cytology alone; mammographic and clinical findings should also be taken into consideration.

Surgical biopsy of palpable lesions

The procedure can be carried out under general or local anaesthetic. The laboratory processing and examination of the tissue may take a few days in difficult cases.

Surgical biopsy of impalpable mammographic lesions

The use of mammography to aid the diagnosis of patients with symptoms or as a screening test presents the problem of diagnosing mammographic abnormalities not associated with a palpable lesion. Special radiological and surgical localization techniques and highly skilled pathology are required for the biopsy of impalpable lesions.

Clinical staging

Before proceeding to surgery when cancer is suspected, it is essential to define as accurately as possible the clinical stage of the disease as this determines whether or not the tumour is operable. Only Stages I and II (see Table 2.1) are considered 'curable' and therefore operable (Baum 1988). As an aid to staging of the disease a chest X-ray should be carried out to look for lung metastases or involvement of the membranes around the lungs. Skeletal radiology or scintography should be carried out to search for bone metastases and, although rarely helpful, some form of biochemical and haematological screen should be performed to detect evidence of liver or bone marrow involvement.

TREATMENT OF BREAST CANCER: EARLY STAGE DISEASE

The management of breast cancer has changed significantly over the past two decades and continues to do so. The most appropriate therapy should be selected in terms of its influence on long-term survival, local recurrence, control of distant spread, patient preference, quality of life, and risk of poor cosmesis.

Almost all women with early breast cancer will be offered some form of surgery. Although the risk of local recurrence is reduced, there is no evidence that either simple mastectomy or more radical surgery, as opposed to local removal of the tumour, leads to longer survival. There has been a recent trend towards more conservative surgery, used alone or in conjunction with radiotherapy, there is little consensus as to what constitutes the optimal local treatment for early breast cancer. Moreover, while there may be no clinical evidence, undetectble metastatic disease may already have occurred at the time of diagnosis, requiring adjuvant systemic therapy in addition to local treatment. Although much research is being directed to identifying which women are most likely to develop metastases, a careful pathological assessment of the axillary nodes remains the most reliable diagnostic method.

Factors determining the choice of local treatment

If the tumour is small (4 cm or less) the options include:

1. Local excision, supported by radical radiotherapy which lessens the risk of local recurrence.
2. For small invasive cancers and *in situ* lesions wide local excision alone may be sufficient treatment, and randomized controlled trials are currently being conducted in Europe and the USA to determine this.

3. Mastectomy, together with radiotherapy if a node sampling procedure indicates positive lymph nodes.

4. Mastectomy with a clearance of the axillary lymph nodes, when no radiotherapy is needed.

For patients where the tumour is over 4 cm in diameter, high in grade, multifocal, or sited in the retroareolar region of the breast, mastectomy will most often be the preferred treatment.

Surgery

In selected cases, where the disease is confined to the breast, surgery alone, either by simple mastectomy or wide local excision of the local tumour, might be sufficient to achieve cure (Baum 1988). In all other cases, surgery has an important role in achieving local control of the disease.

Determining the pathological involvement of the axillary and perhaps the internal mammary lymph nodes is now considered essential for pre-menopausal women in order to determine accurately the outlook for the woman. This is particularly important when considering the need for adjuvant systemic chemotherapy. A complete clearance of the axilla would be guaranteed to produce the best evidence required but this radical dissection adds to the risk of post-operative lymphoedema. A suitable compromise favoured by many surgeons in the UK is a dissection limited to the lower third of the axilla, at the time of total mastectomy, as knowledge of the pathological status of the axilla higher than this level does not significantly help the surgeon to estimate the prognosis.

There are a number of approaches which effectively conserve the breast or at least preserve a relatively normal appearance. The surgeon may remove all the breast tissue from under the skin, preserving the nipple and filling the cavity with a silicone implant, the so-called subcutaneous mastectomy. Alternatively, following a local excision of the tumour, the residual breast and lymphatic fields can be treated by radical radiotherapy. Even more conservatively, the surrounding breast tissue and regional nodes can be treated by radical radiotherapy alone, following diagnosis via needle biopsy or aspiration cytology of the tumour. Treatment of the tumour alone is considered inadequate because, although the disease may appear to be affecting one site within the breast, in 40 per cent or more of cases it is known to represent a multifocal change within the whole breast tissue, with other areas of premalignant or frankly malignant change (Baum 1988).

Not all cases are suitable for breast conservation. Many women with large tumours in normal-sized breasts, average tumours in very small breasts, or tumours that are immediately behind the areola region, will still need to have a mastectomy in order to achieve adequate control of the disease. Furthermore, attempts at conservation in these types of cases often produce poor cosmetic results. A further problem exists in the way women adapt psychologically to breast conservation. In spite of the intuitive belief that breast conservation will avoid most of the psychological damaging sequelae of treatment, this has not been the experience in those studies where a formal attempt has been made to study these outcome measures.

Radiotherapy

There are strong arguments against the use of prophylactic irradiation of the internal mammary chain in women with early stage disease. In node positive women, overall survival is not improved by routine surgical and/or radiotherapeutic treatment of the lymphatic pathways. Administration of radiotherapy in such cases is a life quality issue, not one of survival (Yarnold 1991). Radiotherapy to the chest wall and regional lymph node fields improves the degree of local control of the disease. Radiotherapy should be given to those patients who are thought to have the greatest risk of local recurrence following surgery alone, such as patients with large primary tumours, particularly those demonstrating a highly undifferentiated pattern histologically.

In addition, those patients having less than a full surgical clearance of the underarm region, and those who demonstrate pathological involvement of the lymph node sample, would probably benefit from post-operative radiotherapy to prevent uncontrollable axillary recurrence, even though such treatment would be unlikely to influence long-term survival. When patients have been referred for treatment, it is conventional for the radiotherapist to irradiate the chest wall and regional lymph nodes in the internal mammary chain, the depressions under and over the collar-bone, and the axilla.

Radiotherapy to the axilla following a radical dissection is not prescribed because of the severe lymphoedema of the arm that can result from this combined approach.

Adjuvant systemic therapy

Clinical trials of adjuvant therapy have established that both cytotoxic chemotherapy, the anti-oestrogen tamoxifen, and ovarian ablation can reduce 10-year mortality from breast cancer and increase the period of disease-free survival. A recent overview showed that there was a 12 per cent increase in 10-year survivorship in women with Stage II disease and 6 per cent for Stage I. This meta-analysis of almost all known adjuvant trials of either tamoxifen or chemotherapy concluded as follows (Early Breast Cancer Trialists' Collaborative Group 1992):

1. Tamoxifen given daily for five years as immediate treatment produces a

significant deferment of recurrence both for pre- and post menopausal women.

2. Tamoxifen at a dosage of 20 mg a day taken for two years or more following local therapy produces a reduction in 10-year mortality from breast cancer which is most certain among women aged 50 and over (postmenopausal women).

3. Combination chemotherapy, particularly CMF-based regimens (cyclophosphamide, methotrexate, 5-fluorouracil), produces a 10-year mortality reduction which is most certain among women under 50 (premenopausal women).

4. There is no evidence that continuing CMF treatment for longer than six months is more effective.

5. Both chemotherapy and tamoxifen significantly reduce recurrence rates among both younger and older women. The combination is more effective than either treatment alone for women over 50.

6. Ovarian ablation either by surgery or radiotherapy reduces 10 year mortality in premenopausal women.

Implications for treatment

In general, the data suggest that the smaller the risk of relapse for the individual patient then the smaller would be the absolute benefit of adjuvant

Table 2.3 *Numbers of extra 10-year survivors from treatment of 100 middle-aged women with stage II breast cancer (N.B. absolute benefit might be about half as great in stage I, R. Peto and R. Gray, personal communication)*

Allocated treatment	Numbers of extra 10-year survivors per 100 treated (best estimate)
Age of 50 Tamoxifen alone for 2 years (longer treatment may have more effect)	8
Multiple agent cytotoxic chemotherapy alone (e.g. six months or more of CMF)	5
Tamoxifen + chemotherapy	12
Age under 50 Ovarian ablation alone	11
Multiple agent chemotherapy alone	10
Ovarian ablation + chemotherapy	at least 12
Tamoxifen for 5 years	? 5–8

therapy and so the greater would be the relative importance of any toxic side effects of that therapy.

With this principle in mind, some simple guidelines emerge. About 80 per cent of breast cancer patients in UK are aged 50 or more and among such women tamoxifen has little toxicity and particularly definite benefits.

The choice of which women to treat is made even easier by the fact that the effects of tamoxifen on survival remain statistically significant irrespective of:

1. age (50–9, 60–9 or 70+)
2. stage (I or II)
3. concurrent cytotoxic chemotherapy (given or not)
4. menopausal status (pre or post)
5. whether or not oestrogen receptor protein could be detected in the breast tumour tissue (ER positive or ER poor).

So some years of tamoxifen can now be recommended for almost all postmenopausal breast cancer patients, including those with a relatively good prognosis. And even if 10-year survival is considered unlikely because of age or other diseases, tamoxifen is worthwhile since it also delays breast cancer recurrence substantially. Among younger women the effects of tamoxifen on survival are less definite, but the effects of ovarian ablation and of cytotoxic chemotherapy on survival are highly significant.

Screen-detected lesions

The management of screen-detected impalpable lesions, particularly non-invasive carcinomas or invasive carcinomas less than 1 cm in diameter, is by no means straightforward. For small invasive carcinomas there seems to be little evidence for distinguishing these from slightly larger ones other than the influence on choice of conservation or more extended operations. In general these lesions are treated by some form of conservation therapy with axillary node dissection determining the use of radiotherapy or adjuvant systemic therapy. Radiotherapy can be avoided unless the tumour is of a high grade or the nodes are involved. The use of radiotherapy with these very small lesions is uncertain and must be determined by clinical trials. These lesions in general have an excellent prognosis.

The treatment of ductal carcinoma *in situ* (DCIS) is likely to become an important issue as an increasing number will be diagnosed by screening. There is little consensus yet as to how such lesions should be treated. DCIS detected at mammographic screening has to be considered a new disease entity. We need to accept that we do not understand its natural history and have no real guidelines as to its treatment.

DCIS is a lesion with a great potential to progress and become invasive. It therefore requires some form of definitive therapy although what this might be remains an important research issue. In general, in DCIS treated with excision biopsy alone there will be at least 25 per cent incidence of subsequent invasive cancer (Page *et al.* 1982). Biopsy alone therefore cannot be considered as adequate treatment. Mastectomy in most cases almost guarantees cure, but represents overtreatment in many patients. Treatment options are:

1. complete local excision alone with close follow-up;

2. complete local excision plus radiotherapy and/or tamoxifen;

3. mastectomy.

A trial is currently under way in the UK which aims to evalute complete local excision plus or minus breast radiotherapy and/or long-term tamoxifen.

TREATMENT OF BREAST CANCER: ADVANCED DISEASE

Breast cancer metastasizes most commonly to lymph nodes, the skeleton, lungs, and liver, but spread to any organ may occur. Local infiltration or ulceration over the chest wall may occur, and is very distressing to the patient. Treatment may be local, systemic, or both. Treatment of advanced disease has two objectives: palliation of symptoms and prolongation of life, with the main emphasis being to improve the quality rather than the length of the patient's remaining life (Baum 1988).

Both local surgery and radiotherapy have a useful role to play in advanced disease although appropriate systemic treatment should also be given in order to achieve maximum control of the disease. For painful bony lesions complete relief of symptoms can be achieved by a short course of localized radiotherapy. If the bone pain is more generalized, adequate analgesia is essential. Dyspnoea is controllable by fluid drainage, followed by the introduction of cytotoxic drugs into the pleural cavity. Shrinkage of liver metastases can be achieved by giving either high doses of corticosteroids or wide-field radiotherapy to the liver. Cerebral metastases can be shrunk by dehydration therapy or corticosteroids, in particular dexamethasone. Radiotherapy to the brain may also achieve palliation. For anaemia, blood transfusions may be required in the short term, but for longer-term control large doses of corticosteroids, androgen therapy, or chemotherapy using the vinca-alkaloids may be used (Baum 1988). Pathological fractures will require fixation.

Sequential systemic therapy can be used to produce remission and prolong life. Simple endocrine therapy can produce good results. For premenopausal women this could be either be surgical removal of the ovaries or by tamoxifen, and for postmenopausal women, tamoxifen. Approximately 30 per cent remission rate can be achieved. The use of single agent cytotoxic therapy (for example, cyclophosphamide) produces a similar order of remission but with greater toxicity. The combination of three or more cytotoxic drugs, each with different modes of action, can produce far higher remission rates in terms of the temporary reduction of the tumour bulk, but with potentially much greater side-effects. In general it is better therefore to attempt simple endocrine therapy first, and only proceed to combination chemotherapy if this fails.

ADVERSE EFFECTS OF TREATMENT

Surgery to the breast

However a woman reacts to hearing her diagnosis, most hope to keep their breast. In general, the choice of initial treatment for the affected breast does not influence outcome in terms of survival. Unfortunately only about 30 to 50 per cent of lumps are suitable for treatment by lumpectomy by virtue of their size or proximity to the nipple. Where surgeons feel able to discuss options with the patient, about 30 per cent of women suitable for either operation will choose to have a mastectomy. Although most people realize the need to offer some form of surgery to provide local control of disease, the 1980s have seen a move towards more conservative treatment with an increase in cosmetic acceptability but also an increase in the need for radiotherapy which for some patients is as debilitating as the surgery. Since psychological problems seem to afflict women whatever surgery they have, it is essential that adequate counselling and support is available as soon as treatment begins to be planned. It is often useful to include the partner in these discussions in order to diminish fears and dispel myths about the final cosmetic result. Very few patients nowadays undergo radical mastectomy with its mutilating consequences, particularly lymphoedema of the arm. The sampling of axillary nodes to help stage the disease is in general now preferred to total axillary clearance. Physiotherapy following surgery can be extremely helpful in limiting post-operative oedema and also in reducing muscle stiffness and wasting from disuse. The discomfort of oedema can be lessened with the use of elasticated arm stockings or in more severe cases with a special intermitten flow pump, the Flowtron.

   The length of stay in hospital varies according to the type of surgery performed, but all women should be visited by the specialist nurse counsellor, whom they should already have met in the out-patient clinic, before discharge. Their feelings about the treatment so far, particularly their reaction to the scar, can be elicited and answers given to any queries they might have about further therapy. This is also the time to discuss their views about a prosthesis. While the sutures are still *in situ* or the wound is not fully healed, a permanent external prosthesis is not usually possible but a light-weight temporary prosthesis to be worn inside the bra can help women regain their confidence more quickly. Choosing the right type of permanent prosthesis is extremely important and women need to be given all the available information about what is available both on the NHS and from private suppliers before they make their final choice. It is not uncommon for women to feel very dissatisfied with their prosthesis—worries that it will fall out or slip and make them look uneven, that it is too hot and heavy, or that it is just simply revolting, can result in significant morbidity in terms of body image. In some women, breast reconstruction may be available but this does not always result in a satisfactory cosmetic appearance and certainly is not a panacea for women who are not coping with a prosthesis.

Radiotherapy

The side-effects of radiotherapy have to some extent been overstated in the past and so it remains one of the most feared consequences of a diagnosis of breast cancer. The way in which it is introduced to the patient and the explanation offered for its efficacy is important in reducing the anxiety that most women feel about having to have radiotherapy. That there are adverse physical effects cannot be denied. Skin reactions, malaise, and nausea are all common but can be helped by anticipating the problems before they arise and by advising sensible measures to limit any discomfort. During treatment the skin may redden and flake off leaving a raw area which may take some time to heal. It should not be washed or covered with cream but baby powder can be used to help diminish any irritation. After treatment, zinc and castor oil cream may be used to soothe and soften the skin. Anti-emetics can be used to reduce any nausea although it is often anxiety rather than the radiotherapy itself which is the cause of this problem. Fatigue is a very common complaint and can last for some months after the treatment has ended. Having to visit the hospital so often is in itself tiring, particularly when the waiting period is spent in gloomy departments in the company of other very ill people. Occasionally there are symptoms of radiation damage to deeper organs—oesophagitis, rib necrosis, and lung fibrosis, but as radiotherapy techniques improve, the likelihood of these sequelae diminishes.

Hormonal therapy

Until fairly recently, oophorectomy or irradiation of the ovaries to produce an artificial menopause was the mainstay of adjuvant endocrine therapy. The distressing symptoms that the acute onset of the menopause brought that could not be treated with HRT were for some women worse than having to face a diagnosis of breast cancer and the removal of a breast. Tamoxifen (Nolvadex) can produce a similar therapeutic effect by blocking oestrogen receptors with few accompanying side-effects, particularly in postmenopausal women. Endocrine therapy for advanced disease in the past consisted of adrenalectomy and/or hypophysectomy. Equally reliable results can now be achieved with aminoglutethamide but side-effects are unpredictable.

Chemotherapy

Chemotherapy has the worst reputation of all the treatments available for breast cancer since it invariably produces at least some side-effects in all women. However, these vary from woman to woman and depend on the drugs being used and to some extent the attitude towards the therapy. The most common side-effects experienced are nausea and vomiting, diarrhoea, mouth ulceration, hair loss, cystitis, menstrual irregularities in premenopausal women, infections due to a lowered white cell count, reduced resistance to infection, and depression. Hair loss is responsible for much of the psychological morbidity associated with chemotherapy, and the provision of a suitable wig is mandatory. Good social support is essential if a woman is to have the resources to complete a course of chemotherapy which involves many visits to the hospital over six months to a year, as well as days on end of feeling systemically unwell. The psychological sequelae of chemotherapy is such that the very thought of the next injection is enough in some women to bring on a bout of nausea and vomiting. Careful assessment of the needs of each woman is required to ensure that she is offered appropriate help to counteract any adverse reactions to chemo-therapy. Relaxation therapy and desensitization have both been used with some success in this context.

PSYCHOLOGICAL ASPECTS OF BREAST CANCER

The woman with newly diagnosed breast cancer has to cope with a multitude of problems. Cancer is regarded with almost universal dread and surveys have shown that it is perceived with more alarm than any other disease. Despite the fact that breast cancer has had such a high media profile recently, myths and misconceptions about the disease are still very common. A recent study in a south London breast screening clinic (Fallowfield *et al.* 1990*a*) found that women severely underestimated the risk of getting breast cancer but also thought that most breast lumps were due to cancer. Although most women realize the significance of finding a breast lump, a surprisingly high number delay in seeking medical advice.

Having made the decision to consult a doctor and been referred to the hospital, most women find the period of waiting for the result of the biopsy the most stressful (Maguire 1976; Fallowfield *et al.* 1987). The reason given for the very high levels of anxiety seems to be more associated with the fear of having cancer than the potential loss of a breast (Fallowfield *et al.* 1990*b*). Women may display five different types of response on hearing the diagnosis: denial, fighting spirit, stoic acceptance, anxious/depressed acceptance, and helplessness/hopelessness. In addition, the reaction to discovering that she has breast cancer will be determined for each woman by her own health beliefs as well as her personality and personal circumstances. Her beliefs about the role of heredity, infection, lifestyle, trauma to the breast, stress or punishment for earlier misdemeanours in life (divine retribution) will need to be elicited by those involved in breaking the bad news. She may well have personal experience of the disease from a friend or relative and have particular fears about the loss of a breast, recurrence, the toxicity of chemotherapy, pain, or the effect of the diagnosis on family and friends. These are all important considerations when deciding on management of her disease and in order to be able to counsel her appropriately.

The manner in which the diagnosis is relayed to the woman is obviously extremely important in determining her immediate reaction; it is also likely to have more long-standing effects on the way she views her disease. Although the hospital consultant is most likely to have the major role here, nurse counsellors and psychologists with a special interest in breast cancer are increasingly being appointed in specialist breast clinics. At the time of diagnosis, many women are in such a state of shock that they are unable to take in very much of what has been told to them apart from the fact that they have cancer. The presence of a relative or a close friend during the bad news consultation not only helps in recall of facts but may lessen the subsequent anxiety and depression. Clear and concise communication from the hospital to the general practitioner as soon as possible after the diagnosis is known is extremely important. The GP is likely to be visited either by the patient herself asking for further information about what is going to happen to her, or by members of her family asking for help. This help will be necessary in order to cope with their own distress as well as to support the patient. The GP is in an ideal position to provide continuing care to women with breast cancer, particularly on the psychological front. However, there will also often be a need to answer questions to do with the treatment that is to be undertaken at the hospital such as the pros and cons of lumpectomy versus mastectomy. GPs need to keep up to date with the current treatment regimens at their local breast unit and to have good communication networks with the hospital team.

With the trend towards more conservative surgery, it was hoped that the psychological morbidity associated with breast cancer would diminish. However, several studies have all found that the levels of anxiety and depression are about the same regardless of which treatment has been given (Maunsell *et al.* 1989; Fallowfield *et al.* 1986). Women's fears of recurrence were another area where it was thought that differences might exist between women who had breast conservation and those who had mastectomy. This does not appear to be so as women seem to be more concerned with the fear of cancer itself and the possibility of recurrence rather than the fear of losing a breast. One area where the type of surgery seems to have an effect on psychological well-being, with breast conservation being superior, is body image. This is not surprising but more important is the subsequent effect on sexual functioning. There is very little data available on this specific topic as most studies have combined questions on body image and sexual functioning. Kemeny *et al.* (1988) found that women who had undergone mastectomy were less likely to feel sexually attractive than women who had undergone segmentectomy, but that both groups denied problems in sexual relations. A common trap to fall into is to assume that it is only married women or younger women who worry about their sexual attractiveness. It should be routine to enquire about these feelings in *all* women having breast surgery.

Since at the present time there is no clear advantage in terms of survival between the different surgical treatments, nor are there any major differences in psychosocial functioning, it would seem reasonable to offer women greater involvement when deciding on management wherever possible. The results from studies trying to demonstrate the benefits of this approach are so far inconclusive, with no long-lasting advantage in terms of psychological morbidity in women who choose their treatment (Morris and Royle 1988; Fallowfield *et al.* 1990*b*). Whatever treatment is given there are certain risk factors which predispose to significant psychological distress: inadequate information, adjuvant chemotherapy, complications of treatment, pre-existing psychological problems, lack of social support, and poor personal coping strategies. It is estimated that at least 25 per cent of women treated for breast cancer suffer from significant psychological morbidity and that the majority of these will benefit from either simple counselling or occasionally referral for more specialized help. The GP and other members of the primary care team need to be able to recognize these particularly vulnerable women and to offer suitable intervention either themselves or through referral to an appropriate specialist.

CONCLUSION

There is a substantial morbidity and mortality associated with disorders of the breast. Breast cancer constitutes a major public health problem in the UK. Little progress has been made in the past decades with respect to prospects for primary prevention. By contrast, early diagnosis by mammographic screening in women aged 50 and over offers considerable benefit for reducing population mortality from breast cancer. Improvements in the treatment of breast cancer have been only slight, although the recent results from trials of adjuvant therapy offer real prospects for improving prognosis. All breast disease, both benign and malignant, is associated with significant psychological symptoms.

The general practitioner has a major role to play in the detection, treatment, and long-term care of breast disease. When a woman presents with a breast symptom, however trivial, the GP should reassure her that she was right to attend. Some women have an obvious abnormality which requires referral, others appear to have no significant change. For those women where the position is less clear, it is best to refer for a consultant opinion, or to ensure that the patient keeps an early follow-up appointment with the GP. If there is any doubt, the woman should be referred, if only to put her own mind at rest. Before referral to hospital, the GP should discuss with the woman the possible diagnostic and treatment options.

USEFUL ADDRESSES

BACUP (British Association for Cancer United Patients),
121–123 Charterhouse Street, London EC1M 6AA.
Tel: 071 608 1661.
Breast Care and Mastectomy Association (BCMA),
26 Harrison Street, Kings Cross, London WC1H 8JG.
Tel: 071 837 0908.

CancerLink,
17 Britannia Street, London WC1X 9JN.
Tel: 071 833 2451.

CRC Primary Care Education Group,
University of Oxford, Department of Public Health & Primary Care,
65 Banbury Road, Oxford, OX2 6PE.
Tel: 0865 310457.

Health Education Authority,
Hamilton House, Mabledon Place, London WC1H 9TX.
Tel: 071 383 3833.

REFERENCES AND FURTHER READING

Adam, S. A., Horner, J. R., and Vessey, M. P. (1980). Delay in treatment for breast cancer. *Community Medicine*, **2**, 195.
Austoker, J. (1990*a*). *Breast cancer screening: a practical guide for primary care teams*. NHSBSP, Oxford.
Austoker, J. (1990*b*). Breast cancer screening and the primary care team. *British Medical Journal*, **300**, 1631–4.
Baum, M. (1988). *Breast cancer: the facts*. Oxford University Press.
Benson, E. A. (1982). Breast abscesses and breast cysts. *The Practitioner*, **266**, 1397–401.
Byers, T., Graham, S., Rzepka, T., *et al.* (1985). Lactation and breast cancer. *American Journal of Epidemiology*, **121**, **(5)**, 664–74.
Cancer Research Campaign (1991). *Facts on cancer*. CRC Factsheet 6.
Dent, D. M. and Cant, P. J. (1989). Fibroadenoma. *World Journal of Surgery*, **13**, 706–10.

Day, N. E. (1991). Screening for breast cancer. *British Medical Bulletin,* **47,** 400–15.

Dupont, W. D. and Page, D. L. (1991). Risk factors for breast carcinoma in women with proliferative breast disease. In *The breast: comprehensive management of benign and malignant diseases* (ed. K. I. Bland and E. M. Copeland), pp. 292–8. W. B. Saunders, Philadelphia.

Early Breast Cancer Trialists' Collaborative Group (1992). Systemic treatment of early breast cancer by hormonal, cytotoxic, or immune therapy. *Lancet,* **339,** 1–15, 71–85.

Ellman, R. (1989). Clinical cost–benefit of screening programmes. In *Women at high risk of breast cancer* (ed. B. Stoll), pp. 95–106. Kluwer Academic Publishers, Dordrecht.

Fallowfield, L. J. (1991). *Breast cancer.* Tavistock/Routledge, London.

Fallowfield, L. J., Baum, M., and Maguire, G. P. (1986). Effects of breast conservation on psychological morbidity associated with diagnosis and treatment of early breast cancer. *British Medical Journal,* **293,** 1331–4.

Fallowfield, L. J., Baum, M., and Maguire, G. P. (1987). Addressing the psychological needs of the conservatively treated breast cancer patient: a discussion paper. *Journal of the Royal Society of Medicine,* **80,** 696–700.

Fallowfield, L. J., Rodway, A., and Baum, M. (1990*a*). What are the psychological factors influencing attendance, non-attendance and reattendance at a breast cancer screening centre? *Journal of the Royal Society of Medicine,* **83,** 547–51.

Fallowfield, L. J., Hall, A., Maguire, G. P., *et al.* (1990*b*). Psychological outcomes of different treatment policies in women with early breast cancer outside a clinical trial. *British Medical Journal,* **301,** 575–80.

Greer, S. (1974). Psychological aspects: delay in the treatment of breast cancer. *Proceedings of the Royal Society of Medicine,* **67,** 470–3.

Haagensen, C. D. (1986). *Diseases of the breast* (3rd edn). W. B. Saunders, Philadelphia.

Henderson, B. E., Pick, M. C., and Casagrande, J. T. (1981). Breast cancer and the oestrogen window hypothesis. *Lancet,* **ii,** 363–4.

Henderson, B. E., Pike, M. C., and Ross, R. K. (1984). Epidemiology and risk factors. In *Breast cancer: diagnosis and management* (ed. G. Bonadonna). John Wiley, New York.

Hislop, T. G. and Elwood, J. M. (1981). Risk factors for benign breast disease: a 30 year cohort study. *Canadian Medical Association Journal,* **124,** 283–91.

Hughes, L. E., Mansel, R. E., and Webster, D. J. T. (1987). Aberrations of normal development and involution (ANDI). A new perspective on pathogenesis and nomenclature of benign breast disease. *Lancet,* **ii,** 1316–19.

Hughes, L. E., Mansel, R. E., and Webster, D. J. T. (1989). *Benign disorders and diseases of the breast: concepts and clinical management,* pp. 75–92. Baillière Tindall, London.

Kemeny, M. M., Wellisch, D. K., and Schain, W. S. (1988). Psychological outcome in a randomised surgical trial for treatment in primary breast cancer. *Cancer,* **62,** 1231–7.

Kinlen, L. J. (1991). Diet and breast cancer. *British Medical Bulletin,* **47,** 462–9.

Maguire, G. P. (1976). The psychological and social sequelae of mastectomy. In *Modern perspectives in the psychiatric aspects of surgery* (ed. J. Howell), pp. 390–421. Brunner/Mazel, New York.

Mant, D. and Vessey, M. P. (1991). Epidemiology and primary prevention of breast cancer. In *The breast: comprehensive management of benign and malignant diseases* (ed. K. I. Bland and E. M. Copeland), pp. 235–46. W. B. Saunders, Philadelphia.

Maunsell, E., Brisson, J., and Deschenes, L. (1989). Psychological distress after initial treatment for breast cancer: a comparison of partial and total mastectomy. *Journal of Clinical Epidemiology*, **42**, 765–71.

McPherson, K. and Doll, H. (1991). Oestrogens and breast cancer. *British Medical Bulletin*, **47**, 484–92.

McTiernan, A. and Thomas, D. B. (1986). Evidence for a protective effect of lactation on the risk of breast cancer in young women. *American Journal of Epidemiology*, **124**, **(3)**, 353–8.

Morris, J. and Royle, G. T. (1988). Offering patients a choice of surgery for early breast cancer: a reduction in anxiety in patients and their husbands. *Social Science and Medicine*, **26**, 583–5.

Nichols, S., Waters, W. E., and Wheeler, M. J. (1980). Management of female breast disease by Southampton general practitioners. *British Medical Journal*, **281**, 1450–3.

Nichols, S., Waters, W. E., Fraser, J. D., *et al.* (1981). Delay in the presentation of breast symptoms for consultant investigation. *Community Medicine*, **3**, 217.

Page, D. L. *et al.* (1981). Intraductal carcinoma of the breast: follow-up after biopsy only. *Cancer*, **49**, 751–8.

Phelan, M., Dobbs, J., and David, A. (1991). 'I thought it would go away': patient denial in breast cancer. *Journal of the Royal Society of Medicine* (in press).

Roberts, M. M., Elton, R. A., Robinson, S. E., *et al.* (1987). Consultations for breast disease in general practice and referral patterns. *British Journal of Surgery*, **74**, 1020–2.

Royal College of General Practitioners (1981). Breast cancer and oral contraceptives: findings in Royal College of General Practitioners Study. *British Medical Journal*, **282**, 2089–93.

Royal College of General Practitioners, Office of Population Censuses and Surveys, Department of Health and Social Security (1986). *Morbidity statistics from general practice*. Third National Study 1981–82.

Semiglazov, V. (1991). *Role of BSE in early breast cancer detection: 5 year results of the USSR/WHO randomised study in Leningrad*. Abstract presented to the First EUSOMA International Conference.

Sloane, J. P. (1991). Changing role of the pathologist. *British Medical Bulletin*, **47**, 433–54.

Stewart, H. J. (1991). Adjuvant systemic therapy for operable breast cancer. *British Medical Bulletin*, **47**, 343–56.

UK National Case Control Study Group (1990). Oral contraceptive use and breast cancer risk in young women: subgroup analysis. *Lancet*, **355**, 1507–9.

Vessey, M. P. (1984). Exogenous hormones in the aetiology of cancer in women. *Journal of the Royal Society of Medicine*, **77**, 542–9.

Vessey, M. P., McPherson, K., and Doll, R. (1981). Breast cancer and oral contraceptives: findings in the Oxford FPA contraceptive study. *British Medical Journal*, **282**, 2093–4.

Williams, E. M., Baum, M., and Hughes, L. E. (1976). Delay in presentation of women with breast disease. *Clinical Oncology*, **2**, 327–31.

Yarnold, J. R. (1991). Early stage breast cancer: treatment options and results. *British Medical Bulletin*, **47**, 372–87.

Yelland, A., Graham, M. D., Trott, P. A., *et al.* (1991). Diagnosing breast carcinoma in young women. *British Medical Journal*, **302**, 618–20.

3. Contraception

John Guillebaud

It is only within recent years that the subject of family planning has been included in basic medical training. This is perhaps because it has only recently been appreciated that it is important to have safe, reliable contraception over which women feel they have some control, not only for the prevention of unwanted conceptions but also for the psychological welfare of the women themselves.

In the past, many doctors found themselves ill-equipped to offer advice and most women sought help from Family Planning Association (FPA) clinics, or their successors after 1974 within the National Health Service. The important role of the general practitioner in this aspect of preventive medicine was stressed some years ago in a Royal College of General Practitioners Report (RCGP 1981b), and now the majority of women choose to consult him/her, although some still prefer the anonymity and specialization of the FPA clinic. General practitioners are potentially in the most favourable position to offer good advice, being already familiar with the patient's health and circumstances. They are able to assess her special needs as well as those of her partner and family. But some practices lag behind the standards of the best, in providing little else beyond oral contraception, and in devoting too little time and skill to counselling. There is much to be said for at least one dedicated family planning session each week, in which methods like the intra-uterine device (IUD) and diaphragm can be discussed and fitted without time pressure, and training can take place.

About 95 per cent of the general practitioners of England and Wales offer a contraceptive service for their patients, but many women still choose to go to a family planning clinic, and some will go to both. It is clear that consumer choice needs to be preserved. Although in either context most advice is provided by the doctor, a very important contribution is also made by nurses. The midwife, health visitor, or other domiciliary nurse is well placed to motivate and guide those in need. Much of the routine counselling and follow-up can be fruitfully delegated to a fully family-planning trained (ENB Course 901) practice nurse—with usually a gain rather than a loss in standards. Cap-fitting, pill-teaching, IUD-checking, and cervical smear-taking are all duties which can be appropriately delegated to her, as well as the supervision of those who choose methods based on fertility awareness.

Most couples require contraception for many years and their needs will change over time and with altered circumstances. The general practitioner is in an ideal position to cope with the subtleties and supervision which such a challenge presents. Because of this, many have found it worthwhile to undertake the postgraduate training for the certificates of the Joint Committee on Contraception (JCC). The RCGP Report (1981*b*) recommends that all vocational trainees should take the basic certificate, which includes theoretical teaching and practical experience as well as consideration of the often complex psychological and emotional factors involved in the use of all non-surgical techniques. There is also valuable (seminar-based) further training available through the Institute of Psychosexual Medicine—though all clinicians should have 'sensitive antennae', in order to receive often hidden signals about psychosexual aspects in any family planning consultation. Since 1991 the training for IUD insertion and the management of problems such as 'lost threads' has also been placed within a separate course, so that the relevant certificates will in future signify a higher level of training in the necessary practical skills.

Women are exposed to the risk of pregnancy throughout their reproductive life, potentially about 40 years between the menarche and the menopause, during which they have to face the problems of contraception. Not only are the available methods imperfect, there are also innumerable factors which influence the acceptability of both the principle and the ways and means of family planning. Psychological and emotional feelings often originating in family background, race, religion, and culture can be powerful, and increasing public anxiety concerning the risks of contraception further complicate the problems. Exaggerated press reports can cause unjustified alarm, upsetting the equanimity of some patients who are happily using a certain method and preventing others from starting it. When reassuring reports are published comment is usually brief at best.

Doctors should formulate their own assessment of the risks and benefits of each method for the individual patient based on up-to-date opinion and information and then back their counselling with good literature. The latest UK Family Planning Association (FPA) leaflets are ideal in this respect, user friendly (contrast most package inserts) yet accurate and adequately comprehensive: thereby providing strong medico-legal back-up for practitioners who may later be asked to justify their actions in the increasingly likely event of litigation. FPA leaflets may thus be regarded as an essential supplement to, but by no means as a replacement for, the counselling time by doctor and/or nurse; who must also invariably keep accurate and contemporary records.

TRENDS IN CONTRACEPTIVE USAGE

The methods of contraception used by couples have changed over the years and there have been changes within the social classes. Oral contraceptive usage declined in response to intermittent 'pill scares', but appears now to have steadied at a little over 3 million users (FPA figures 1991). Among other methods sterilization has become far more prevalent according to survey data summarized in Table 3.1. In 1987 this was the method used by at least 42 per cent of women aged 35 to 44 in Great Britain. About half relied on female and half on male sterilization. Usage of the condom has also increased somewhat in the younger age groups, especially under 25, but in the view of most authorities nowhere near as much as would be desirable to control hetero-sexual spread of the human immunodeficiency virus (HIV).

CHOICE OF METHOD

The majority of women who seek contraception are healthy and young, and present fewer problems than the over-35s, teenagers, and those with intercurrent disease. Considerable misunderstanding and ignorance still exist concerning the available varieties. There is an increasing tendency for sterilizing procedures to be demanded at a too-early age. Deferment or even avoidance of surgery is often possible by careful discussion and explanation of alternatives, particularly injectables or the modern IUDs (see below). Some women find difficulty in asking for advice and too often the very young do not do so until after they have actually been pregnant. Older women are often particularly unwilling to discuss this topic if they are embarrassed or doubt the propriety of sex except for procreation, or its indulgence over the age of 40.

Since the first edition of this book there is a new and urgent concern, to advise sexually active women of all ages on how they may minimize their personal risk of sexually transmitted viruses, especially the human im-munodeficiency virus (HIV). Monogamy is a behaviour pattern always worthy of encouragement (on medical grounds), supplemented, in the real world, by enthusiasm for the condom—usable often in addition to a recognized non-barrier contraceptive.

The practitioner may feel the need to offer unsolicited advice on some occasions and needs also to assess the strength of motivation of all women who request contraception. Unless used correctly and consistently, suc-cessful use of any method is unlikely if its effectiveness depends upon the user. But condemnation of, for example, coitus interruptus does not guarantee either adoption of or successful use of a theoretically more effective method. Indeed it may regrettably lead to non-use in 'emergency' situations even of this, a very far from totally ineffective method. With 'so far successful' users it may instead be worth exploring with the couple the use of a simple contraceptive pessary as an adjunct to the withdrawal method. It is safe to say that 'any method is better than none, but some are better than others'.

Table 3.1 *Women aged 18–44: trends in contraceptive use in Great Britain 1976, 1983, 1986, and 1989*

Current usual method of contraception	Survey			
	FFS 1976	GHS 1983	GHS 1986	GHS 1989
	%			
Users[1]	68	75	75	72
Pill	29	28	26	25
IUD	6	6	8	6
Condom	14	13	13	16
Cap	2	1	2	1
Withdrawal	5	4	4	4
Safe period	1	1	2	2
Other	1	1	1	1
Female sterilization	7	11	11	11
Male sterilization	6	10	12	12
Non-users	31	25	25	28
Sterile after another operation	2	2	2	3
Pregnant/wanting to get pregnant	7	7	8	9
Abstinence/no partner	–⎱23	–⎱16	12⎱16	14⎱18
Other	–⎰	–⎰	4⎰	4⎰
Base = 100 per cent[2]	5231	4444	4879	4776

[1] Abstinence is not included as a method of contraception. Those who said 'going without sex to avoid getting pregnant' was their only method of contraception are shown with 'others' as not using a method.

[2] Percentages add to more than 100 because some women used more than one method or had more than one reason for not using a method.

Sources: Family Formation Survey 1976, OPCS; General Household Survey 1983, 1986, 1989.

If a woman does not enjoy sex it is difficult for her to prepare for it. Her fear of pregnancy is used as a defence and she will probably find some reason why she cannot use any method, reacting badly to any one she tries. Religion still exerts a powerful influence concerning both the principle and practice of contraception. One Catholic girl overcame her conscience by giving up the Pill for Lent. Menstrual bleeding confers restrictions for orthodox Jewish women, Muslims and Hindus. (For Muslims both the husband and wife must agree to the use of birth control; but the genitals can only be touched with the left hand, making diaphragm usage difficult.) Hence, the prolonged loss associated with the IUD or the irregular cycles common with the progestogen-only pill weigh against the acceptability of these methods for such women.

Fashions also change. During the last 20 years male barriers and the Pill have been the most widely used reversible methods. The IUD and diaphragm are chosen by a small but varying proportion. There is a growing interest in the use of the fertility awareness methods, and withdrawal is still practised by a surprising number throughout all sections of society. At the time of writing it remains to be seen what impact the newest methods will have: namely the female condom, the progestogen-only ring, and Norplant.

The special needs, wishes, and circumstances of each individual have to be considered. Identification and resolution if possible of any anxieties that she or her partner harbour will help to select the most appropriate method. Once the patient makes her choice and the presence of absolute contra-indications has been excluded, then the general practitioner has the re-sponsibility to prescribe the method correctly, teach it carefully, and then supervise progress (perhaps indirectly through the nurse, but personally if relative contraindications apply).

There are also important related problems which may confront the doctor. They may be physical, psychological, or psychosexual, and unless they are considered in an understanding and flexible manner, the couple may have great difficulty with the use of contraception and unwanted pregnancies may then occur. In one chapter it is possible to highlight only the more common and most important problems. More detailed information is contained in the books *Contraception—science and practice* (Filshie and Guillebaud 1989), *Contraception—your questions answered* (Guillebaud 1989), and *Handbook of family planning* (Loudon 1985). Each method will be discussed in turn and then the special needs of particular types of women will be considered.

Relative reliability of contemporary methods

For the majority of women it proves very easy to conceive and much more difficult to contracept. Priorities vary, in that what appears no problem to one couple may be very much so to another.

Potential reliability is of paramount important to most couples when selecting a method. To give realistic estimates, however, is not easy, because the theoretical effectiveness of each gives little indication of its likely reliability in practice, which will depend on the ability of the couple to use it correctly and consistently. Even the IUD, which depends for its success primarily on the skill of the practitioner, requires the woman's involvement in feeling the strings and attending for checks at appropriate intervals if it is to produce its best results.

Widely varying limits are frequently quoted because the results of any study are bound to be influenced by the age, motivation, and sexual activity of the population concerned, and by the enthusiasm of the investi-gator, and the degree and duration of follow-up achieved.

Table 3.2 gives an updated (1991) indication of reliability ranges which can be quoted to couples.

HORMONAL CONTRACEPTION

The combined oral contraceptive (COC)

The following subjects demand brief discussion:

(1) benefits versus risks;
(2) choice of users ('safer women');
(3) choice of pills ('safer pills'), taking account of:
   (a) biological variation in the pharmacology of contraceptive steroids;
   (b) endometrial bleeding as a possible 'threshold bioassay' of their blood levels;
(4) supervision and follow-up, including implications of the monthly pill-free week.

Benefits versus risks
Capable of providing virtually 100 per cent protection from unwanted pregnancy, taken at a time unconnected with sexual activity, the Pill provides enormous reassurance through the associated regular, short, light, and usually painless withdrawal bleeding at the end of the 21-day pack. Inevitably, most of this section will be on possible risks and hazards associated with taking the Pill, but the positive aspects should not be forgotten; they are listed in Table 3.3. Although some of these findings await full confirmation, such good news is rarely mentioned while the suspected risks are widely publicized and often over-stressed.

Understanding of potential side-effects is based chiefly on the reported findings and analyses of two valuable prospective studies in this country, that of the RCGP and the Oxford FPA Study which both commenced in 1968. The first compares morbidity, mortality, and pregnancy outcomes in users and non-users while the second has either IUD-users or diaphragm-users as controls. The main findings have been confirmed by numerous case–control studies. Space does not allow full discussion of all the work which has been published in the 30 years during which the Pill has been available in this country. Practitioners can formulate their own opinion of the risks by more extensive reading, but the following points help to summarize present medical opinion upon which contemporary prescription of the Pill is based.

Tumours.   No medication continues to receive so much scrutiny and investigation as the Pill. For some time fears have been expressed about its possible connection with breast and cervical cancers.

Table 3.2 *User-failure rates for different methods of contraception per 100 woman-years (1991)*

	Range in the World Literature[1]	Oxford/FPA Study[2]—all women married and aged above 25		
		Overall (any duration)	Age 25–34 (≤2 years use)	Age 35+ (≤2 years use)
Sterilization				
Male	0–0.2	0.02	0.08	0.08
Female	0–0.5	0.13	0.45	0.08
Injectable (DMPA)	0–1.0			
Levonorgestrel implant (Norplant)				
Combined pills				
50 µg oestrogen	0.1–3	0.16	0.25	0.17
<50 µg oestrogen	0.2–3	0.27	0.38	0.23
IUD				
Ortho-Gyne T200	> 2			
Nova-T/Multiload Cu 250	1–2			
Cu-T 380 (Slimline)	0.3–1.0			
Multiload Cu 375	0.3–1.0			
(375 designed for longevity appears marginally more effective than 250)				

Progestogen-only pill ⎫ Levonorgestrel vaginal ring ⎬	0.3–4.0	1.2	2.5	0.5
Diaphragm	2–15	1.9	5.5	2.8
Condom	2–15	3.6	6.0	2.9
(Female condom no data, believed comparable)				
Coitus interruptus	8–17	6.7		
Spermicides alone	4–25	11.9		
Fertility awareness	6–25	15.5		
Contraceptive sponge	9–25			
No method, young women	80–90			
No method at age 40	40–50			
No method at age 45	c. 10–20			
No method at age 50 (if still having menses)	c. 0–5			

[1] Excludes atypical studies giving particularly poor results and all extended-use studies.

[2] Vessey *et al.* 1982.

Notes: 1. Ranking of efficacy, but overlap of ranges in the first column.
2. Influence of age: all the rates in the fourth column being lower than those in the third column. Lower rates still to be expected above age 45.
3. Much better results obtainable in other states of relative infertility, such as lactation (see below).

Table 3.3   *Beneficial effects of the combined pill*

Contraceptive

1. Highly effective

2. Highly convenient, non-intercourse-related

3. Reversible

Non-contraceptive

4. A reduction in the rate of most disorders of the menstrual cycle:
   (a) less heavy bleeding; therefore
   (b) less anaemia;
   (c) less dysmenorrhoea;
   (d) regular bleeding; and timing can be controlled (for example, no pill-taker need have 'periods' at weekends);
   (e) less symptoms of premenstrual tension overall;
   (f) no ovulation pain

5. Fewer functional ovarian cysts—since abnormal ovulation prevented

6. Fewer extra-uterine pregnancies—since normal ovulation inhibited

7. Less pelvic inflammatory disease (PID)

8. Less benign breast disease

9. Possible reduction in the rate of endometriosis

10. Fewer symptomatic fibroids

11. Possibly less thyroid disease (both overactive and underactive syndromes according to RCGP study)

12. Fewer sebaceous disorders (oestrogen-dominant COCs)

13. Possibly fewer duodenal ulcers—this effect is not well established and could be due to anxious women avoiding COCs

14. Possibly less *Trichomonas vaginitis*

15. Possibly less toxic shock syndrome

16. A beneficial effect on some cancers—see text

17. No toxicity if overdose is taken

18. Obvious beneficial social effects.

Recent studies have not confirmed the previously-reported protection against rheumatoid arthritis by modern low-dose pills.

The incidence of *breast cancer* is high and therefore this disease must inevitably be expected to develop in women whether they take COCs or not. Since the recognised risk factors include early menarche and late age of first birth, use by young women was rightly bound to receive scientific scrutiny.

The book edited by Mann (1990), which was the Proceedings of a meeting at the Royal Society of Medicine attended by almost all the researchers in this field, summarizes the literature to that date—which is copious, complex, confusing, and contradictory! Research is complicated by the problems related to: *latency, changes in formulation, time of exposure, and high risk groups*. A major cause of discrepancies may be the fact that long-term use of the COC by young women is a relatively recent and variable phenomenon between populations.

The largest case–control study on this emotive subject (the Cancer and Sex Hormones or CASH study) based in Atlanta, USA, was repeatedly reported during the 1980s as not finding any excess risk of breast cancer, whenever in life the Pill exposure occurred (Vessey 1989). However a reanalysis by Peto (1989) of CASH data reveals a significant excess risk, for all women aged 20–44 at diagnosis, if they used the COC before the first full-term pregnancy. Thus CASH now seems compatible with those other studies (references in Mann 1990) which indicated some degree of excess risk in various young categories of women.

To the latter must now be added the UK National Case Control Study (NCCS) (1989), which reported an excess of early Pill use among women developing breast cancer under age 36. The significant increased risk was duration dependent, whether exposure was before the first-term pregnancy or after it, and reached 74 per cent at eight years. Sub-50 μg dose oestrogen pills seemed to have a lower risk.

Yet, UK cancer registration data show no increase at all in any of the age groups who have had access to the Pill (including the under-forties). It is not yet clear whether this is because the register is seriously incomplete for young women, or whether the NCCS is wrong for some unexplained reason.

NCCS's interpretation of the literature to date is that the risk is for breast cancer occurring at a young age, and it may not persist into older ages. The RCGP found the risk only among pill-users aged 30–35 at diagnosis and not above 35, consistent with transient risk. The other prospective studies are also reassuring. But the risk could yet be found to persist. We await the findings of a new study by NCCS on older women aged 36–45.

In explaining this to women, one may say: the first NCCS report implies that three in 1000 COC-users for more than four years (sitting, say, in a large concert hall) would be under treatment for breast cancer by age 36. Of these, two could not blame the Pill (background rate 2:1000). And it is possible the third was predisposed to develop the disease at a later age.

Clinical implications

1. First, we can least be confident that 'use of oral contraceptives in the middle of the fertile years (say between the ages of 25 and 39) has no effect whatsoever on breast cancer risk' (Vessey *et al.* 1989).

2. The breast cancer issue should now normally be addressed, in a sensitive way, as part of routine pill counselling for younger women, but opportunely (i.e. not necessarily at the first visit if not raised by the woman). This will include mentioning the protective effects against at least two malignancies (ovary and endometrium, see below). The known contraceptive and non-contraceptive benefits of COCs may seem so great to many (but not to all) as to compensate for almost any likely lifetime excess risk of breast cancer.

3. No study has shown any greater increment of risk caused by COC use in women with benign breast disease (BBD), or with the family history of a young first-degree relative with breast cancer, than in the generality of women. But since these are circumstances in which there is already a predisposition to the disease, perhaps each should now (despite the protective effect of the Pill in reducing the risk of developing BBD in the first place) be considered reasons for special caution (i.e. *relative contraindications*). If the woman chooses the COC it should be a low-oestrogen formulation, for a limited duration, with specific counselling and extra surveillance.

4. If the COC does truly increase breast cancer risk in certain categories of women, dose-dependency has been shown at least for oestrogen and it is likely the risk will be minimized by the use of modern low-dose brands causing least metabolic disturbance. It remains acceptable to prescribe such formulations for the young, including teenagers, without an arbitrary time limit.

5. Women's breasts should be checked prior to the prescription of COCs, and self-examination taught. If a woman develops carcinoma of the breast, COCs should be discontinued and not given again. Women with a history of this cancer should normally avoid COCs (see p. 67).

For *cervical cancer* the picture is also unclear. A prospective study (Vessey *et al.* 1983) showed a twofold increase of cervical neoplasia in long-term users of the Pill compared with IUD-users. This finding was to some extent confirmed by the WHO study of invasive disease (WHO 1985). Studies on cervical cancer are complicated by the problem of getting accurate information relating to different patterns of sexual activity both for women and their partners. The prime carcinogen is clearly sexually transmitted, probably a virus or combination of viruses.

The COC may act, at worst, as a weak co-factor, certainly weaker than cigarette smoking, and possibly speeding transition through the pre-invasive stages (Drife and Guillebaud 1986). Long-term users of oral contraceptives should have regular cervical smears, but three yearly is still considered adequate unless there are other risk factors. The COC may continue to be prescribed in cases under treatment and/or monitoring for pre-invasive lesions (see 'Relative contraindications' below).

The benign *liver tumours* are rare conditions but do occur more frequently in COC users—with an extremely low incidence estimated at around one in 100 000 users (Vessey *et al.* 1989). The risk is believed to increase with duration of use of older high-dose products and all cases had significant liver enlargement. Rarely, long-term use of the Pill may also be associated with primary liver cancer, the association being strongest where there is no cirrhosis or Hepatitis B infection (Vessey *et al.* 1989).

Two cancers are *less* frequent in COC-users (Drife and Guillebaud 1986), namely *carcinoma of the ovary* and of the *endometrium*. Numerous studies have shown that, in round terms, for both cancers there is a reduction to one-half in the incidence among all users; to one-third in long-term users; and a protective effect can be detected in ex-users for up to 10–15 years. Suppression of ovulation and of normal menstruation in COC-users probably explains the similarity of the findings.

Choriocarcinoma was more common among women given the Pill in the presence of active trophoblastic disease (with elevated hCG) in some studies—but not in others from the USA. Other cancer links have been mooted but not confirmed. For further discussion, see Vessey *et al.* (1989). The 'bottom line' when counselling women is as follows: *Populations using the Pill may develop different benign or malignant neoplasms from control populations, but there is no proof that the overall risk of either type of neoplasia is increased.* (It could even be reduced, though there is no proof of that either.) This is also the conclusion from all the scientifically most likely data inputs into Vessey's computer model (1990).

Cardiovascular disease.   Considerably larger quantities of both oestrogen and progestogen were used in the published studies than are used today.

The 1977 Report of the RCGP study showed a fourfold risk of Pill-takers' dying from cardiovascular disease. Reporting again in 1981 and 1983, observations on larger numbers confirmed this finding but allow clarification of the risk for certain women (Table 3.4).

It can be seen that the extra risk to non-smokers under the age of 35 is very small indeed, and that at all ages smoking considerably increases the risks. It is the fatal arterial event attributable to the use of the Pill which is heavily concentrated in smokers. The risk at a given age among smokers is not reached until about 10 years later by non-smokers (Table 3.4)—implying that 'smoking ages the arteries'. Arterial diseases are not only commoner among smoking pill-takers, the case-fatality rate is also much

Table 3.4   *Circulatory disease mortality*

Age		Number of deaths reported		Ever users versus controls		
		Ever users	Controls	Excess risk per 100 000 woman-years	Relative risk	
15–24	Non-smokers	0	0		– ⎫	Non-smokers
	Smokers	1	0		⎬	1:77 000
25–34	Non-smokers	2	1	1.7	1.6 ⎱	Smokers
	Smokers	6	1	10.0	3.4 ⎰	1:10 000
35–44	Non-smokers	7	2	15.1	3.3	1:67 000
	Smokers	18	3	48.2	4.2	1:2000
45+	Non-smokers	4	1	40.9	4.6	1:2500
	Smokers	17	2	178.8	7.4	1:500

From RCGP study, reported 1981, *Lancet*, **1**, 541 (approx. 23 000 pill-takers, 23 000 controls).

higher (RCGP 1983). Venous thrombo-embolism does not appear to be related to smoking at all (Vessey 1982).

Cardiovascular deaths in the 1981 RCGP study were mostly as a result of subarachnoid haemorrhage or myocardial infarction. The death rate from subarachnoid haemorrhage in England and Wales has not increased since 1959 although the Pill has been available since 1961 and about 3 million women take it daily. It has been pointed out (Thorogood *et al.* 1981) that any risk is small and is probably associated with a hypertensive effect. The other chief cause of death was from myocardial infarction and a study (Adam *et al.* 1981) of women between the ages of 15 and 41 who died from this condition in 1978 showed that in the absence of predisposing factors the risk for women on the pill was increased about twofold.

More recently neither the RCGP study (Croft and Hannaford 1989) nor the Oxford/FPA study (Vessey *et al.* 1989) have been able to detect any increased risk in non-smokers. This means on the most pessimistic interpretation that the risk of using modern low-oestrogen brands must now be very small if not absent for women free of risk factors.

Recognized risk factors.   These are listed below and classified in more detail in Table 3.5:

1. Abnormal (atherogenic) lipid profile or (thrombogenic) coagulation profile. The trigger for investigation should be any relevant family history of arterial or venous disease at a young age.
2. Diabetes mellitus.

Table 3.5 *Risk factors for Cardio-Vascular System (CVS) disease*

Risk factor	Absolute contraindication	Relative contraindication	Remarks
Family history (FH) CVS disease (arterial or venous) in a first-degree relative ≤45	Known atherogenic lipid profile or pro-thrombotic haemostatic profile—or tests not available	Normal blood profiles or first attack in relative >45	NB: If FH of *arterial* disease must test BOTH for lipids and haemostasis
Diabetes mellitus (DM)	Severe or diabetic complications present (e.g. retinopathy, renal damage)	Not severe/labile, and no complications, young patient with short duration of DM	POP usually a better choice hormonal method
Hypertension	Diastolic BP ≥ 95 mmHg on repeated testing	Diastolic BP 85–95 mmHg see text	POP often better choice
Cigarette smoking	40+ cigarettes/day	5–40 cigarettes/day	
Increasing age	≥45 non-smokers (older in selected cases, see text)	35–45 non-smokers	Smokers should avoid/discontinue COCs 10 years earlier
Excess weight	>50% above ideal for height	20–50% above ideal	
Migraine	Focal, crescendo or ergotamine treated	Uncomplicated/acceptable to the woman	Relates to stroke risk. Consider tricycling if non-focal type headaches mainly in pill-free interval

Note: Some of the numbers selected are a little arbitrary and perhaps too strict if they are the sole problem (for example the COC might actually be allowed reluctantly to a current healthy 25-year-old admitting to two packs of cigarettes a day). They also relate to use solely for contraception. Use of COCs for medical indications often entails a different risk benefit analysis, i.e. the extra therapeutic benefits may outweigh expected extra risks.

3. Hypertension. Important if either pre-existing or pill-induced (see below). Avoid or stop the COC altogether if blood pressure (BP) exceeds 160/95 (either figure) on *repeated measurements*.

4, 5. Age/smoking. According to a US FDA Committee, there is no upper age limit for COC use in selected healthy, risk-factor free women (Fortney 1990). See Table 3.5, further discussion on p. 84, and 'The older woman' (page 110–13).

6. Gross obesity (>50 per cent ideal weight).

7. Migraine. Relates to stroke risk.

Note the absence of uncomplicated varicose veins in this list.

The COC is preferably prescribed only to women free of risk factors (the 'safer women'); otherwise additional monitoring is required (see below). Like all relative contraindications they are synergistic, and become absolute if more than one is present (e.g. smoking plus diabetes).

Progestogens of the norethisterone group and levonorgestrel, when given in other than the lowest available doses (which latter are acceptable), tend to lower high-density lipoprotein cholesterol (specifically HDL_2–cholesterol). This effect, not shown by desogestrel, gestodene, or norgestimate, is believed to signify an increased liability to arterial disease in long-term use. Oestrogens have the opposite effect. However, numerous studies have shown that the effects of oestrogens on haemostasis tend to increase the probability of intravascular thrombosis—and this may not only occur in veins but also in arteries especially when there is pre-existing arterial wall disease (Stadel 1981). The obvious conclusion is to reduce the biological effect of *both components* to the acceptable minimum (see below) producing hopefully 'safer pills'.

Comparative risks.   From the available epidemiological evidence practitioners will have formed their own ideas on the risk/benefit ratio of oral contraception. The patient, however, wants to know what the risk is to her and would like to be able to compare it with that of pregnancy. It has been said that 'living can be hazardous to health', and in contemporary living conditions there are many dangers and any estimate must be approximate. As far as the Pill is concerned, Table 3.6 can prove very reassuring.

Patients with intercurrent disease.   There are some conditions in which the combined pill is absolutely contraindicated (see above) but others which are positively benefited or at least not affected. There are persistent myths about some of the latter and it is unfortunate that women are unnecessarily deprived of this method for reasons now shown to have no link—like thrush and uncomplicated varicose veins.

It is impossible to list every other known disease which might have a bearing on pill-prescribing, and for many the data are unavailable or contradictory. In most serious chronic conditions, unless they affect the risk of circulatory disease, the patient can be reassured that the COC is not known to have any effect, good or bad; but it should then be used only with the most careful monitoring and alertness for the onset of new risk factors. Reliable protection from pregnancy is often particularly important when other diseases are present.

Table 3.6 *Comparative risks: estimates*

	Risk of death/100 000 at risk	Odds
Hang gliding	200	1 in 500
Coal mining	20	1 in 5000
Car driving	17	1 in 6000
Struck by a vehicle (UK)	6	1 in 17 000
Playing soccer	4	1 in 25 000
Home accidents	3	1 in 33 000
Pill: Non-smokers/under 35	1.3	1 in 77 000
Smokers/under 35	10	1 in 10 000
Death from pregnancy/childbirth:		
UK	8	1 in 12 500
Latin America	270	1 in 370
Africa	640	1 in 156

After Guillebaud (1991).
Sources: B. D. Dinman (1980). *Journal of the American Medical Association*, **244**, 1226–8.
RCGP (1981). *Lancet*, **1**, 541–6. Anon (1991). *British Medical Journal*, **302**, 743.

Sickle cell disorders. Sickle cell trait has no bearing on the COC. The situation regarding the homozygous conditions (SS and SC genes) is more uncertain. Both sickle cell disease and the COC individually lead to an increased risk of thrombosis, possibly superimposed during the arterial stasis of a crisis (Evans 1984). Hence many authorities and most manufacturers have for many years included the frank sickling diseases among the absolute contraindications to the COC. However, Serjeant (1985) reviewing studies in West Africa and the West Indies suggests that sickle cell disease should only be considered a weak relative contraindication—especially when balanced against the particularly serious risks of pregnancy. In this country injectables (see page 86) or the POP are normally better choices.

Hypertension. Hypertension is, itself, an important risk factor for heart disease and for both types of stroke. In most women on the Pill there is a slight increase in both systolic and diastolic blood pressure within the normotensive range. Approximately 1–2 per cent become clinically hypertensive. The rate increases with age and duration of use.

Predisposing factors for COC-induced hypertension include a strong family history and any tendency to water retention and obesity. Past pregnancy-induced hypertension does not predispose to hypertension during COC use; but it is a risk factor for myocardial infarction, very markedly so if the woman also smokes (Croft and Hannaford 1989). The COC is therefore relatively contraindicated.

Diabetes.   See Tables 3.5, 3.8, and p. 115.

Choice of pills and users

Initial choice of preparation.   Having excluded those women with absolute contraindications (Table 3.7), and proceeding with due caution/extra monitoring in the presence of relative contraindications (Table 3.8), the practitioner is faced with a bewildering variety of formulations (Tables 3.9 and 3.10). Which should be chosen?

For a start, there are in reality only five groups or 'ladders' of progestogens, since norethisterone acetate and ethynodiol acetate are converted *in vitro* with great efficiency to norethisterone.

Secondly, although much has been written about matching pills to particular hormonal profiles, the systems have no practical value for the initial selection of the low-dose pills now in use. Few would disagree with the general recommendations of the National Association of Family Planning Doctors (NAFPD) which are as follows: 'The pill of choice should be the one containing the lowest suitable dose of oestrogen and progestogen which:

(1) provides effective contraception;

(2) produces acceptable cycle control (a concept expanded below);

(3) is associated with fewest side-effects;

(4) has the least known effect on carbohydrate and lipid metabolism and haemostatic parameters.' (NAFPD 1984)

Table 3.7 *Absolute contraindications to combined oral contraception*

A. *Past or present circulatory disease*

1. Any arterial or venous thrombosis

2. Ischaemic heart disease or angina

3. *Severe* or *combined* risk factors for arterial disease. See Table 3.5

4. Atherogenic lipid disorders

5. Known prothrombotic abnormality of coagulation/fibrinolysis—including the congenital thrombophilias with abnormal levels of individual factors, development of the lupus anticoagulant, and post-splenectomy if the platelet count is above 500×10^9/litre[1]

6. Other *conditions predisposing to thrombosis*—including blood dyscrasias; polyarteritis nodosa; Keppel Trenaunay syndrome; from four weeks before until two weeks following mobilization after elective major or leg surgery, during leg immobilization, or varicose vein treatments (offer instead POP or injectable); and residence above 4000 m, which is associated with raised

Table 3.7 *(contd.)*

blood viscosity due to haemoconcentration in the short term. (The subsequent polycythaemia would be a relative contraindication to COCs).

7. Focal and crescendo migraine; migraine requiring ergotamine treatment (see p. 74)

8. Transient ischaemic attacks even without headache

9. Past cerebral haemorrhage—which can be secondary to cerebral venous thrombosis, also to avoid hypertension if past subarachnoid bleed

10. Most types of valvular heart disease (discuss with cardiologist); pulmonary hypertension

B. *Disease of the liver*

1. Active liver disease (i.e. whenever liver function tests currently abnormal, including infiltrations and cirrhosis), recurrent cholestatic jaundice, or a history of cholestatic jaundice in pregnancy. Dublin–Johnson and Rotor syndromes. (NB. after any viral hepatitis—COC-taking may be resumed 3 months after liver function tests have returned to normal.)

2. Liver adenoma, carcinoma

3. Gallstones (but COC may be used after cholecystectomy)

4. The porphyrias

C. *History of serious condition affected by sex steroids or related to previous COC use*

Chorea
COC-induced hypertension
Herpes gestationis
Haemolytic uraemic syndrome
Otosclerosis (some authorities permit supervised COC use)
Stevens–Johnson syndrome (erythema multiforme), if COC-associated trophoblastic disease *but only until βhCG levels are undetectable.* In the USA this is considered a relative contraindication even when hCG present.

D. *Pregnancy*

E. *Undiagnosed genital tract bleeding*

F. *Oestrogen-dependent neoplasms*
Especially breast cancer (but some oncologists permit COC in selected cases in prolonged remission). Past breast biopsy showing premalignant epithelial atypia is usually also considered an absolute contraindication.

G. *Woman's anxiety re COC safety unrelieved by counselling*

Note: Several of the above (e.g. D, E, G) are not necessarily permanent contraindications.

[1] S. Machin, 1987, personal communication.
[2] M. Ward, Alpinist, 1986, personal communication to NAFPD.

Source: Guillebaud (1989).

Table 3.8   *Relative contraindications*

1. First see Table 3.5. Risk factors for arterial disease are all relative contraindications: provided normally that only one is present, and not to so marked a degree that it would absolutely contraindicate this method.

2. Homozygous sickle cell disease (see below).

3. Long-term partial immobilization (e.g. in a wheelchair).

4. Sex steroid-dependent cancer. Seek the specialist's advice: most will permit COC use after treatment for melanoma. A history of breast cancer is almost invariably considered an absolute contraindication.

5. Oligo-/amenorrhoea should be investigated but the Pill may subsequently be prescribed.

6. Hyperprolactinaemia: this is now considered only a relative contraindication for patients under specialist supervision.

7. Very severe depression, if likely to be exacerbated by COCs; but unwanted pregnancies can be very depressing!

8. Chronic systemic diseases. Crohn's disease is now considered a relative contraindication, as are diabetes and chronic renal disease. In both the latter HDL-Cholesterol is lowered.

9. Diseases requiring long-term treatment with drugs which might interact with the Pill (see text for special management).

10. *New relative contraindications* now include:
    (a) if a young first-degree relation has had breast cancer;
    (b) the presence of established benign breast disease;
    (c) during the monitoring of mildly abnormal cervical smears;
    (d) during and after definition treatment for cervical intraepithelial neoplasia, CIN.

(After counselling the decision may well be taken to prescribe the COC. Women in categories (c) and (d) need monitoring—at least by annual smears.)

Each doctor needs to be familiar with the composition of the available preparations. Women may react unpredictably and several types may have to be tried before a suitable one is found. Some women are never suited. This is hardly surprising. Individual variation in motivation and tolerance of minor side-effects is well recognized. But there is also marked individual variation in blood levels of the exogenous hormones and in responses at the end organs, especially the endometrium (Guillebaud 1989). Thus it is a false expectation that any single pill will suit all women.

The NAFPD guidelines need to be individualized. Prescribers should try to identify, if necessary over a series of initial visits as about to be described, the lowest dose for each woman which is effective—(1) above—and does

Table 3.9 *System of summarizing pills according to progestogen content ('ladders')*

Pill		μg	μg
		Levonorgestrel	*Ethinyl oestradiol*
1. Ovran (Wyeth)		250*	50
Eugynon 30		250	30
Ovran 30 (Wyeth)		250	30
Ovranette (Wyeth)		150	30
Microgynon (Schering)		150	30
Trinordiol (Wyeth) (triphasic) ⎫	6 tablets	50	30
Logynon (Schering) (triphasic) ⎬	5 tablets	75	40
⎭	10 tablets	125	30
Logynon ED = Logynon + 7 inert tablets			
		Norethisterone	*Mestranol*
2. Norinyl-1 (Syntex)		1000	50
Ortho-Novin 1/50 (Ortho-Cilag)		1000	50
		Norethisterone	*Ethinyl oestradiol*
Norimin (Syntex)		1000	35
Neocon (Ortho-Cilag)		1000	35
Binovum (Ortho-Cilag)		7 × 500; 14 × 1000	35
Trinovum (Ortho-Cilag)		7 × 500; 7 × 750; 7 × 1000	35
Trinovum ED = Trinovum + 7 inert tablets			
Synphase (Syntex)		7 × 500; 9 × 1000; 5 × 500	35
Ovysmen (Ortho)		500	35
Brevinor (Syntex)		500	35
		Norethisterone acetate	*Ethinyl oestradiol*
3. Loestrin 30 (Parke Davis)		1500	30
Loestrin 20 (Parke Davis)		1000	20
		Ethynodiol diacetate	*Ethinyl oestradiol*
4. Conova 30 (Searle)		2000	30
		Desogestrel	*Ethinyl oestradiol*
5. Marvelon (Organon)		150	30
Mercilon (Organon)		150	20

* *Contained* in 500 μg dl norgestrel.

Table 3.9   *(contd.)*

	Gestodene	Ethinyl oestradiol
6. Femodene (Schering)	75	30
Minulet (Wyeth)	75	30
Femodene ED = Femodene + 7 inert tablets		
Triadene (Schering)/Tri Minulet (Wyeth)	6 × 50; 5 × 70; 10 × 100	6 × 30; 5 × 40; 10 × 30
	Norgestimate	Ethinyl oestradiol
7. Cilest (Ortho-Cilag)	250	35

not cause the annoying symptom of breakthrough bleeding (BTB)—(2). It is believed that this will minimize adverse side-effects—both serious and minor (3), and should also reduce the measurable metabolic changes (4).

More specifically, the first choice of pill should *normally* be made from those in Table 3.10, with a tendency not to choose the more complicated triphasics and 20 μg pills for teenagers, nor the levonorgestrel/norethisterone pills for women with CVS risk factors.

Note that the well-known formulation Microgynon/Ovranette is under a slight cloud and no longer in the 'preferred' table. This is because a clear majority now of research studies show statistically significant potentially adverse lipid changes (specifically suppression of HDL_2-cholesterol). This pill remains acceptable for younger women free of all known arterial disease risk. This is *not* because it has 'become unsafe' for the remainder, but only because there are now options which appear *on present evidence* to be preferable metabolically. This is the same principle which earlier led to reduced prescribing of previous pills which were in their day the market leaders, notably Minovlar and more recently Eugynon 30/Ovran 30.

Similar metabolic (lipid) considerations explain the omission of other low oestrogen pills from Table 3.10. Thrombotic risk is not to be considered less important however (see page 64); this seems to be primarily oestrogen-dose dependent, meaning, for example, that Mercilon might be a good choice for the overweight woman.

During follow-up, the aim is to give long term the *lowest acceptable* amount of both hormones. To achieve this the following important concepts need to be brought together:

1. *Individual* variation in absorption and metabolism causes blood levels of all contraceptive steroids to vary tenfold (Back *et al.* 1981). There are also variable end-organ responses.

2. It is hypothesized that those with the highest blood levels are likely to be the most affected metabolically, and also more at risk of both major and minor side-effects.

Table 3.10 *Preferred group of low-dose COCs (less than 50 μg of oestrogen, inducing the more acceptable blood lipid profiles)*[1]

Pill	μg	μg
	Levonorgestrel	*Ethinyl oestradiol*
Logynon/Trinordiol	6 × 50; 5 × 75 10 × 125 [92]	6 × 30; 5 × 40 10 × 30 [32]
	Norethisterone	
Binovum[2]	7 × 500; 14 × 1000 [833]	35
Trinovum	7 × 500; 7 × 750 7 × 1000 [750]	35
Synphase[2]	7 × 500; 9 × 1000 5 × 500 [714]	35
Brevinor/Ovysmen	500	35
	Desogestrel	
Marvelon	150	30
Mercilon	150	20
	Gestodene	
Femodene/Minulet	75	30
Triadene/TriMinulet	6 × 50; 5 × 70; 10 × 100 [79]	6 × 30; 5 × 40; 10 × 30 [32]
	Norgestimate	
Cilest	250	35

[1] Mean daily dose of phased brands in square brackets.
[2] Confusing to the user, so Trinovum usually preferred.

3. It is also probable that women with the lowest blood levels tend to manifest this by BTB—as do women whose blood levels are lowered by enzyme-inducers.

4. Absence of BTB signifies either high or adequate blood levels of the administered steroids.

How then can we avoid giving to any woman who tends to have the highest blood levels a stronger formulation than she requires? Pending the availability of direct measurements in the clinic or surgery, we can 'titrate' the dose given against the occurrence of BTB, using the endometrium as an approximate *'threshold bioassay'*. The aim should be that each woman receives the least long-term metabolic impact that her uterus will allow— i.e. the lowest dose of contraceptive steroids which is just, but only just, above her own bleeding threshold. In practice this means:

If there is good cycle control, at the time of repeat prescription, the possibility of trying a lower dose brand (if available) should always be considered. On the other hand:

If BTB occurs and is unacceptable or persists beyond two cycles, provided that none of the important alternative explanations applies (Table 3.11), the next strongest brand up the 'ladder' in Table 3.9 should be tried. Especially if the complaint is absent withdrawal bleeding, phased pills may be particularly useful for purposes of cycle control. The excessively progestogen dominant (less 'lipid-friendly') brands Eugynon 30/Ovran 30 and Conova 30 are best avoided unless indicated for therapeutic reasons; but if cycle control can only be achieved by a 50 μg oestrogen pill, for that particular woman the latter need not be considered a 'strong' brand.

Obviously this 'titrating' process is not helped by the lack of provision by the manufacturers of a good range of doses, especially for the newer progestogens.

Table 3.11   *Checklist in cases of possible 'breakthrough bleeding' (BTB) in pill-takers. A note of caution: first eliminate other possible causes!*

Disease—**Examine** the cervix. It is not unknown for bleeding from an invasive cancer to be wrongly attributed to BTB. *Chlamydia* can cause a sanguineous discharge.

Disorder of pregnancy causing bleeding (e.g. abortion, trophoblastic tumour).

Default—missed pill(s). Remember that the BTB may start two or three days later and be very persistent thereafter.

Drugs—especially enzyme-inducers; see text.

Diarrhoea with **vomiting**—diarrhoea alone has to be very severe to impair absorption significantly.

Disturbance of absorption—likewise has to be very marked to be relevant, e.g. after *massive* gut resection. (Ileostomy cases studied have had no demonstrable absorption problems.)

Diet—gut flora involved in recycling ethinyloestradiol may be reduced in *vegetarians*. Could sometimes be a factor in BTB, but not usually an important effect.

Duration too short—minimal BTB which is tolerable may resolve after two to three months.

Finally, after the above have been excluded:

Dose ● if she is taking a monophasic, try a phasic pill

   ● increase the progestogen component

   ● try a different progestogen

   ● consider using a 50 μg pill such as Ovran.

Adapted from Sapire (1990).

Second choice if there are non-bleeding side-effects. The use of contemporary pills has reduced the reporting of so-called 'minor' side-effects. When symptoms do occur it is generally bad practice to give further prescriptions, such as diuretics, anti-migraine treatments, or antidepressants for weight gain, headaches, or depression respectively. For the last of these, pyridoxine 50–100 mg daily may be beneficial. Otherwise there are two preferred, if empirical, courses of action, namely:

1. decrease the dose of either hormone, if still possible—in the limit, oestrogen can be eliminated by a trial of the progestogen-only pill

2. change to a different progestogen (Table 3.10).

Otherwise, more specific guidance for side-effects and conditions associated with a relative excess of either steroid may be obtained from Tables 3.12 and 3.13.

Cervical erosions are common and can be treated by cryocautery if, and only if, they are the cause of symptoms. Modern pills do not appear to increase the incidence of monilial infection which is common in all women, although some women with recurrent thrush state they have less problems off the Pill, in which case it is worth listening to the patient.

Supervision and follow-up

Although each packet contains an insert, the wording can cause anxiety. Each woman needs individual teaching, backed by a good instruction leaflet (ideally those produced by the UK FPA). Starting on day 1 avoids the requirement to take extra precautions, and indeed new studies show this to be acceptable up to day 4 (see Table 3.14). It is important to remind the woman that pills must be taken in the correct order and the packet

Table 3.12 *Which second choice of pill? (relative oestrogen excess)*

Symptoms	Conditions
Nausea	Benign breast disease
Dizziness	Fibroids
'Premenstrual tension' and irritability	Endometriosis
Cyclical weight gain (fluid)	
'Bloating'	
Vaginal discharge (no infection)	
Some cases of breast tenderness	

Treat with progestogen-dominant COC, such as Loestrin 30, Eugynon 30 (but with caution regarding lipids, see p. 64). Mercilon 20 is the best oestrogen-deficient option.

Table 3.13 *Which second choice of pill? (relative progestogen excess)*

Symptoms	Conditions
Dryness of vagina	Acne/seborrhoea
Some cases of:	Hirsutism
sustained weight gain	
depression	
loss of libido	
lassitude	

Treat with oestrogen-dominant COC, such as Cilest or Marvelon; then Dianette (an acne treatment which is also contraceptive, containing 35 μg of ethinyloestradiol combined with 2 mg cyproterone acetate); or possibly Norinyl-1.

completed regardless of bleeding. Protection is afforded during the seven tablet-free days provided another packet follows. If taken correctly, each new pack is started on the same weekday.

It is important to record the patient's *blood pressure* before starting the pill and to check it after three months and subsequently at intervals of six months or one year as the risk of hypertension continues to be present. A moderate increase in blood pressure may also act as a marker for an increased risk of thrombosis, especially in the presence of any other risk factor.

Migraines are of special relevance to pill-monitoring. If migraines are focal (i.e. include any symptoms like asymmetric loss of vision, motor power, or sensation, or dysphasia, which are interpretable as due to transient cerebral ischaemia), the oestrogen of the COC should be stopped for fear of superimposed thrombosis causing a permanent ischaemia (i.e. a thrombotic stroke). Most authorities would likewise avoid/discontinue the COC if the woman's first ever attack occurred while taking it; and in all women with severe or 'crescendo' migraines, especially if ergotamine treatment were required. The oestrogen-free contraceptive methods are not however contraindicated.

Breast self-examination and awareness should be taught. *Cervical screening* should be performed regularly according to local guidelines.

Importance of the pill-free week.   This promotes a reassuring withdrawal bleed (WTB)—and indeed if this does not occur in two successive cycles, it is best to exclude pregnancy. However, its importance might be greater than that, in allowing some degree of recovery from systemic effects of the Pill. In one study, for example, HDL-cholesterol suppression by the COCs

Table 3.14 *Starting routines*

	Start when?	Extra precautions for 7 days?
1. Menstruating	At or after 5th day of period	YES
	1st day/before day 4	No[1]
2. Post-partum		
(a) no lactation	Day 21 post partum (low risk of thrombosis by then, first ovulations reported day 28+)	No
(b) lactation	Not normally recommended at all (POP preferred)	
3. Post-induced abortion/ miscarriage	Same day	No
4. Post-trophoblastic tumour	One month after no hCG detected (see p. 67)	As (1)
5. Post-higher or same dose COC	Instant switch[2]	No
6. Post-lower dose COC	After usual 7-day break	No
7. Post-POP	1st day of period	No
8. Post-POP with POP-related amenorrhoea	Any day (end of packet)	No
9. Other secondary amenorrhoea (*pregnancy excluded*)	Any day	YES

See text.

[1] Except in the case of Logynon ED and Femodene ED—here the starting routine entails the taking of a variable number of placebos; hence extra precautions are recommended *for 14 days*.

[2] This advice is because of reports of rebound ovulation occurring at the time of transfer, if the usual 7-day break is taken.

studied was eliminated by the end of the pill-free interval (Demacker *et al.* 1982). Hence it is probably wise only to cut out the gap between packets either in the short term (upon request to avoid a 'period' on special occasions*), or for special indications, such as the occurrence of regular *hormone-withdrawal headaches*. The tricycle regimen is often used, in which three or four packets of a monophasic pill are taken in succession, followed by a pill-free gap. This leads to only four WTBs and, in this

* Phasic pill-users who wish to postpone withdrawal bleeds must use the final phase of a spare packet, or pills from an equivalent formulation to that phase (e.g. 'Neocon' in the case of 'Trinovum').

Table 3.15 *Indications for the tricycle regimen (using a monophasic pill)*

1. Headaches including non-focal migraine, and other bothersome symptoms occurring regularly in the withdrawal week.
2. Unacceptably heavy or painful withdrawal bleeds.
3. Paradoxically, to help women who are concerned about absent withdrawal bleeds (this concern thereby arising less often!)
4. Epilepsy: this benefits from relatively more sustained levels of the administered hormones (see also below for another reason related to the anti-epileptic treatment).
5. Endometriosis: a progestogen-dominant monophasic pill may be tricycled for maintenance treatment after primary therapy.
6. Suspicion of decreased efficacy (see text, p. 78).
7. At the woman's choice.

Note: In view of the possibility that the monthly pill-free interval is beneficial (see p. 74–5), one of these special indications should normally apply.

example, only four headaches per year. Other important indications are in Table 3.15 and discussed further below.

Biochemical and ultrasound data also demonstrate return of pituitary and ovarian follicular activity during the pill-free time in about one-quarter of pill-takers, in some women to a marked extent. Therefore breakthrough ovulation is most likely to follow any lengthening of the pill-free interval. Such lengthening may result from omissions, malabsorption, and drug interaction *involving pills either at the start or at the end of a packet.*

Clearly the advice to the woman who has missed pills, which is still given in some package inserts, to take extra precautions to the end of her packet, is wrong since it fails to allow for ovarian activity returning in the pill-free time. Smith *et al.* (1986) showed, admittedly in a study involving small numbers, that even if only 14 or even as few as seven pills had first been taken, no women ovulated after seven pills were subsequently missed—implying at the very least that three or four pills may be missed mid-packet with impunity! This and other work may be summarized:

1. Seven consecutive pills are enough to 'put the ovaries to sleep' (therefore pills 8 to 21 in a packet simply 'keep them asleep').
2. Seven pills can be omitted without ovulation, as in the regular pill-free week.
3. More than seven pills missed *in total* increases the risk.

The 7-day 'Rule', as now used by the UK FPA and also the UK Manufacturers, states (wording adapted slightly):

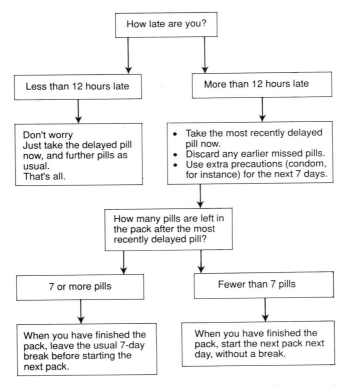

Fig. 3.1 What to do if you have forgotten to take pills. (From *Family planning today* 1991.)

1. If you are more than 12 hours late in taking any pill, or miss more than one, the pill may not work. As soon as you remember, continue to take your pills normally, but you may not be protected for the next seven days so either avoid sex or use another method (the condom, for example).

2. If you have more than seven pills left in the pack, continue taking them and start the next pack as you would normally do after the usual gap between packs.

3. If you have less than seven left, so your packet of pills runs out during the next seven days, this means you should start the next pack as soon as you have finished the present one—in other words, do not have a gap between packs (and skip any dummy 'reminder tablets').

The last part of the advice is critically important and can be explained as: 'it would be silly to let your ovaries have another break from the effect of your contraceptive so soon after the break you made by mistake (by the pills you missed)'.

The woman should, of course, be asked to return if she has no bleeding in the next pill-free break.

Vomiting and diarrhoea.   Extra contraceptive precautions should start from the onset of vomiting which occurs within three hours of taking a tablet and continue for seven days after the illness ends, with elimination of the pill-free interval as indicated by the above advice. Diarrhoea alone is not a problem, unless it is of cholera-like severity!

Women who have had a previous combined pill failure.   They may claim perfect compliance or may perhaps admit to omission of no more than one pill. Either way, since surveys show that most women miss tablets quite frequently but very few conceive, the ability to do so selects out those who are likely to have low levels of the COC hormones, or ovaries with above-average return to activity in the pill-free interval. So all women in this group should in my view be advised to take three (or four) packets in a row, the so-called tricycle regimen, followed by a shortened pill-free gap. Often six days is a good choice in these cases since it is easy to remember— each tricycle's start day now being identical to the finish-day—but the gap may be shortened further in a 'high risk' case.

Drug interaction.   (See Back and Orme 1990 or Guillebaud 1989 for more details and references.) This may reduce the Pill's efficacy mainly in two ways. The first and by far the more important is by induction of liver enzymes, which leads to increased elimination of both oestrogen and progestogen. Alternatively, disturbance by certain broad spectrum anti-biotics of the gut flora which normally split oestrogen metabolites arriving in the bowel can reduce in a very small—but unknown—minority of women the reabsorption of reactivated oestrogen. (Note: this effect on the entero-hepatic cycle is not a factor in the maintenance of *progestogen* levels and so is irrelevant to the progestogen-only pill.) See Table 3.16 for the most important drugs and the clinical implications.

Short-term use of any interacting drug/long-term use of broad spectrum antibiotic.   Extra contraceptive precautions are advised for the duration of the treatment and then as the 'seven-day rule' above, according to when in the pill packet the last potentially less effective pill was taken. *Rifampicin* is such a powerful enzyme-inducer that even if it be given only for two days (as, for instance, to eliminate carriage of the meningococcus), increased elimination by the liver must be assumed for four weeks thereafter (Orme 1991, personal communication). Extra contraception or a stronger pill with elimination of one or more pill-free intervals (see below) should be recommended to cover that time. With *broad spectrum antibiotics* there is the useful fact that the large bowel flora responsible for recycling oestrogens are reconstituted with resistant organisms in about two weeks. In practice therefore, if the COC is commenced in a woman who has been taking a tetracycline long term (for acne, for example) there is no need to advise extra contraceptive precautions. There is a potential problem only in the reverse situation, when the tetracycline is first introduced to treat a long-term pill-taker. Even then, extra precautions need to be sustained only for 2 weeks (plus, if indicated by Fig. 3.1, no break before the next pack).

Long-term use of enzyme-inducers.   This chiefly applies to epileptics and women being treated for tuberculosis (Table 3.16). Especially for patients treated with rifampicin, an alternative method of contraception such as an intra-uterine device or depot medroxyprogesterone acetate with a shortened (eight-week) injection interval should be offered.

But if the combined pill is preferred it is appropriate to prescribe initially a 50 μg oestrogen-containing preparation of which only three remain on the market (Table 3.9) and also recommend that the *tricycle regimen* described above be used (Table 3.15). This reduces the number of contraceptively 'risky' pill-free intervals (PFIs). It is particularly appropriate for epileptics since the frequency of attacks is often reduced by the maintenance of steady hormone levels. At the Margaret Pyke Centre we recommend that the PFI is also shortened at the end of each tricycle to five or four days according to the perceived conception risk.

If the preferred progestogen is not marketed as a 50 μg pill, a logical if expensive alternative is to use combinations of tablets, e.g. one Mercilon and one Marvelon daily. If so, careful records are essential since this is outside the current recommendation of the Data Sheets.

Breakthrough bleeding may be the first clue to a drug interaction; and should also be used as an indication to make appropriate alteration to the pill prescription, or to advise a change of method. If the long-term user of an enzyme-inducer develops BTB, the first step is to give two or more tablets a day, if necessary to provide a combined oestrogen content of 80 or 100 μg (maximum), titrated against the BTB.

In this way the usual policy, giving the minimum dose of both hormones to finish just above the threshold for bleeding, can be followed. The woman can be reassured that she is metaphorically 'climbing a down escalator'. In other words, her increased liver metabolism means that her system is still basically receiving a low-dose regimen. She is exposed to more metabolites, but this is not known to be harmful (and for some women the available alternatives are just not acceptable).

Discontinuing enzyme-inducers.   Enzyme induction may take numerous days to reach its peak when the drug is introduced, and it may be 4 to 8 weeks before the liver's level of excretory function reverts to normal when it is withdrawn. Hence if any enzyme-inducer has been used for a month or

Table 3.16 *The more important drug interactions with COCs*

Class of drug	Approved names of important examples	Main action	Clinical implications for COC use
Drug which may reduce COC efficacy			
Anticonvulsants	barbiturates (esp. phenobarbitone) phenytoin primidone carbamazepine	Induction of liver enzymes, increasing their ability to metabolize *both* COC steroids.	Tricycling preferred, as in text, using 50 μg oestrogen COCs, increasing to max 100 μg if BTB occurs. *Sodium valproate* and *clonazepam* are anticonvulsants *without* this effect.
Antibiotics			
(a) Antitubercle	rifampicin	*Marked* induction of liver enzymes.	Short term, see text. Long term, use of alternative contraception is preferred, e.g. Depo-Provera with 8-week injection intervals (p.89). Otherwise as for anticonvulsants with 4-day gaps after each tricycle.
(b) Antifungal	griseofulvin	Enzyme inducer	As for anticonvulsants.

(c) Broad spectrum ampicillin and relatives tetracyclines	Change in bowel flora, reducing enterohepatic recirculation of ethinyloestradiol (EE), only, after hydrolysis of its conjugates.	Short courses—wisest to use additional contraception during illness and follow 7-day rule—see text. Long-term low-dose tetracycline for acne—no apparent problem, probably because resistant organisms develop, within about 2 weeks. POP is unaffected by this type of interaction.
Hypnotics glutethimide dichloral phenazone *Tranquillizers* meprobamate	Induction of liver enzymes probable.	Avoid these drugs in COC-users (alternatives available).
Drugs which may increase COC efficacy ascorbic acid paracetamol	Competition in bowel wall for conjugation to sulphate. If either of these drugs present, more EE available for absorption.	Only applies to mega-doses (0.5–1 g daily) of vitamin C. Effectively results in the patient taking a high oestrogen COC No effect on the progestogen Advise: at least two hours separation of either drug from the time of pill-taking.
co-trimoxazole	Inhibits EE metabolism in liver.	None, if short course given to low-dose COC user.

more (or *at all* in the case of rifampicin) it is recommended (Orme 1986, personal communication to NAFPD) that there is a delay of about four weeks before the woman returns to a standard low-dose pill regimen. This should be increased to 8 weeks after more prolonged use of rifampicin or barbiturates. And logically there should then be no gap between the higher- and the low-dose packets.

Effects of COCs on other drugs

(See Back and Orme 1990.) COC steroids are weak inhibitors of hepatic microsomal enzymes. They thus slightly lower the clearance of, for example, diazepam and prednisolone. This may perhaps increase the risk of side-effects, seriously in the case of the drug cyclosporin—but otherwise the change is very unlikely to be noticed clinically.

As COCs tend to impair glucose tolerance, sometimes cause depression and raise the blood pressure, they naturally tend to oppose the action of antidiabetic, antidepressant, and antihypertensive treatments. If the latter treatments are required, however, the COC is relatively not absolutely contraindicated.

Practitioners who detect possible interactions (of any type) are asked to complete a yellow card for the Committee on Safety of Medicines.

Reasons to stop the Pill

Pill-takers should be advised of those symptoms listed in the FPA leaflet which mean they should immediately stop the Pill, pending investigation and treatment:

1. Painful swelling in the calf.
2. Pain in the chest or stomach.
3. Breathlessness or cough with blood-stained sputum.
4. A bad fainting attack or collapse, or focal epilepsy.
5. Unusual or severe and very prolonged headache/migraine.
6. Disturbance of speech (dysphasia).
7. Loss of sight in either eye or either field of vision.
8. Numbness, severe paraesthesiae or weakness of limb(s) on one side.

Numbers (4) to (8) may be caused by transient cerebral ischaemia. They mean that *oestrogen* should be stopped, but any progestogen-only method may be started immediately. Other reasons for stopping are usually less urgent:

9. Detection of a sustained BP above 160/95 on repeated measurement, or perhaps at lower values if there are other risk factors for CVS disease.
10. Appearance of a new risk factor, e.g. onset of diabetes or the diagnosis of frank breast cancer.

11. Onset of jaundice.

12. Four weeks before elective major or leg surgery, or at once with heparinization if admitted as an emergency (see Table 3.7).

13. Immobilization, e.g. after orthopaedic injury or operation.

14. Personal choice, e.g. because pregnancy is desired.

15. When contraception is no longer needed (no partner, sterilization, or after the menopause has been established).

The first period after stopping the Pill is often delayed. Amenorrhoea for six months should always be investigated, whether or not it occurs after stopping the Pill.

Congenital abnormalities and fertility

There are many conflicting reports in the world literature not helped by small numbers studied and confounding factors such as smoking, alcohol, and other drugs which have not always been considered. Two per cent of all full-term fetuses have an important malformation.

The conclusions of a WHO Scientific Group (1981) have not been materially challenged subsequently. These were:

(1) no established evidence for any adverse effects on the fetus of oral contraceptives used prior to the conception cycle;

(2) with regard to oral contraceptive use after conception, the evidence for an increased risk of congenital malformations is unclear; but if such a risk exists, it must be very small.

It is always wise to warn women against taking any medication if they believe themselves to be pregnant. If the general practitioner is asked the question, 'Should I come off the pill for two to three months before getting pregnant?', there is no dogmatic answer. It should certainly do no harm; but there is no objective evidence that it is worth the effort. Certainly any woman finding herself pregnant less than three months after stopping the COC should be strongly reassured. In relation to fertility, conception may be delayed by a few months on average on stopping the Pill, but there is no evidence that the Pill causes long-term irreversible infertility.

There is no benefit to be achieved by taking short breaks of six months or so every few years, as was once recommended. One-quarter of young women taking such short breaks had unwanted conceptions in one study. Moreover a pill-taker can be reminded that she has regularly given her body 'breaks' from the COC totalling 13 weeks in each year (see p. 74 above).

Duration of use

Though still uncertain, it remains possible that increased duration of use may adversely affect the risk of circulatory disease in users, though reassuringly it clearly now does not do so in ex-users (Stampfer *et al.* 1988).

Pending more information therefore it may be prudent to restrict total *accumulated* duration of use to a maximum of 15 years in those with risk factors. In the remainder the new ruling of the FDA's Advisory Committee (p. 63 above) removes any strict upper limit. Some women may therefore choose to continue to age 50 with over 30 years' use—and even then switch to HRT (see p. 112–13).

Summary

The combined pill provides highly acceptable contraception for many. Individuals vary, however, and some are suited to only one formulation. Presentation of multiple side-effects in spite of the prescription of low doses would indicate the need for a different method, but excessive anxiety about consequences should first be suspected and possible psychosexual aspects discussed. No matter how carefully those with contraindications are excluded, a few women will experience adverse effects. Supervision is essential, especially of blood pressure and headaches, and it is important that the woman feels able to report back (often to the practice nurse) at any time.

Oral contraception is easy and a preferred method for many. If the combined pill is not suitable, the progestogen-only ('oestrogen-free', 'POP', or 'mini') pill is a good alternative.

Progestogen-only pill (POP)

There are six varieties available (Table 3.17).

This is an under-used and often abused method which requires maximum motivation by both patient and doctor. Taken absolutely regularly each day within a couple of hours, without breaks and regardless of bleeding

Table 3.17

				Number of tablets
Noriday	(Syntex)	350 μg	norethisterone	28
Micronor	(Ortho)	350 μg	norethisterone	28
Femulen	(Searle)	500 μg	ethynodiol diacetate	28
Neogest	(Schering)	75 μg	dl norgestrel	35
Microval	(Wyeth)	30 μg	levonorgestrel	35
Norgeston	(Schering)	30 μg	levonorgestrel	35

(NB: 75 μg dl norgestrel is equivalent to 37.5 μg levonorgestrel.)
The choice of POP is largely empirical, though Neogest has been superseded (by the last two in Table).

patterns, it can provide protection from pregnancy not far short of the combined pill, especially above age 30. The Oxford/FPA Study reported a failure rate of 3.1 per 100 woman-years at age 25–29, but this improved to 1.0 at 35–39 and as low as 0.3 for women over 40 (Vessey *et al.* 1985).

NB: The same database suggests but does not prove the possibility that *the failure rate is higher in women who weigh above 70 kg (11 stone)*, as already established for progestogen rings and implants. Such women should be warned of this possibility, and unless this risk is refuted by future studies they might reasonably be offered two POPs daily.

Mechanism of action and maintenance of efficacy

This is complex because of variable interaction between the administered progestogen and the endogenous activity of the woman's ovary (Guillebaud 1989). Fertile ovulation is prevented in at least 60 per cent of cycles. In the remainder there is reliance mainly on progestogenic interference with mucus penetrability, backed by some anti-nidatory activity at the endometrium. The former effect is at its minimum at the time each new dose is taken, hence the most usual time for intercourse is the *worst* regular time for a woman's pill-taking.

The starting routines are summarized in Table 3.18. Where there is interference with contraceptive activity due to missed pills, vomiting, or drug interaction, this is believed to start within as little as *3 hours*; but to be adequately corrected as far as the mucus is concerned if renewed pill-taking is combined with extra precautions for just *48 hours*. (Note: at the time of writing discussions are in progress, involving the manufacturers and family planning bodies, which may lead to extension of this recommendation to *7 days*. As always with the POP there is a paucity of good data. But seven days would be logical with regard to the antiovulatory effect in over

Table 3.18 *Starting routines with the POP*

	Start when?	Extra precautions?
Menstruating	1st day of period	No
Post-partum		
(a) no lactation[1]	Any time before the 4th week	No
(b) lactation[1]	Usually 4 weeks after delivery	No
Induced abortion/miscarriage	Same day	No
Post-combined OC	Instant switch	No

[1] Bleeding irregularities minimized by starting at or after the 4th week.

half of any population of POP-users; which by analogy with the COC might be expected to take a week to be restored, see p. 76.)

Antibiotics do not interfere with the effectiveness of the POP (see Table 3.16)—apart from the enzyme-inducers rifampicin and griseofulvin. Another contraceptive method would normally be advised for users of interacting drugs in that category; though a trial of two POPs per day has also been proposed if nothing else is acceptable.

There is no real basis on which to decide which POP to use, though that will change once one of the new more 'lipid-friendly' progestogens is available as a POP. The choice depends mainly on the doctor's (and the woman's) preference. Though with all POPs the dose to the infant is believed to be harmless, it appears that the least amount of administered progestogen gets into the breast milk if a levonorgestrel preparation is used.

Indications

1. Side-effects with, or recognized contradictions to, the combined pill, in particular those believed to be oestrogen-related.
2. Older women—especially *smokers* above age 35.
3. Diabetes—see p. 115.
4. Hypertension—either COC-related, *or* other varieties controlled on treatment.
5. Migraine, including focal varieties. The woman may continue to suffer the migraines but the fear of an oestrogen-promoted thrombotic stroke is eliminated.
6. Lactation—the combination is as effective as the COC is in non-breast-feeders. The COC may be recommenced when periods return with weaning.
7. Sickle cell disease.
8. At the woman's choice.

Contraindications

Absolute contraindications are few (and the last four are not necessarily permanent):

1. Past or current *severe* arterial disease, or very high risk thereof.
2. Any serious side-effect on the COC not certainly related solely to the oestrogen, e.g. progestogen allergy, liver adenoma.
3. Undiagnosed genital tract bleeding.
4. Actual or possible pregnancy.
5. Recent trophoblastic disease—until HCG is undetectable in blood as well as urine, since there is no certainty it is not the progestogen that

increases the likelihood of chemotherapy being required, in some studies. (See p. 61.)

6. The woman's unrelieved anxiety about the POP method. To these can be added two strong relative contraindications specific to the POP, namely:

1. Previous ectopic pregnancy.
2. Past *symptomatic* functional ovarian cyst formation.

The first of these is clearly the stronger contraindication, especially in nulliparae, since the POP sometimes allows ovulation with the risk of implantation in the possibly already-damaged remaining fallopian tube. But the frequency of symptomatic cysts is also greater, leading to a problem in differential diagnosis among POP-users with abdominal pain. NB: asymptomatic persistent follicles or cysts which are very commonly picked up on a routine ultrasound scan (Tayob *et al.* 1985) do not have this relevance.

The remaining *relative contraindications* are:

1. Risk factors for arterial disease, including as above under 'Indications'. The presence of more than one risk factor can be permissible, unlike with the COC.
2. Sex-steroid-dependent cancer. Seek the agreement of the relevant hospital consultant.
3. Current liver disorder with persistent biochemical change.
4. Enzyme-inducer drugs (see above).
5. Chronic severe systemic diseases (see p. 64–5). If pregnancy is known to cause deterioration, the POP has the disadvantage of lesser efficacy than the COC. But if hormones were one day shown to aggravate the particular condition the tiny dose in the POP should have less effect.
6. Overweight (see above).

Problems and management

Negligible changes to most metabolic variables have been reported, presumably because of the low dose coupled with the counteracting effect of endogenous oestrogen still produced by the woman's incompletely-suppressed ovaries. This may not be true in POP-users with long-term amenorrhoea and the concern that this might cause adverse lipid effects or osteoporosis is still debated. If available, it would be reasonable to check an oestradiol level in such cases and consider a change of method if it is low (less than 100 pmol/litre).

Apart from the occasional complaint of breast tenderness, which is usually transient but may be recurrent and can sometimes be overcome empirically by changing from one progestogen to another, the main problem presented is that of menstrual irregularity. With advance warning this is usually well tolerated. It is often helpful if the woman keeps a record chart in early months, as this quickly highlights the type of problem and usually demonstrates improvement. Premenstrual and some climacteric symptoms are often relieved. More than half the women will have a cycle between 25 and 35 days.

Even when cycles are short, between 21 and 24 days, complaints are rare provided the bleeding is not too heavy. Two or three days' light bleeding twice a month is another common and acceptable pattern. A few women will experience prolonged and heavy bleeding and if this is not relieved by changing the brand of pill another method should be selected.

Prolonged spells of amenorrhoea occur most often in older women. Once pregnancy is excluded, the amenorrhoea must be due to anovulation so signifies very high efficacy. Unless there is evidence of hypo-oestrogenism (see above) the method can be continued. Diagnosing the menopause in these cases poses a difficulty discussed on page 113.

Blood pressure needs to be regularly monitored but where raised during administration of the combined pill, it usually reverts to normal on the POP. Indeed if it does not do so the woman most probably has essential hypertension.

Because it is thought not to affect blood-clotting mechanisms it may be used for women with a past history of thrombo-embolism. Good counselling and record-keeping are essential in these situations, as most manufacturers' leaflets still recommend against this use.

The acceptability of the POP depends largely on the practitioner's attitude and confidence based on experience.

The progestogen-only contraceptive vaginal ring ('Femring')

This is made of Silastic from which there is the sustained daily release of levonorgestrel. There is therefore no peak load of hormone reaching the liver and the 20 μg dose is about the same as finally reaches the blood after a tablet of Microval or Norgeston (see Table 3.17) has passed through the GI tract and liver.

In most respects this vaginal ring is like the POP, except for aspects relating to its route of administration and the advantage of not having to remember to take tablets every day. Practically everything above about the POP applies to Femring, including its mechanisms and variable interactions with each woman's menstrual cycle, its similar effectiveness, its minimal effects on metabolism, its advantages, and its side-effects. Specific contraindications are marked vaginal prolapse and untreated vaginitis, and alternative contraception should be used with some vaginal medications notably clotrimazole and povidone iodine.

The prospective user is shown how to squeeze the ring and insert it into the vagina, waiting until the first day of her period. Unlike the diaphragm it does not need to be located in any special position related to the cervix. It is then left for 90 days, after which a replacement is required. If preferred by either partner it may be removed during intercourse, but preferably for no more than about one hour at a time. Indeed, if three hours have elapsed, as with the POP extra precautions are necessary for the next 48 hours. But there is no problem with the ring's effectiveness during an attack of vomiting or diarrhoea—another advantage.

If the ring slips out into the toilet bowl it should simply be retrieved, washed in clean water, and reinserted. If this keeps recurring the woman should return for examination (exclude prolapse, pelvic tumour, or constipation).

There is a strong suspicion that Femring is less effective under age 25 and in women weighing above 70 kg (11 stone). Another method may then be preferable—unless there is reduced fertility (during lactation or above age 40, for example) or the woman can manage to lose the excess weight.

The ring can sometimes cause a specific problem: vaginal irritation or discharge. But as with the POP the commonest side-effect is irregular bleeding, or amenorrhoea, about which forewarned is forearmed. Functional cysts also occur and can be symptomatic, resulting in the usual problem of excluding an ectopic pregnancy.

At the time of writing, plans to market this new option have been postponed.

Injectables

There are two available: Depo-Provera (depot medroxyprogesterone acetate or DMPA), 150 mg every 12 weeks; and Noristerat (norethisterone oenanthate), 200 mg every 8 weeks, given in either case by deep intramuscular injection, within the first five days of the menstrual cycle. Only Depo-Provera is currently licensed by the Committee on Safety of Medicines, for long-term contraceptive use in women for whom other contraceptives are contraindicated or otherwise unsatisfactory. It has been repeatedly endorsed by the expert committees of prestigious bodies, including WHO and the gynaecological subcommittee of the US Food and Drug Administration (though it is still, even in 1992, not available in that country for contraceptive use). For use-effectiveness it is second to none among reversible methods (0–1 per 100 woman-years), primarily through causing anovulation. If enzyme-inducers are required, especially rifampicin or antiepileptics, the injection interval is shortened (to 8–10 weeks).

Why is DMPA not far more widely used in general practice since there are, surely, very many women in the category 'other reversible contraceptives found wanting'? Anxiety has been generated worldwide and in many quarters by animal research of very doubtful relevance to humans. Recent human studies are compatible with a co-factor effect on breast cancer in young women similar to that suggested for the COC (see p. 59); but this is unproven and should not in my view affect practice when prescribing the method to women free of other risk factors for breast cancer. It is also true that the effects, whether wanted (contraceptive) or unwanted, are not reversible for the duration of the injection. This is the critical point to be explained to prospective users during counselling, backed by the approved manufacturer's leaflet. However, a consensus view is that DMPA is actually a safer drug than the combined pill, despite the adverse publicity it receives.

After the last dose conception is commonly delayed (median delay 9–10 months, which is of course 6 months ex-use of the method). But a study in Thailand showed that almost 95 per cent of previously fertile users had conceived by 28 months after their last injection (Pardthaisong *et al.* 1980). This study refutes allegations of permanent infertility caused by the drug.

Side-effects

These include irregular bleeding or amenorrhoea and, in long-term users, weight gain. Preliminary warning saves anxiety about these. Excessive bleeding may resolve if the next injection is given early—but not less than four weeks since the last—or if oestrogen (e.g. Premarin 1.25 mg or ethinyloestradiol 20 μg alone or from a pill formulation) is given daily for 21 days. Post-partum bleeding problems are minimized if the first dose is delayed for five to six weeks, but much earlier use is permissible for some women's convenience after delivery. Menstrual abnormalities remain the greatest obstacle to any large increase in the method's popularity.

Absolute contraindications are those listed above for the POP. The relative contraindications are almost identical too, except that there needs to be a little more caution because the dose is larger, some studies do show a reduction in HDL-cholesterol levels, and there is that built-in lack of immediate reversibility. Unlike with the POP, the frequency of ectopics and ovarian cysts is *reduced*.

The main *indication* for an injectable is the woman's desire for a highly effective method which is independent of intercourse, when other options are contraindicated or disliked. It may be used despite past thrombosis (see comments above for the POP), and is ideal for many women wanting effectiveness while on the waiting list for major or leg surgery (see Table 3.7). Blood pressure is checked before each dose, though most studies fail to show any hypertensive effect. It is positively beneficial in endometriosis, in sickle cell anaemia, and for women at risk of pelvic inflammatory disease (PID) since the attack frequency is reduced. Faced with a nulliparous single woman who keeps forgetting her pills, a useful slogan is: 'When you think IUD, discuss instead Depo-Provera.'

Post-coital contraception or 'emergency contraception'

The need for an emergency measure to prevent pregnancy after an un-expected exposure to the risk is well-recognized. The use of large doses of oestrogen is now outmoded as it was associated with severe nausea and vomiting.

Two methods have now been shown to be effective (Table 3.19). A high oestrogen dose (50 μg) combined pill—Ovran, or the package known as PC 4, taken as two pills stat and repeated after 12 hours—will prevent implantation in about 98 per cent of cases. This hormonal therapy is effective for up to 72 hours after the *earliest* act of unprotected intercourse. Contraindications are those suggesting any significant risk of arterial or venous thrombosis, or any other contraindication to oestrogen (*not* progestogen whose significance relates only to long-term therapy). *There is no age limit* if sufficient conception risk is deemed to be present.

Table 3.19 *Methods of post-coital contraception*

	Pill	IUD
Method	PC 4 or Ovran Two pills stat Two pills 12 hours later	Nova T, CuT380 Slimline, or Multiload
Timing after intercourse	Up to 72 hours	Up to 5 days after calculated date of *ovulation*
Efficacy	98 per cent	Almost 100 per cent
Side-effects	Nausea and vomiting	Pain, bleeding, infection risk
Contraindications	Pregnancy +: Those relating to oestrogen	Pregnancy +: As for IUDs generally

Insertion of a medicated IUD up to five days after the calculated ovulation day prevents implantation in almost 100 per cent of women, even in cases of multiple exposure. There are risks of pain, bleeding, or infection as with any IUD so that this option is not often advisable for the nulliparous woman. Cervical swabs (e.g. for *Chlamydia*) and antibiotic 'cover' may sometimes be appropriate and the device can always be removed following the next period. On the other hand, it can be ideal in many parous women for the device to be retained as the long-term method.

The following points should be covered at counselling:

1. Careful assessment of menstrual/coital history and hence appropriateness of the treatment.
2. Discussion of mode of action and ethics, if this is a concern.
3. Discussion of medical risks, especially: *failure rate* (2 per cent or up to 5 per cent with mid-cycle exposure, but close to nil if IUD method used); *teratogenicity* (believed negligible—though no proof—since the

hormones will not reach the blastocyst before implantation); and *ectopic pregnancy*. If the latter occurs it would almost certainly have done so anyway, without this (pre-implantation) treatment. But a past history of ectopic remains a strong relative contraindication to both methods.

4. Advice regarding nausea and vomiting. Anti-emetics are not very useful and are not routinely prescribed at the Margaret Pyke Centre. If either dose is vomited within three hours, the woman may be given two further tablets or, in a high risk case, an IUD inserted.

5. Discussion of contraception—in the current cycle (in case the hormonal method merely postpones ovulation) and long term. IUD insertion deals with both these aspects. If the COC is chosen it should be started as soon as the woman is convinced her next period is normal, and if this is no later than day 4 additional contraception need not be recommended thereafter.

All this implies the importance of (a) a good rapport with maximum good faith in obtaining the coital and menstrual history; (b) vaginal examination at the first visit as a rule, to exclude concealed clinical pregnancy or overt infection, and to establish a baseline size and shape of the uterus; and (c) effective arrangements for follow-up. A repeat examination at the follow-up visit is required only if there is clinical uncertainty.

Special indications apply to coital exposure when there has been:

1. Omission of more than two COC tablets after and therefore lengthening the oral contraceptive-free interval (see p. 75–6 above). After the emergency regimen the woman may return immediately to the COC with 7 days' condom use in addition, subject to her 100 per cent agreement to return for follow-up, in this case four weeks later. NB: In view of the slogan on p. 76, *midpacket pill-omissions after seven tablets have been taken never indicate emergency treatment*, unless, say, at least four have been missed. And towards the end of a packet, omission of the next pill-free interval will suffice.

2. Omission of two or more POP tablets, implying complete loss of the mucus effect. Again, the POP is restarted immediately after the emergency regimen, with 7 days' condom use in addition.

3. Removal or expulsion of an IUD prior to the time of implantation (see p. 98) if another IUD cannot be inserted for some reason.

Research continues and alternatives such as mifepristone or danazol may supersede the current methods in due course.

INTRA-UTERINE CONTRACEPTIVE DEVICES (IUDs)

The best modern devices can be expected to give failure rates of less than one per 100 woman-years (see Table 3.2). Women who are happily suited by this method love it, the rest hate it, and sadly their views are more vigorously expressed. In reality it is a method that is beginning to make an overdue 'come-back', now specifically for the older parous woman who wants a user-friendly effective reversible alternative to the Pill for some years—perhaps prior to but often instead of sterilization.

All users will experience longer and usually also heavier bleeding and the acceptability and tolerance of this varies. While irregular, intermenstrual, or post-coital bleeding may be associated, gynaecological causes must be excluded—especially ectopic pregnancy and in the older woman genital malignancy.

It cannot be overemphasized that *the overall effectiveness and acceptability of this method depends primarily on the skill of the practitioner who inserts it.* This cannot be learnt from books. The JCC's 'apprenticeship' training scheme is ideal, practising with the aid of small pelvic models and diagrams or videos before patients are actually fitted with a minimum of 10 devices of at least two designs. Considerable and ongoing experience is an absolute essential for good technique. Among other sequelae, inadequately inserted devices are prone to be expelled or malpositioned (a cause of failure, or of 'lost threads'). Perforation of the uterus may occur, especially when it is soft (post-partum or post-abortion), during lactation, or if its acutely anteverted or retroverted position is not identified and allowed for with use of atraumatic holding forceps during insertion. See Table 3.20, column H.

Types of device

More than 100 devices have been designed since their introduction.

Inert devices
Lippes Loop, four sizes (size C was most commonly used). These were withdrawn in 1986 but may still be retained in some women. There is no upper limit for duration of use.

Medicated devices
Since the last edition of this book, several devices have been withdrawn in this country—based primarily on the medico-legal climate of the USA and for financial reasons rather than on drug regulatory grounds:

Gravigard—Copper 7.

Minigravigard—Mini-Copper 7 (small, was especially suitable for emergency use in nulliparae).

Progestasert (vertical arm contained progesterone—needed annual renewal). The LNG-IUD is similar but releases 20 µg of levonorgestrel daily

Table 3.20 *Problems and complications of IUDs—a summary*

	Main hazards	A Directly or indirectly threatens fertility?	B Linked with symptomatic pain?	C Linked with symptomatic bleeding?	D May present as 'lost threads'?	E Special problem in the young nullipara?	F Frequency with increasing age	G Frequency with increasing duration of use	H Can be caused by poor insertion technique?
1. Intra-uterine pregnancy (device *in situ*)	Miscarriage Infection, see 6	Yes	Yes	Yes	Yes	Yes	→	→	Yes, as result of 5
2. Extra-uterine pregnancy	Significant mortality Loss of tubal function	Yes	Yes	Yes	No	Yes	↑ (Little effect)	↑	Yes[1]
3. Expulsion	Pregnancy, then as 1, 6	Yes	Yes	Yes	Yes	Yes	→	→	Yes
4. Perforation	Pregnancy Risks of IUD removal Adhesion formation	Yes	Yes	No	Yes	No	=	=	Yes
5. Malposition	Predisposes to 1, 3, 7, 8 One cause of 'lost threads'	Yes	Yes	Yes	Yes	Yes	=	=	Yes
6. Pelvic infection	Loss of tubal function	Yes	Yes	Sometimes	No	Yes	→	→	Yes[1]
7. Pain	Underlying cause may be overlooked, see column B	—	—	Often	No	Yes	=	→	Yes, as result of 5
8. Uterine bleeding	Underlying cause may be overlooked, see column C; also uterine cancer	—	Often	—	No	No	↑	→	Yes, as result of 5

[1] If insertion either introduces or exacerbates (pre-existing and undiagnosed) pelvic infection, leading to tubal damage.

and has many advantages including reduced or absent menstruation and a five-year duration of use (Guillebaud 1989). Not yet available in UK, but will hopefully be before 1994.

Currently marketed
   Ortho-Gynae T-380 Slimline (approved for 4 years).

Multiload   Cu 250 } (approved for 3 years).
             Cu 250 short
             Cu 375 (approved for 5 years).

Novagard Nova T (approved for 5 years).

Ortho-Gyne T   Cu T-200 (approved for 3 years). This has a higher failure rate than the others listed and little to recommend it.

NB: The approved durations of use have no bearing on the true longevity of modern copper devices. No study has shown a defined upturn in pregnancy rates after a certain number of years, as might be expected if insufficient copper remained. Hence the authoritative statement of the Family Planning Association and the National Association of Family Planning Doctors, namely that: 'Less frequent replacement would reduce the risks of pelvic inflammatory disease, uterine perforation, expulsion, and other complications that mainly occur soon after insertion . . . We recommend that for routine management the modern copper-bearing IUDs . . . should be assumed to have an active lifespan of five years or more.' (Newton and Tacchi 1990). Moreover 'any device fitted after the age of 40 may be safely left in place until the menopause' (Szarewski and Guillebaud 1991).

The above statements supply strong medico-legal safeguards for what is manifestly better for our patients, regardless of the Data Sheets. It must however be clearly documented that the woman has not been promised any greater efficacy in the next year, if beyond those licensed, than existed in the preceding year.

Choice of device

Practitioners will have their own favourite devices based on their own experience. For most parous women the Copper T-380 has the advantage of a long effective duration of use—now established as over eight years (justifying the words 'or more' in the FPA/NAFPD statement above). The Multiload is the simplest to insert correctly which is very relevant for practitioners with infrequent opportunities to maintain their expertise. The 375 model appears to perform appreciably better as well as lasting longer and is preferred. It also has a low expulsion rate if there is a past history of that problem, or when inserted at the time of termination of pregnancy. (Even better for resistance to expulsion and also for patient comfort, it seems, will be the innovative Cu-Fix or Flexigard, a device under study with six bands of copper bonded straight on to a nylon thread bearing a knot, which is embedded by the stylet-introducer in the fundal myometrium.)

Although the IUD method is not recommended for nulliparous women, in those cases where it is indicated the (smaller) Nova-T should be used. Insertion is more difficult and often associated with some degree of cervical shock. Premedication with mefenamic acid 500 mg and a low threshold for use of paracervical lignocaine anaesthesia is helpful. The method is less reliable in nulliparae, there is a greater expulsion rate, and dysmenorrhoea is exacerbated. The risk of pelvic infection and subsequent fertility problems has been shown to be considerable. See below and Table 3.20.

Menstrual problems may occur with any IUD, but heavy bleeding is less frequent with the smaller devices (one advantage permitted by the use of copper). If the bleeding proves excessive and if intra-uterine contraception is preferred or badly needed, mefenamic acid treatment may be helpful (see p. 181). Unfortunately it does not help the more common and often more annoying 'spotting' or intermenstrual bleeding. An alternative is to remove the device and insert another preferably smaller design. Those women who tolerate very heavy loss because of the convenience of the method must be checked for anaemia. *Pain may be* an acceptable side-effect of the method, but the safe slogan is *'pain +/− bleeding has a serious cause until proved otherwise'*. See columns B and C of Table 3.20.

Absolute contraindications
These may be classified as:

Permanent
  1. Past history of tubal ectopic pregnancy.*
  2. Past history of tubal surgery, or other high ectopic risk.*
  3. Distorted uterine cavity, or cavity sounding to less than 5.5 cm depth.
  4. Known true allergy to a constituent (e.g. copper).
  5. Known infection with the human immunodeficiency virus (HIV). This is chiefly because of the increased risk of severe pelvic infection in the immunocompromised.

Temporary
These imply a delay before possible later insertion:
  6. Undiagnosed, irregular genital tract bleeding.

---

* Considered relative contraindications in selected parous women.

7. Suspicion of pregnancy.
8. Active pelvic infection, or pelvic tenderness not yet diagnosed.
9. High risk of genital sexually transmitted disease (e.g. recent attack of *Chlamydia*, or after rape) or marked purulent discharge.
10. Immunosuppressive treatment.*

Other contraindications are *relative* and mostly related to the risk of impairing future fertility (the main issue in all counselling about the method).

Relative contraindications
1. Past history of treatment for pelvic infection.
2. Suspected subfertility.
3. Lifestyle risking sexually transmitted disease.
4. Nulliparity and young age, especially less than 20. The reason here is both increased *likelihood* of infection (see below) and also the more serious *implications* thereof. Absolute contraindications if (1) to (3) also apply.
5. Valvular heart disease. (Prosthetic heart valve: absolute contraindication).

Such women should preferably use another method—because of the increased risk of bacterial endocarditis. If the method were selected, the fitting should be done by an expert, with antibiotic cover. Most cases with minor heart lesions may be given the Brompton Hospital regimen of an oral sachet of amoxycillin 3 g one hour before, repeated eight hours after the procedure. Otherwise the recommendations of the British National Formulary should be followed. The patient would also need to be warned even more carefully than other IUD-users to seek prompt medical advice should she develop pelvic pain, deep dyspareunia, or excessive discharge.

6. Fibroids or congenital abnormality *without* serious distortion of the uterine cavity.
7. Severely scarred uterus, or severe cervical stenosis.
8. Heavy periods before insertion for any reason, including anticoagulation.
9. Anaemia.
10. Severe primary dysmenorrhoea.
11. Endometriosis.
12. Wilson's disease, especially if penicillamine used to treat. (There are one or two anecdotes of *in situ* pregnancy in copper IUD-users given this drug.)

---

* Considered relative contraindications in selected parous women.

NB: When available, the LNG-IUD will be the preferred device if almost any of the above relative contraindications applies.

Timing of insertion and removal

It is customary to insert devices in the closing days of or immediately after a period. The presence of a pregnancy is thereby excluded, the procedure is easier, and any associated bleeding is accepted as part of normal loss. Recent data suggest increased risks, particularly of expulsion, if IUDs are inserted during the main flow. At the Margaret Pyke Centre we normally plan to insert between days 4 and 14.

Insertion no later than five days from the calculated day of ovulation prevents nidation and is increasingly offered as a post-coital method. It is of course possible to insert a device at any time, once existing implanted pregnancy is excluded. In cases of amenorrhoea (e.g. post-partum) a very practical tip is to use the most sensitive modern pregnancy tests twice, before and after 14 days during which time the couple agree to practise 'brilliantly good' birth control or abstinence.

After a recent delivery, in general practice IUDs should be inserted at 4–6 weeks, extended to 6–8 weeks after a caesarean section. Extra care is needed, especially during lactation, to minimize the risk of perforation.

Where possible the result of a cervical test for *Chlamydia* infection should be available (see below). It must be documented that the woman gave her informed verbal consent based on her reading and understanding the current leaflet of the UK FPA or equivalent.

Removal except in cases of emergency—for example, when severe pelvic infection is present (in which case consider hormonal post-coital contraception)—should only be carried out during a period, or inter-menstrually if the IUD has not been relied on by the patient for the preceding seven days. The method is now known to work mainly by preventing fertilization (WHO 1987—a highly recommended review), but it undeniably can also operate by altering the endometrium, rendering it unsuitable for implantation. Therefore, once any device is removed an already fertilized ovum could embed in the same cycle, and pregnancy continue.

Problems and management

The list of IUD problems is short enough to be summarized in one Table (3.20)—contrast the COC. Mortality is very low, but moderate to severe morbidity relatively common. The table draws attention to the important interrelationships of the problems: symptoms such as pain and bleeding mean 'trouble' until proved otherwise; 'lost threads' has a number of explanations as further classified in Table 3.21. Selection and adequate

Table 3.21 *Differential diagnosis of 'lost threads' with IUDs*

Main diagnoses A. Not pregnant	Clinical clues	B. Pregnant	Clinical clues
1. **Device in uterus** Threads cut too short, or caught up around device during original insertion or avulsed at a previous removal attempt; or device itself malpositioned	(a) Periods likely to be those characteristic of IUD *in situ* (b) Uterus normal size	4. **Device *in situ* + pregnancy**	(a) Amenorrhoea (b) Pregnancy test likely to be positive, with clinically enlarged uterus (sufficient to pull up thread)
2. **Unrecognized expulsion**	(a) Recent periods as woman's normal pattern (b) Uterus normal size	5. **Unrecognized expulsion + pregnancy**	(a) Amenorrhoea, following one or more apparently normal periods (i.e. unmodified by IUD) (b) Signs of pregnancy variably present (may be too early on first presentation)
3. **Perforation of uterus**	As 2 plus (rarely) mass or actual IUD palpated on bimanual examination	6. **Perforation of uterus + pregnancy**	As 5 plus (rarely) mass or actual IUD identified on bimanual examination

instruction of potential users is emphasized by columns E–G of Table 3.20; and the paramount importance of correct insertion is re-emphasized by column H.

Pregnancy

There have been cases of serious and even fatal mid-trimester septic abortion when an IUD has been left in the pregnant uterus. Paradoxically therefore, early removal (before the strings disappear) is always recommended. While this may lead to abortion, leaving the device *in situ* at least doubles the rate—as well as predisposing to ante-partum haemorrhage, premature labour, and stillbirth. If the threads have already gone missing the whole pregnancy must be considered *at high risk and steps taken to ensure discovery/recovery of the device after delivery.*

There is no evidence that the presence of copper on the device has a damaging effect on the fetus.

Ectopic pregnancy may occur. A history of a previous extra-uterine pregnancy must be considered as an absolute contraindication to the use of an IUD in any woman who may wish to have further children. The ratio of ectopic to intra-uterine pregnancies in IUD users ranges from about 3–9 per cent (WHO 1987): in non-IUD users it is now about 1 to 100. Some studies suggest the actual risk per 1000 users may actually be reduced as compared with non-users, meaning that the higher ratio just given is caused by the success of IUDs in causing *an even greater reduction in the denominator of pregnancies in the uterus.* Clinically, though, the implications are the same as if the IUD were causative: if pelvic pain occurs in an IUD-user this diagnosis must always be excluded.

Lost strings: expulsion and perforation

Expulsion most commonly occurs during bleeding, soon after insertion, and with less than one-third of instances beyond the first year. Even with accurate insertion some women seem prone to expulsion, especially at reinsertion with immediately preceding removal. A most useful test for partial expulsion at follow-up is to pass a sound (or a readily-available sterile throat swab) up to the level of the internal os.

Women should be taught how to check the strings and if not felt there are several other possible explanations (see Table 3.21). These are summarized by the maxim 'lost strings means the woman is pregnant or at risk of pregnancy until proved otherwise'. All such women therefore need to be advised to use an alternative contraceptive method until the protective presence of an IUD has been established. Above all, they need full explanations and supportive counselling throughout the management.

I recommend the following very practical scheme. Diagnosis and treatment are simultaneous in most cases, with minimum use of hospital facilities:

1. *Exclude implanted pregnancy.* Take a careful menstrual history, do a bimanual examination, and as indicated perform the most sensitive pregnancy test available. If the woman is pregnant, the management is primarily that of the pregnancy itself.

In the absence of pregnancy, it is entirely appropriate (even in a general practitioner's surgery) to proceed as follows:

2. *Insert long-handled Spencer–Wells forceps or equivalent into the endocervical canal.* If the jaws are gently opened and shut the threads can be retrieved in about half of all intra-uterine-located devices. If the IUD is judged still to be correctly located, no further action need be taken. But since disappearance of the threads may be a sign of malposition it is usually advisable to remove and replace the device. If the threads are not found, the woman should be asked whether she would prefer thread retrieval as below (which should also quickly establish if there actually is a device *in utero*); or imaging first, as at step 5 below. Early recourse to imaging partly depends on her pain threshold, but is also much kinder than chasing a device which has actually been expelled or perforated.

3. *Try the use of thread-retrievers,* ideally with mefenamic acid pretreatment and local anaesthesia (LA) (as for insertion in nulliparae, see above). In the UK the most established is the Emmett Retriever, which is available presterilized and disposable. It has a handle to which is attached a thin plastic strip with multiple notches designed to trap the threads, and comes with instructions for use. Most practitioners will prefer to arrange hospital referral if this fails, but if convinced that the device is located in the uterus some may feel confident enough to continue—now definitely with use of LA.

4. *Next try small, blunt IUD-removal hooks* (Grafenberg pattern) or various resterilizable forceps, with short jaws or claws (e.g. the IUD Removing Forceps supplied by Rocket), opening wholly in the uterine cavity. In skilled hands these metal devices will nearly always retrieve the device.

5. *Arrange appropriate imaging, and referral thereafter as appropriate.* If the facilities are available, an ultrasound (u/s) scan may confirm *correct* intra-uterine location within a non-pregnant uterus. This can enable the woman to continue using the same device, with periodic re-scanning; but if there is any suspicion that it is malpositioned, appropriate steps should be taken for its removal as at 4 above—preferably under local, rarely under general, anaesthesia. If the u/s scan shows unequivocally that the uterus is empty, and non-pregnant, an X-ray is then required to differentiate between expulsion and perforation. A uterine marker (such as another IUD) may often be useful.

Perforation

The incidence is about one in 1000–2000 insertions. They are often post-partum and always insertion-related: to quote Jack Lippes, 'Devices do not perforate; for this to occur we need a practitioner.' If perforation has occurred removal should be arranged and this can usually be effected by laparoscopy. Copper-carrying devices provoke considerable adhesions so proceeding to laparotomy is not unusual.

Cases have been reported where strings are still protruding through the cervix although the device is actually in the Pouch of Douglas or embedded in bladder or bowel.

Infection

Although not presenting as often as heavy or frequent bleeding, the occurrence of pelvic infection is the most serious problem. Many studies have been reported as showing a greater risk of pelvic inflammatory disease in IUD-users than in non-users. In many of these the controls were inappropriate: e.g. pill-takers who are at reduced risk (see p. 58).

The risk clearly links with risk of sexually transmitted infections, and shows a similar decline with increasing age. In 1980 (Booth *et al.*), a report from the Margaret Pyke Centre revealed among 871 nulliparous women that after two years the 16 to 19-year-olds had an infection rate more than 10 times that of the 30 to 49-year-olds. It appeared that the lifestyle of the young women, or their partners, increased the likelihood of exposure to sexually transmitted infection. In good studies (WHO 1987) there was no increased risk of the most serious sequel, namely tubal infertility, among women who used an IUD but reported having only one sexual partner. Moreover, the proportion of women still infertile at two years after IUD removal for planned pregnancy is not different from that among women discontinuing other reversible methods.

However, because the superimposed foreign-body effects of an IUD may worsen an attack, and because bilateral monogamy is not common in most modern societies, overall the method is better avoided in the young and nulliparous woman.

Management of an attack will depend on the circumstances of the individual case. In parous women it may be possible to retain the device. It is, however, preferable to remove it, ideally after first establishing the antibiotic therapy. Reinsertion should be delayed at least six months; some authorities would say indefinitely.

Severe cases or those where there is a diagnostic problem (especially in excluding ectopic pregnancy or pelvic appendicitis) should be referred for hospital assessment. Full-dose antibiotic therapy is indicated, selection being modified on the result of an endocervical swab. *Chlamydia* is often the primary causative organism, with secondary infection including anaerobes frequently superimposed. A broad spectrum antibiotic, preferably a tetracycline, is therefore best given together with metronidazole while laboratory reports are awaited.

The woman should always be counselled particularly about the dire risk of tubal occlusion should her lifestyle lead to recurrences: rising to 23 per cent with just one further attack and to above 50 per cent with three or more in all. Contact tracing is also important though so often overlooked.

Actinomyces-like organisms (ALOs). These are sometimes reported on routine cervical smears in asymptomatic women who have had an IUD in place for some years, more frequently the longer the device has been in use. While frank actinomycosis is exceptionally rare, and a very small component of IUD-associated pelvic infection, its consequences can be disastrous so caution needs to be exercised. A study by Mao and Guillebaud (1984) showed that IUD removal led to clearance of this finding from subsequent cervical smears, even if (surprisingly) a new copper device were inserted at the same time. In asymptomatic women this simple replacement is reassuring to all concerned and is now our standard practice, after counselling and with subsequent cytology (at 3 months then annually). The device itself should be sent for bacteriology.

It is also acceptable for the woman simply to be appropriately advised and monitored thereafter. But if she has or develops pelvic pain, dyspareunia, or excessive discharge, and if tenderness is noted on examination, the knowledge that ALOs are present should markedly lower the threshold for IUD removal. If bacteriology ever shows infection rather than merely 'carriage' of the organism, penicillin is the antibiotic of choice—but in high dose and for at least three months.

Routine follow-up/duration of use

Correct location of IUDs should be confirmed 4–6 weeks after insertion, sounding the cervical canal with (for example) a throat swab being a valuable check for partial expulsion. Annual follow-up is then sufficient *provided* the IUD-user is fully informed of the danger-signs in Tables 3.20 and 3.21 and has open access to return promptly to the surgery if they occur. Devices are removed as indicated for complications, for planned pregnancy, or one year after the menopause. Otherwise Table 3.20 column G supports a flexible policy to 'leave well alone'.

BARRIER METHODS

'Old fashioned' as these methods may be, they are once again in fashion. In spite of well-known disadvantages they all (notably the sheath) provide useful protection against sexually transmitted diseases (see Chapter 13).

All users of this type of method should be informed in advance about emergency contraception, in case of lack of use or failure in use. It is also not widely enough known that vegetable and mineral oil-based lubricants, and the bases for some prescribable vaginal products, can seriously damage rubber: baby oil, for example, destroys up to 95 per cent of a condom's strength within 15 minutes. The Durex Information Service (1991) has produced a useful leaflet listing common vaginal preparations which should be regarded as safe and unsafe to use with condoms and diaphragms. See Table 3.22.

Table 3.22   *Vaginal preparations which are safe/unsafe to use with barrier methods*

Safe	Unsafe
Aqueous enemas	*Arachis Oil Enema*
Aci-Jel	*Baby Oil*
Betadine	*Cyclogest*
Canesten	*Ecostatin*
Clotrimazole	*Fungilin*
Delfen Foam	*Gyno-Daktarin*
Double Check	*Gyno-Pevaryl*
Durex Duracreme	*Monistat*
Durex Duragel	*Nizoral*
Durex Lubricating Jelly	*Nystan Cream*
Durex Senselle	*Petroleum Jelly*
Glycerine	*Orthodienoestrol*
Gynol II	*Ortho-gynest*
K-Y Jelly	*Premarin cream*
Nystan Pessaries	*Sultrin*
(not cream)	*Vaseline*
Ortho-Creme	
Ortho-Forms	
Ortho-Gynol	
Ovestin Cream	
Pevaryl	
Staycept Jelly	
Staycept Pessaries	
Travogyn	
Two's Company	

Source: Durex Information Service for Sexual Health 1991.

Sheaths/condoms

These are the only proven barrier to transmission of HIV and are being used increasingly with another contraceptive as well as alone. Yet unbelievably, and sadly, at the time of writing it still remains impossible for most couples to obtain this life-saver free of charge either at or via their GP Surgery. Readers are urged to lobby for this facility, and in the interim to find some means, as some practitioners have done, to utilize the AIDS budget to this end.

Condoms are everyone's second choice, second in usage to the Pill under 30 and to sterilization above that age. Most couples have had some experience of their use. Failure can practically always be attributed to incorrect use, mainly because of escape of a small amount of semen either before or after the act. One general practitioner was able to report a failure rate as low as 0.4 per 100 woman-years, but 5–15 is more representative. The print on the packet is too small for the learner to read in the heat of the moment and a clear explanation of the basics is always appreciated. Particularly when the COC has to be stopped after many years on medical grounds, couples need to be taught just how 'dangerous' a fluid semen will now become.

Some couples are entirely satisfied with the sheath, others use it as a temporary or a back-up method. For some, however, 'spoilt' by non-intercourse-related alternatives, it is completely unacceptable. Some older men, or those who have any sexual anxiety, complain that its use may result in loss of erection. But allergy can also be real and is often solved by use of the special 'Allergy' sheaths with no spermicide and reduced allergenic residues from the manufacturing processes. For those women who dislike the smell or messiness of semen, the sheath solves their problem.

Research is in progress into loose-fit lubricated plastic condoms, intended to overcome the most intractable problem of the method, that undeniable interference with penile sensation during the penetrative phase of intercourse.

Femidom

This is the only version of the female condom expected in the UK and it is likely to be marketed during 1992. It is a polyurethane sac with an outer rim at the introitus and a loose inner ring, whose retaining action is similar to that of the rim of a diaphragm. It thus forms a well-lubricated secondary vagina and it is considerably less likely than the male condom to rupture in use. Reports about its acceptability are mixed, but as the first female-controlled method with high potential for preventing HIV transmission it must surely be welcomed to the range of contraceptive options.

The cap or diaphragm

Many women express surprise at the simplicity of this method when first tried and complain because it had not been offered to them earlier. Some who found it unacceptable early in their lives find it much easier after experience with tampons and when sexual activity takes on a relatively regular pattern. Protecting the cervix from infection and semen, and inserted as a routine well ahead of coitus, it can be used without spoiling spontaneity. There is little reduction in physical sexual sensitivity as the clitoris and introitus are not affected and cervical pressure is still possible. Spermicide is essential as no mechanical barrier is complete, though more research is required to prove the point. The jelly vehicles (gels) may provide useful lubrication for the older woman, for those in the postnatal period, and others slow to lubricate as a result of sexual arousal.

Although many substances are well absorbed from the vagina there is no proof of systemic harm from the use of current spermicides, chiefly those using Nonoxynol-9 or its close relatives. Experience now spans over 60 years. A review by Bracken (1985) of 14 studies published to date concludes that, in particular, no association with congenital malformations or spontaneous abortion has been demonstrated. Occasionally a sensitivity to spermicide arises but rubber allergy is exceptionally rare. Direct local irritation does also occur, particularly if Nonoxynol-9 is used very frequently as by prostitutes; this effect has recently ended the advice to use it as an adjunctive virucide, though in normal use it remains entirely acceptable as a *spermicide*.

The acceptability of the diaphragm depends upon the manner in which it is offered. Its failure rate makes it an unsuitable choice for most young women who would not accept a pregnancy. But it is capable of excellent protection especially over the age of 35 (Table 3.2) provided it is correctly and consistently used. Correct fitting is important, and can only be learnt by practical 'apprenticeship'; the complaint of discomfort implies wrong fitting. Even more important is skill in teaching placement and the vital secondary check that the cervix is covered. As for the IUD, there is no substitute for one-to-one training in this process of fitting and teaching, in which one can perhaps learn most from the older generation of skilled family-planning trained nurses. The FPA leaflet should be provided as it includes all the (somewhat arbitrary) 'rules' of the method.

When it is apparent that a woman has great difficulty in inserting anything into her vagina, be it tampon, pessaries, or a cap, obviously the method is not suitable. Sometimes this problem may be connected with some psychosexual difficulty and this may first present during the teaching of the method. Permission to discuss associated fears and anxieties may prove helpful. Simple lack of anatomical knowledge is often involved.

When a vaginal barrier is rejected on account of 'messiness' this also may be due to such a problem. The offer of a less wet-feeling alternative for the spermicide (see below) may help: especially Delfen foam, or the option of C-film moistened and applied to the upper (cervical) surface of their diaphragm (Loudon *et al.* 1991).

If either partner complains of feeling the barrier during coitus, the fitting must be urgently checked. It could be too large, or too small; the retro-pubic ledge might be insufficient to prevent the front slipping down the anterior vagina; or most seriously the diaphragm may be being regularly placed in the anterior fornix. The arcing-spring diaphragm is particularly useful when this last problem is identified.

Chronic cystitis may be exacerbated by pressure from the anterior rim and sufferers may do better with a vault or cervical cap; though spermicide-related changes to the vaginal flora may also be a factor. The smaller non-diaphragm caps are now rarely used, yet some women cannot otherwise be suited or find them more comfortable to use than the ordinary diaphragm.

Diaphragms should be checked annually, post-partum, and if there is a 4 kg change in weight—gain or loss. If the size remains constant, how often a new one is needed will vary. Some get misshappen, very discoloured and worn by one year, and some appear pristine after two years.

Female barriers can be used happily and very successfully by many women, but high motivation is essential. Routine nightly insertion is practised by many, thereby allowing complete spontaneity of sexual activity. A good sense of humour helps the acceptability of this method!

SPERMICIDES

While invaluable as adjuncts to caps and sheaths, by themselves creams, jellies, pessaries, and foams are usually not acceptably reliable; but even used alone pregnancy rates under 10 per 100 woman-years have been obtained.

The *contraceptive sponge* is best considered as a carrier for spermicide, hence primarily appropriate for women whose natural fertility is reduced (namely age over 45, during lactation or secondary amenorrhoea). Spermi-cides in any acceptable form may also be useful as a supplement in couples who consider their only contraceptive option to be the withdrawal method; or for child-spacing.

FERTILITY AWARENESS: THE 'DOUBLE-CHECK' (SYMPTOTHERMAL) METHOD

At one time the rhythm or safe period method was generally despised and only adopted by staunch Roman Catholics. Modern versions are increasingly demanded by those who prefer to use a so-called 'natural' method, even although it is necessarily restrictive and presupposes the highest possible motivation. It can only result in maximum reliability if intercourse is confined to the premenstrual days following evidence of ovulation such as a rise in basal temperature which has been sustained for 72 hours at least 0.2°C above the preceding six days' values. The thermometer is prescribable on FP10 and temperature charts are available.

Temperature estimations are difficult when some cycles are anovulatory, especially in the post-partum period, during lactation, and in the climacteric years. At all times the use of basal body temperature changes is best combined with observations of the mucus discharge as detected at the vulva. This becomes increasingly fluid, glossy, transparent, slippery, and stretchy, like raw egg-white, under the influence of follicular oestrogen. The peak mucus day can be recognized retrospectively as the *last* day with such features before the abrupt change to a thick and tacky type (under the influence of progesterone). The infertile phase is defined as beginning on the evening of the fourth day after the peak mucus day, provided this is *also* after the third higher morning temperature reading.

Reliance only on the *later* of both the above signals for the onset of the post-ovulatory phase for unprotected intercourse can give acceptable failure rates of 1–6 per 100 woman-years. The pre-ovulatory phase is less effective. The indicators are:

1. The first sign of mucus, detected either by sensation or appearance.
2. Calendar calculation of the shortest cycle minus 19, where at least six cycle lengths are known, and the woman did note a high temperature phase in the preceding cycle to indicate that ovulation did occur in that cycle.

Whichever of these two indicators comes *first* indicates the requirement to abstain.

Use of both phases is only to be recommended to 'spacers', since calculations and mucus observations do not reliably predict ovulation far enough ahead to eliminate the capricious survival (sometimes for seven days) of sufficient sperm to cause a pregnancy.

Any who wish to use this method deserve careful explanation and teaching. An invaluable book for prospective users is by Anna Flynn and Melissa Brooks (see 'Further reading for patients'). Useful instruction leaflets can be obtained from:

(1) The FPA, 27–35 Mortimer Street, London W1N 7RJ;
(2) The Natural Family Planning Service, Catholic Marriage Advisory Council, 1 Blythe Mews, Blythe Road, London W14 0NW;
(3) The Natural Family Planning Centre, Birmingham Maternity Unit, Queen Elizabeth Medical Centre, Edgbaston, Birmingham B15 2TG.

Personal teaching may be arranged through (2) and (3) above.

STERILIZATION

There is a tendency for couples to expect sterilizing procedures to solve all problems and to be free of any associated risk, complications, or consequences. While providing maximum reliability, failures are occasionally reported and the rate usually quoted is two per 1000. A lower rate of one case in 2000–7000 was quoted for *late* failures of vasectomy by Philip *et al.* (1984) but it is important to recognize that these followed two azoospermic semen analyses.

General anaesthetics carry their own very small risk, but modern techniques have considerably reduced the severity of the operation and the length of hospitalization required. Psychological and physical consequences have been reported, of both tubal ligation and vasectomy, and the need for careful preliminary discussion with both partners is absolutely essential if ultimate satisfaction is to result.

Although sterilization is usually undertaken as a permanent procedure, requests for reversal do occur. In a series published by Winston (1980) reporting on 103 women who requested reversal between 1975 and 1976, 87 per cent were under age 30; 63 per cent had been sterilized after delivery; and no less than 75 per cent had been unhappily married. He reported a 58 per cent pregnancy rate after microsurgery when the 37 per cent who had had a completely irreversible operation had been excluded. With increasing experience of such specialist surgeons and the wider use of clips and rings, reversal successes have improved. Even though modern surgical techniques can be used to reverse some sterilizations, such operations demand skill, are difficult to get, are often expensive, and are not always successful. It is still wise therefore, to consider sterilization to be irreversible and only to proceed when both partners can accept this. Couples sometimes feel differently after the passage of time. Regret is more likely if the decision is made at a time of crisis or stress, and as a general rule post-partum and post-termination sterilizations should simply not be done.

The psychological sequelae of sterilization have been looked at. Earlier studies showed considerably higher rates of psychiatric morbidity, psychosexual dysfunction, and regret than a prospective study (Cooper *et al.* 1982) in which women were interviewed four weeks prior to elective sterilization and followed up at 18 months. In this latter study considerable regret was felt by 2 per cent at six months and by 4 per cent at 18 months, and post-operative psychiatric disturbance and dissatisfaction were largely associated with pre-operative psychiatric disturbance. The poorer results in other studies may be related to several factors including that, previously, patients were more likely to have been sterilized in association with a termination or immediately post-partum.

Most of these studies on sequelae of sterilization were hospital-based but a small general practitioner study (Curtis 1979) identified 61 sterilized women. A control group of patients were asked similar questions about their experiences since their last pregnancy. These questions covered the area of menorrhagia, hysterectomy, libido changes, and showed little difference between the two groups. As far as patient satisfaction with the sterilization was concerned, 45 had no regrets and 16 had some regrets, but only two of these seemed to be really serious. Many other studies give similar results.

Some couples seek sterilization in the hope that it will solve their sexual difficulties. Other couples who find it impossible to use contraceptive methods may be using the fear of pregnancy as a defence against sexual activity. This defence is removed by tubal ligation or vasectomy. For most couples, however, an irreversible step is just what they want, and once this decision is reached then the most appropriate procedure needs to be identified after discussion.

As compared with vasectomy, tubal occlusion is a more invasive procedure even when performed, as it now readily can be, under local anaesthesia. It confers immediate sterility while it may be several months before the semen is clear of sperm after the male operation. More importantly, especially once she passes the age of 40 the woman is unlikely to wish for restoration of her fertility, even with any future new partner. Following vasectomy, however, after death of the wife or marriage breakdown the man (even if past 50) nearly always finds a new and younger partner, and *she* makes him then more likely to regret his sterility. So although the male procedure is very simple and safe medically, with occasional haematomas the main complication, this difference from the female operation needs to be faced by older couples during counselling.

After female sterilization, the later development of menstrual problems is often reported. Since these and the operation in women are both common, a chance association is likely. It is never possible to anticipate any woman's menstrual future and indeed there are many published series which refute any connection, including one that measured menstrual blood loss before and two years after surgery.

Over the years vasectomy has stood accused of various long-term effects, notably accelerated arteriosclerosis and cancer either of the testis or of the prostate. So far none has been confirmed in a voluminous literature. So at present it is not thought to be good medicine to mention any of these postulated risks proactively during counselling: any questions raised by the man himself should of course be answered reassuringly and honestly, conceding the difficulty of proving no effect.

THE OVER-35-YEAR-OLD WOMAN

Most women of this age have achieved their desired family size and/or established themselves in some form of career or working life. Conception to them—especially in the fifth and sixth decades—may well be catastrophic: psychosocially, and also through the ever-increasing risk of maternal mortality, perinatal mortality, and fetal abnormality. Those (relatively few) women who continue menstruating regularly are likely to be fertile. But for the remainder, during the ten years before the menopause, menstrual cycles become irregular.

Older women are not easily convinced that episodes of amenorrhoea along with less frequent intercourse mean that conception is actually much less likely to occur. Yet as we have seen simpler methods like contraceptive sponges or foam have acceptable efficacy above age 45. The cap or diaphragm can be extremely reliable—though is usually acceptable only if already in use since a younger age—and the spermicide compensates for diminishing lubrication. There is now agreement that any copper IUD fitted after the 40th birthday may be left *in situ* until the menopause. These are all good reversible options for any older woman.

Hormone methods

Until recently many practitioners have considered these (apart perhaps from the POP) as off-limits for the older woman. This rigid view is now outdated. For a start, post-coital oestrogen–progestogen (the Yuzpe regimen) is clearly not contraindicated on the grounds of age alone, at any time up to the menopause, if conception is likely (see p. 91). *But what about much longer use of an oestrogen plus progestogen regimen?* In these premenopausal years there are many potential non-contraceptive advantages, such as the reassurance of regular bleeds and the sexual benefits: avoiding intercourse-related methods and preventing oestrogen deficiency with associated skin ageing, poor vaginal lubrication, and loss of libido. Symptoms of the so-called 'normal' menstrual cycle (especially the premenstrual syndrome and frequent, heavy, painful periods) are controlled. Even more important is the reduced risk of gynaecological pathology. Pelvic infection, extra-uterine pregnancy, fibroids, dysfunctional haemorrhage, endometriosis, functional ovarian cysts, and carcinoma of the ovary and uterus are all less frequent in long-term users of combination oestrogen/progestogen therapy. The principal, entirely acceptable, alternatives are either neutral (e.g. barriers, sterilization); or, *though they may in many individuals be entirely satisfactory*, they have the potential to exacerbate menstrual cycle-linked problems (e.g. intra-uterine devices, progestogen-only methods). If the latter occur, the risks of some treatments (whether medical with lipid-altering drugs like danazol, or surgical by hysterectomy) may well be considerably greater than those of the Pill.

Moreover, hot flushes and early osteoporosis may begin before the actual menopause. In short, age alone no longer rules out a modern contraceptive/hormone replacement regimen. *In selected healthy non-smokers above age 45* the many therapeutic/preventive benefits outweigh in my view the small though definite increased risks of prescribing a modern 'lipid-friendly' pill. This view receives strong support from the US Food and Drug Administration's Fertility and Maternal Health Drugs Advisory Committee, which on 26 October 1989 *recommended to the FDA that there should be no upper age limit* for oral contraceptive use by healthy non-smoking women (Fortney 1990).

Since this historic pronouncement, at the Margaret Pyke Centre we generally prefer an appropriate ultra-low dose pill to 'ordinary' hormone replacement therapy for conception-risking women who need supplementation for their diminished ovarian function. Scrupulously careful supervision is essential. And pending more data, *smokers above age 35* requesting hormonal contraception should use a progestogen-only method. An IUD or sterilization may be even better.

Various new combined options are or will soon be available which may, unlike most current methods of hormone replacement, be reliably contraceptive, including: oestrogen plus progestogen skin patches; vaginal rings; or, perhaps best, a progestogen-releasing intra-uterine device to protect the uterus from hyperplasia (while minimizing systemic side-effects of the progestogen) plus oestrogen by any chosen route. The possibility looms, as shown in the USA for unopposed oestrogen used when contraception is no longer required, of actually reducing the possibly-fertile older woman's risk of arterial disease.

Further research is required to prove that the benefits of these new regimens truly outweigh the risks, particularly of breast cancer. But we must escape the absurdity of prescribing to older women hormone replacement pill regimens among which some, by containing a relatively high dose of the progestogens norethisterone or levonorgestrel, may adversely affect lipids and are unlikely to be any safer than their previous contraceptive pills. Yet they only stopped the latter years earlier because doctors told them they were 'too old'!

Finally, use of present fertility awareness methods is almost impossibly difficult because of cycle irregularity, anovulatory spells, and altered vaginal secretions. Improved technology for predicting ovulation (far enough ahead) might change that view. And though sterilization of either party solves the problems of many, it may prove unnecessary with good presentation of alternatives.

When to stop contraception

There is no simple answer to the question which many patients will ask: 'Have I stopped ovulating yet?' Most authorities would still advise them to discontinue all contraception only after the occurrence of complete amenorrhoea for 12 months (or two years if under age 45). Long spells of amenorrhoea in women under 40 may indicate the arrival of a premature menopause, but they may be due to other spontaneously reversible or treatable causes requiring investigation (see Chapter 7 on the menopause). After the age of 40, particularly if the amenorrhoea is associated with hot flushes, the diagnosis of menopausal infertility is increasingly likely.

If the combined pill is now usable until the menopause, how may that be diagnosed? The 'standard' teaching as above, to switch to a non-hormonal method and wait many months, prevents the use of HRT (whose withdrawal bleeds like those of the combined pill will indefinitely mask the menopause, and which is not safely contraceptive) at the very time when vasomotor symptoms may be most pronounced. An alternative protocol is the following: arbitrarily at age 50 the woman switches to a simple method ('Delfen' foam or the 'Today' sponge being adequate at this age) and records any subsequent bleeds and vasomotor symptoms. The latter will follow in less than one month if she has been relying on the COC for her oestrogen (the situation is comparable to sudden loss of ovarian oestrogen by oophorectomy). A high FSH result after one to three months is very suggestive of final ovarian failure at this age. After advice that the risk of later ovulation cannot be completely excluded, the woman may then discontinue contraception, whether or not she chooses to commence HRT.

If however the woman has a normal FSH result and/or menstruates while off hormones, she should assume some residual fertility and use a simple contraceptive, again whether or not she decides to take HRT.

For POP users the following protocol to diagnose menopausal infertility appears to work well: if prolonged amenorrhoea occurs as a new phenomenon above age 45 along with symptoms suggestive of the menopause, the woman may have her FSH measured while still taking the method. If it is low she still needs the POP. If it is high, vasomotor symptoms combined with a repeat high FSH value when off treatment provide confirmation that she may now discontinue contraception (Guillebaud 1989). However younger women and any who want more complete reassurance may if preferred continue a simple contraceptive method, as usual, until one year after the last non-hormonally-induced bleed.

It is important to remember that many unwanted pregnancies occur in women over 45, as evidenced in Table 3.23. In 1988 the number of therapeutic abortions came to 47 per cent of the total conceptions (excluding miscarriages). Although these numbers are small in comparison with other age groups, it can be safely assumed that many of these conceptions would have been associated with much anxiety and stress, better avoided by the use of contraception.

THE WOMAN WHO HAS JUST BEEN PREGNANT

Ovulation may occur as early as 10 days after abortion and by about day 28 after delivery. Early contraception is therefore important. In women who

Table 3.23   *Birth statistics 1988, England and Wales*

Age	Live births	Legal abortions	%
40–44	8520	5047	37
45–49	440	393	47
50+	67	19	21
All above 40	9027	5459	37
cf. All ages	693 577	168 298	19

do not breast-feed the COC should be started no earlier than day 21 in order to minimize any extra risk of venous thrombosis.

The COC may inhibit lactation and does enter the milk in small quantities. The progestogen-only variety is preferable. This does not interfere significantly with lactation and although traces may enter the milk the quantity would be so small that it has been equated to a baby getting the equivalent of one pill in two years. This is considerably less than the progesterone level found in dried cow's milk. The natural childbirth movement nevertheless advises against its use. If a woman is unhappy about this type of contraception she should use an alternative method. See Tables 3.14 and 3.18 for starting routines with oral contraceptives.

The IUD is easily inserted at four to six weeks post-partum but the uterus is still soft and great care is necessary particularly if the woman is lactating. Earlier insertion is more likely to lead to expulsion. If any infection (endometritis) is present, insertion is better delayed.

The sheath method is useful until other methods are established. Caps and diaphragms may be refitted at five to six weeks and this is necessary even after Caesarean section. Use of the fertility awareness approach is very difficult at this time.

Sterilization procedures performed at abortion or in the post-partum period carry extra operative and emotional risks; surgery is now usually, and preferably, delayed for a few months.

THE VERY YOUNG

Although early cycles after the menarche are assumed to be anovulatory, very early conceptions are being reported, and surveys show that around half of the total female population under 16 years of age have had intercourse. This represents a major category of technical law-breaking, not by the girl but by all those male partners.

A modern low-oestrogen, lipid-friendly, *combined pill* usually proves the most suitable method. As far as we know once periods are established it poses no special problems in teenagers, as compared with women in their twenties. *Injectables* are preferable to IUDs because of their protective effect against pelvic infection, though the latter are not absolutely contra-indicated. The *ideal IUD* will probably be the levonorgestrel-releasing variety mentioned above, when available, since it also appears to reduce the risk of infection as well as relieving dysmenorrhoea. But since this age group may now be the most at risk of all sexually transmitted agents including HIV it is essential to promote *use of the condom in addition*, often, to the selected main contraceptive.

Any general practitioner faced with an under-16-year-old needs first, opportunely and non-patronizingly, to raise the advantages both psycho-logical and physical of delaying intercourse until later (and then of mutual loyalty). S/he must also study the revised DHSS *Memorandum of guidance* (DHSS HC[FP]86). Although involvement of at least one parent is vastly preferable, this lists the circumstances in which it is good practice to proceed to prescribe the Pill without it. At all times the young woman must be assured of confidentiality.

WOMEN WITH INTERCURRENT DISEASE

Such a woman usually requires maximum possible protection from preg-nancy. Female sterilization, however, is not always indicated. Depending on factors like her expectation of life, her healthy partner's kind offer to have a vasectomy may be best not accepted. The Pill may be associated with additional risks, but it is particularly good at preventing pregnancy which is often dangerous. Clearly, each couple has to be considered indi-vidually and discussion with the consultant in charge is often mandatory, especially in cancer cases. Diabetes is a good example of many of the principles to be applied.

Diabetes

See Tables 3.5 and 3.8. The combined pill using a 'lipid-friendly' progestogen can be valuable for limited periods, under careful supervision and provided there is no arteriopathy or retinopathy or neuropathy or renal damage (or smoking!), and preferably if the duration of the diabetes has been short. The progestogen-only pill is acceptable and usually very reliable. The greater risk of any infection to diabetics argues somewhat against the IUD, though it can be a satisfactory choice after childbearing (preferably backed by regular spermicide use since these are also germicides). Barriers would be the reversible methods of choice, ideally followed by sterilization when-ever the family is complete.

Other conditions

Clearly if any condition is a recognized absolute contraindication, as listed above for each method, the latter should be avoided. Regarding the remainder which are relative contraindications whose importance varies, see p. 64–5 above and the excellent chapter in Sapire (1990) entitled 'Sexuality, contraception and disease'.

THE FUTURE

In spite of the availability of a full, comprehensive contraceptive service, the requests for termination of unwanted pregnancies continue to increase. For some women it proves very difficult to get contraceptive advice, and others seem unable to use any method successfully. New pills, vaginal rings, intra-uterine devices, injectables, and implants (notably 'Norplant') will undoubtedly be marketed in the near future, and new varieties of vaginal barriers are being tested. Sensitive understanding of the innumerable factors which influence the acceptability of family planning is vital if women are to be helped to avoid unwanted conceptions. There is still a need for more understanding by the very young concerning the ease of conception and by the older woman of the persistence of fertility. Too often women conceive because they do not believe it will happen to them or because they do not intend to indulge in sexual activity but get 'swept off their feet'. Physicians in whatever field they work have a responsibility to make it easy for their patients to ask for advice and then to have the skill to help them use their own choice, happily and effectively.

REFERENCES AND FURTHER READING

Adam, S. A., Thorogood, M., and Mann, J. I. (1981). Oral contraception and myocardial infarction revisited: the effects of new preparations and prescribing patterns. *British Journal of Obstetrics and Gynaecology*, **88**, 838–45.

Back, D. J., Breckenridge, A. M., Crawford, F. F., *et al.* (1981). Interindividual variation and drug interactions with hormonal steroid contraceptives. *Drugs*, **21**, 46–61.

Back, D. J. and Orme, M. L. 'E. (1990). Pharmacokinetic drug interactions with oral contraceptives. *Clinical Pharmacokinetics*, **18**, 472–84.

Booth, M., Beral, V., and Guillebaud, J. (1980). Effect of age on pelvic inflammatory disease in nulliparous women using a Copper 7 intrauterine contraceptive device. *British Medical Journal*, **ii**, 114.

Bracken, M. B. (1985). Spermicidal contraceptives and poor reproductive outcomes: the epidemiological evidence against an association. *American Journal of Obstetrics and Gynecology*, **151**, 552–6.

Cooper, P., Gath, D., Rose, N., *et al.* (1982). Psychological sequelae to elective sterilisation: a prospective study. *British Medical Journal*, **284**, 461–4.

Croft, P. and Hannaford, P. C. (1989). Risk factors for acute myocardial infarction in women: evidence from the Royal College of General Practitioners' oral contraception study. *British Medical Journal*, **298**, 165–8.

Curtis, D. M. (1979). The sequelae of female sterilisation in one general practice. *Journal of the Royal College of General Practitioners*, **29**, 366–9.

Demacker, P. M., Schade, R. W., Stalenhoef, A. F., *et al.* (1982). Influence of contraceptive pill and menstrual cycle on serum lipids and high-density lipoprotein cholesterol concentrations. *British Medical Journal*, **284**, 1213–15.

Drife, J. O. and Guillebaud, J. (1986). Hormonal contraception and cancer. *British Journal of Hospital Medicine*, **35**, 25–9.

Durex Information Service for Sexual Health (1991). Warning: oil-based lubricants and ointments can damage condoms and diaphragms. *LRC Leaflet*, 1–4.

Evans, D. I. (1984). Sickle cells and hormonal contraception. *British Journal of Family Planning*, **10**, 80–1.

Filshie, M. and Guillebaud, J. (ed.) (1989). *Contraception—science and practice*. Butterworths, London.

Fortney, J. A. (1990). Oral contraceptives for older women. *International Planned Parenthood Federation Medical Bulletin*, **24**, 3–4.

Guillebaud, J. (1989). *Contraception—your questions answered*. Churchill Livingstone, Edinburgh.

Loudon, N. (ed.) *Handbook of family planning*. Churchill Livingstone, Edinburgh.

Loudon, N. B., Barden, M. E., Hepburn, W. B., *et al.* (1991). A comparative study of the effectiveness and acceptability of the diaphragm used with spermicide in the form of C-film or a cream or jelly. *British Journal of Family Planning*, **17**, 41–4.

Mann, R. D. (ed.) (1990). *Oral contraceptives and breast cancer*. Parthenon, Carnforth.

Mao, K. and Guillebaud, J. (1984). Influence of removal of intrauterine contraceptive devices on colonisation of the cervix by actinomyces-like organisms. *Contraception*, **30**, 535–45.

National Association of Family Planning Doctors (NAFPD) (1984). Interim guidelines for doctors following the pill scare. *British Journal of Family Planning*, **9**, 120–2.

Newton, J. R. and Tacchi, D. (1990). Long-term use of copper intrauterine devices. *Lancet*, **336**, 182.

Pardthaisong, T., Gray, R. H., and McDaniel, E. B. (1980). Return of fertility after discontinuation of depot medroxyprogesterone acetate and intrauterine devices in Northern Thailand. *Lancet*, **i**, 509.

Peto, J. (1989). Oral contraceptives and breast cancer: is the Cash Study really negative? *Lancet*, **i**, 552.

Philp, T., Guillebaud, J., and Budd, D. (1984). Late failure of vasectomy after two documented analyses showing azoospermic semen. *British Medical Journal*, **289**, 77–9.

RCGP (Royal College of General Practitioners) (1977). Mortality among oral contraceptive users. *Lancet*, **ii**, 727–31.

RCGP (1981*a*). Further analyses of mortality in oral contraceptive users. *Lancet*, **i**, 541–6.

RCGP (1981*b*). Report from General Practice 21. *Family planning—an exercise in preventive medicine*.

RCGP (1983). Incidence of arterial disease among oral contraceptive users. *Journal of the Royal College of General Practitioners,* **33,** 75–8.

Sapire, K. E. (1990). *Contraception and sexuality in health and disease.* McGraw-Hill, London.

Serjeant, G. R. (1985). Pregnancy and contraception. In *Sickle cell disease* (ed. G. R. Serjeant), pp. 287–8. Oxford University Press.

Smith, S. K., Kirkman, R. J., Arce, B. B., *et al.* (1986). The effect of deliberate omission of Trinordiol (R) or Microgynon (R) on the hypothalamo-pituitary-ovarian axis. *Contraception,* **34,** 513–22.

Stadel, B. V. (1981). Oral contraceptives and cardiovascular diseases. *New England Journal of Medicine,* **305,** 612–18, 672–7.

Stampfer, M. J., Willett, W. C., Colditz, G. A., *et al.* (1988). A prospective study of past use of oral contraceptive agents and risk of cardiovascular diseases. *New England Journal of Medicine,* **19,** 1313–17.

Szarewski, A. and Guillebaud, J. (1991). Regular review: contraception, current state of the art. *British Medical Journal,* **302,** 1224–6.

Tayob, Y., Adams, J., Jacobs, H. S., *et al.* (1985). Ultrasound demonstration of increased frequency of functional ovarian cysts in women using progestogen-only oral contraception. *British Journal of Obstetrics and Gynaecology,* **92,** 1003–9.

Thorogood, M., Adams, S. P., and Mann, J. I. (1981). Fatal subarachnoid haemorrhage in young women: role of oral contraceptives. *British Medical Journal,* **ii,** 762.

UK National Case Control Study (1989). Oral contraceptive use and breast cancer risk in young women. *Lancet,* **i,** 973–82.

Vessey, M. P. (1982). Oral contraceptives and cardiovascular disease: some questions and answers. *British Medical Journal,* **i,** 615.

Vessey, M. P. (1989). Oral contraception and cancer. In *Contraception, science and practice* (ed. M. Filshie and J. Guillebaud), pp. 52–68. Butterworths, London.

Vessey, M. P. (1990). The Jephcott Lecture, 1989: an overview of the benefits and risks of combined oral contraceptives. In *Oral contraceptives and breast cancer* (ed. R. D. Mann), pp. 121–35. Parthenon, Carnforth.

Vessey, M. P., Lawless, M., and Yeates, D. (1982). Efficacy of different contraceptive methods. *Lancet,* **i,** 841–2.

Vessey, M. P., Lawless, M., McPherson, K., *et al.* (1983). Neoplasia of the cervix uteri and contraception: a possible adverse effect of the pill. *Lancet,* **ii,** 930–4.

Vessey, M. P., Lawless, M., Yeates, D., *et al.* (1985). Progestogen-only oral contraception. Findings in a large prospective study with special reference to effectiveness. *British Journal of Family Planning,* **10,** 117–21.

Vessey, M. P., Villard-Mackintosh, L., McPherson, K., *et al.* (1989). Mortality among oral contraceptive users: 20 year follow-up of women in a cohort study. *British Medical Journal,* **299,** 1487–91.

WHO Scientific Group (1981). The effect of female sex hormones on fetal development and infant health. *Technical Reports Series,* No. 657. WHO, Geneva.

WHO Collaborative Study of Neoplasia and Steroid Contraceptives (1985). Invasive cervical cancer and combined oral contraceptives. *British Medical Journal,* **290,** 961–5.

WHO Scientific Group (1987). Mechanism of action, safety and efficacy of intrauterine devices. *Technical Reports Series,* No. 753. WHO, Geneva.

Winston, R. M. L. (1980). Reversal of tubal sterilisation. *Clinical Obstetrics and Gynaecology,* **23,** 1261–8.

The IPPF (International Planned Parenthood Federation) produces much useful literature for doctors and also a *Directory of contraceptives* which gives names of the pills available in all countries.

Further reading for patients

Guillebaud, J. (1991). *The Pill* (4th edn). Oxford University Press.
Rakusen, J. and Phillips, A. (1989). *The new our bodies, ourselves*. Penguin, Harmondsworth.
Flynn, A. and Brooks, M. (1990). *A manual of natural family planning*. Unwin Hyman Paperbacks, London.

Useful patient leaflets concerning all methods can be obtained from the FPA, 27–35 Mortimer Street, London W1N 7RJ. Leaflets and pill instructions in other languages are obtainable from the FPA and the IPPF, 18–29 Lower Regent Street, London SW17 4PW, and also through some manufacturers of oral contraceptives.

4. Unwanted pregnancy and abortion

Katy Gardner and Lis Davidson

(Based on the chapter by Judith Bury in the second edition of this book)

Most general practitioners will be familiar with the clinical situation of a woman who is unhappy about her pregnancy but some will find it arouses uncomfortable feelings. The doctor may feel uneasy at being asked to provide a service—referral for abortion—rather than being asked to exercise the classical medical skills of diagnosis or treatment. In addition, the doctor's attitude to abortion may make it difficult to respond to the woman's needs. In this chapter we hope to show that, whatever the views of the doctor, there is a great deal that can be done to help and there are useful skills that can be developed. In fact, the role of the general practitioner in this area can be just as rewarding as in any other medical situation. But first some background.

THE BACKGROUND

Terminology

This is not a chapter simply about abortion. To talk only about abortion would be to pre-empt the decision that the doctor and the woman with an unwanted pregnancy must make. There will, however, be a strong emphasis on abortion, not because it is always the most appropriate outcome for an unwanted pregnancy, but because it is the area that is most likely to involve the general practitioner rather than the social services.

We have chosen the term 'unwanted' rather than 'unplanned' or 'unintended' pregnancy. A pregnancy may have been planned and intended, yet for a number of reasons may be unwanted; on the other hand an unplanned pregnancy may yet be wanted. However, the term 'unwanted' is not without problems; in particular, it hardly does justice to the ambivalence that many women feel.

Abortion legislation

History of the law in England and Wales
The 1861 Offences Against the Person Act made abortion illegal in all

circumstances, although in practice an exception was made when the woman's life was in danger.

In 1938 interpretation of the law was made more liberal by Judge Macnaghten in the Bourne case when he stated that it was lawful to terminate a pregnancy not only to save a woman's life but also 'if the doctor is of the opinion . . . that . . . the continuation of the pregnancy would make the woman a physical or mental wreck' (*British Medical Journal* 1966).

In spite of the Bourne judgement, the limits of the law remained unclear; and the need for clarification was one of a number of factors that led to attempts to change the law. After the war there was a gradual liberalization of views on certain social issues such as homosexuality and divorce as well as on abortion. In the case of abortion this was partly due to concern about the prevalence of illegal abortion with its often dire results. During the 1950s and 1960s the demand for abortion seemed to be increasing; with more effective contraception, many women were choosing to delay or limit their childbearing and take on other roles. Many women were also less willing to accept an unplanned pregnancy than in the past, when the opportunity to control fertility had been more limited. The thalidomide tragedy in the early 1960s further underlined the need for a change in the law. Alongside these factors, the advent of new methods and the use of more effective antibiotics meant that abortion was becoming safer.

The 1967 Abortion Act. The 1967 Abortion Act was the seventh attempt to reform the law on abortion; it came into effect in April 1968.

In 1974 the Lane Committee, which was set up to report on the working of the Abortion Act, concluded that '. . . the gains facilitated by the Act have much outweighed any disadvantages for which it has been criticised' (Lane 1974).

The 1967 Abortion Act did not repeal the 1861 Act but defined exceptions to that Act in which abortion would be legal. These defined exceptions are:

if two registered medical practitioners are of the opinion, formed in good faith—
(a) that the continuance of the pregnancy would involve risk to the life of the pregnant woman, or of injury to the physical or mental health of the pregnant woman, or any existing children of her family, greater than if the pregnancy were terminated; or (b) that there is a substantial risk that if the child were born it would suffer from such physical or mental anormalities as to be seriously handicapped.

In determining the risk of injury to health the Act states that 'account may be taken of the pregnant woman's actual or reasonably foreseeable environment.'

Abortions not covered by these exceptions remained illegal and a time limit was laid down, not by the 1967 Act but by the 1929 Infant Life (Preservation) Act. This states that abortion is illegal (except to save the woman's life) once the fetus has become 'capable of being born alive' which for many years was assumed to be 28 weeks' gestation.

There have been numerous attempts to restrict the 1967 Act but the only alteration has come from the 1990 Human Fertilization and Embryology Act which reset the time limit for abortion at 24 weeks' gestation. However, it also allows that this limit does not apply where there is risk of grave permanent injury or death to the mother or a substantial risk of serious handicap in the child. In fact, the 1990 Act is an example of statute law falling in line with existing practice since very few abortions, 23 in 1989 in England (Hall 1990), were being performed after 24 weeks gestation, and these were being done for reasons permitted under the 1990 Act. It is unlikely therefore that this Act will lead to any radical change in practice.

Abortion laws in Scotland

The 1861 and 1929 Acts did not apply in Scotland. Before 1967 abortion was a common law offence but there were no prosecutions in cases of therapeutic abortion carried out without secrecy by a gynaecologist. By the 1960s a few gynaecologists were openly performing abortions on married women with many children but most gynaecologists were reluctant to test the law.

When the Abortion Act passed into Scottish law in 1968, some feared it might act restrictively but this was not the case. As in England and Wales, many doctors became increasingly willing to perform abortions. Although the absence of the 1861 and 1929 Acts from the statute books does not affect the availability of abortion in Scotland, some differences between England and Scotland remain (see 'Statistics', p. 123).

Abortion laws in Northern Ireland

The 1967 Abortion Act did not extend to Northern Ireland but the 1861 Act does apply there, so abortion remains illegal except to save the woman's life. Every year more than 1000 women travel from Northern Ireland to England for a private abortion.

The changing role of the general practitioner

Before 1938, when a woman consulted her doctor about an unwanted pregnancy, the doctor had little option but to persuade her to continue the pregnancy and to help her through this and through adoption if appropriate. Doctors were rarely involved in helping women to procure an abortion and when they did so they were usually acting illegally. Yet most doctors practising at that time would have been only too familiar with the sight of an ill, infected, and partially exsanguinated woman suffering the results of a backstreet or self-induced abortion.

Over the next 30 years a few women were able to obtain a more or less legal abortion but even then the general practitioner was rarely involved.

The abortion was usually performed privately and the woman usually referred herself. Although the numbers began to increase during the 1960s, the availability of abortion depended above all on the woman's knowledge and her ability to pay.

Estimates of the number of illegal abortions before 1968 vary widely; inevitably we cannot know the numbers accurately as, by their very nature, illegal abortions were clandestine and usually unreported. However, there is ample evidence that illegal abortion was widespread before 1968 and has declined dramatically since (Potts *et al.* 1977).

Since 1968 the role of the general practitioner has changed enormously. The Abortion Act leaves the decision about abortion to doctors and it gives them far more opportunity than before to help a woman decide for herself about the future of her pregnancy. Although GPs differ in their interpretation of the law, the vast majority support the 1967 Act and recognize the improved health that has resulted from it. However, gynaecologists also differ in their interpretation of the law with the result that the availability of NHS abortion varies from one part of the country to another (see Table 4.4). Thus the Abortion Act has not ensured that women can obtain help regardless of where they live and their ability to pay. But it has encouraged women to consider their situation, and to seek help, openly. The GP, who will often know the woman and her family, and who can ensure adequate follow-up, is ideally placed to offer help.

Statistics

It is not easy to calculate the number of pregnancies that are unwanted. Some are terminated but some are not, so that abortion statistics do not give a true indication of the scale of unwanted pregnancy. For example, Cartwright (1987) found that in 1984, 28 per cent of women having their third child and 38 per cent having their fourth child regretted their pregnancies (i.e. were 'sorry it had happened at all' or 'would rather it had happened later'). The proportion of women who described their pregnancy as unintended was 27 per cent in 1975, and in 1984 was 22 per cent of legitimate births and 27 per cent of all births.

More precise statistics are available for legal abortions (OPCS Abortion Statistics and Scottish Health Statistics). After the implementation of the Abortion Act in 1968 the number of legal abortions rose rapidly in the late 1960s and early 1970s, finally slowing down in 1974 when the number of abortions fell for the first time. The introduction of a free contraceptive service seems to have had an important effect, the rate of abortions falling from 11.4 in 1973 to 10.4 in 1977 per 1000 women aged 15–44. Since then, the overall numbers and rates have increased slowly with only the occasional dip. Various explanations such as decreased use of the contraceptive pill, initially following 'pill scares' and more recently following

Table 4.1   *Legal abortions in Britain (resident women): numbers and rates 1969–90*[1]

	Abortions in England & Wales (resident women)		Abortions in Scotland[2]	
	Number	Rate[3]	Number	Rate[3]
1969	49 829	5.3	3556	3.5
1971	94 570	10.0	6856	6.2
1973	110 568	11.4	8566	7.4
1975	106 224	11.0	8354	7.1
1977	102 677	10.4	7139	7.0
1979	119 028	12.0	7754	7.2
1981	128 581	12.4	9007	8.3
1983	127 375	11.9	8459	7.6
1985	141 101	13.0	9189	8.2
1987	156 191	14.1	9460	8.4
1989	170 463	13.4	10 159	9.1
1990	173 900	13.6	10 219	9.1

[1] For clarity, alternate years only are shown.
[2] Figures do *not* include Scottish women having abortions in England (approximately 1000 each year or 1 per 1000 Scottish women aged 15–44 years).
[3] Per 1000 women aged 15–44.
Sources: OPCS Abortion Statistics 1990; Scottish Health Statistics 1990.

increased use of condoms in relation to AIDS, have been suggested. However, the reasons are likely to be somewhat more complex (Bone 1982; Ashton 1983).

The abortion rate in Scotland has been consistently lower than in England and Wales (Table 4.1). This is due, at least in part, to the greater difficulty of obtaining an abortion in some parts of Scotland than in England. Thus each year nearly 1000 Scottish women travel south to obtain an abortion in England.

In 1987 approximately one in five pregnancies in England and Wales and one in eight pregnancies in Scotland ended in abortion. However, Britain still has one of the lowest abortion rates of any country with a liberal abortion legislation (see Table 4.2).

Over half of all abortions are now performed on women who are single, nulliparous, and under 25 years of age. However, young single women are more likely to bypass their own doctor and go direct to the private sector, so general practitioners will see a disproportionate number of older, married parous women requesting abortion.

In most areas of Britain the NHS has not kept pace with the increase in the number of abortions. While the *number* of NHS abortions has in-

Table 4.2 *Abortion rates: some international comparisons in 1987 (unless otherwise stated)*

	Rate[1]
England and Wales	14.2
Scotland	9.0
Cuba (1988)	58.0
Czechoslovakia	46.7
China	38.8
Singapore	30.1
USA (1985)	28.0
Sweden	19.8
Australia (1988)	16.6
Finland	11.7
The Netherland (1986)	5.3

[1] Rate per 1000 women aged 15–44.

Source: Henshaw (1990).

creased since 1969, the *proportion* of all abortions performed by the NHS has fallen, from 67 per cent in 1969 to 50 per cent or below since 1974 (Table 4.3). Some NHS authorities now make arrangements with private abortion clinics to carry out abortions on NHS patients on an agency basis. In 1989, 41 per cent of abortions on resident women in England and Wales were carried out in NHS hospitals and 5 per cent were performed in the private sector on an agency basis. Of the remaining 55 per cent of abortions for which women had to pay, just under half were performed by the charitable organizations, such as British Pregnancy Advisory Service and Pregnancy Advisory Service.

The provision of NHS abortion varies greatly from one part of the

Table 4.3 *NHS provision of abortion in England and Wales 1969–90*

	Total abortions on resident women	Abortions in NHS hospitals	Abortion in NHS hospitals as percentage of total abortions
1969	44 829	33 728	67
1974	109 445	56 320	51
1979	119 028	54 868	46
1984	136 388	64 823	48
1989	170 463	70 722	41
1990	173 900	73 517	42

Source: OPCS Abortion Statistics, 1990.

Table 4.4   *Regional variations in NHS provisions of abortion in 1989*

Region	% of abortions on women resident in that region performed in NHS hospitals	% performed by NHS agency
North	83	0
East Anglia	76	0
South West	65	0
Trent	58	0.07
Wales	57	0
NE Thames	46	0.02
Oxford	43	0
Mersey	42	0.02
ENGLAND (average)	41	5
Wessex	38	7.6
North West	38	0.02
Yorkshire	36	4
SE Thames	34	1.7
NW Thames	32	0
SW Thames	30	10
West Midlands	14	20
Scotland	98	0

Source: OPCS Abortion Statistics 1989; Scottish Health Statistics 1989.

country to another (Table 4.4). This regional variation is due mainly to the difference in the attitudes of gynaecologists (Maresh 1979).

In Scotland 98 per cent of abortions are performed within the NHS but this is more a reflection of the lack of a private sector in Scotland than an indication of superior NHS resources or of a more liberal interpretation of the law.

In 1972 approximately 80 per cent of abortions had been performed by the 12th week of pregnancy. By 1989 this had risen to approximately 88 per cent, with only 1.4 per cent being performed after 20 weeks.

Methods of abortion

Traditionally methods used in performing abortions divide into those used in the first trimester and those used later in pregnancy (see Fig. 4.1). The arrival of RU 486 (mifepristone) will widen the choice of methods available for abortion, especially very early abortion, and this will be described first.

RU 486 (mifepristone)
This is a steroid hormone, similar in structure to progesterone, which binds to progesterone receptors in the uterus blocking the effect of progesterone.

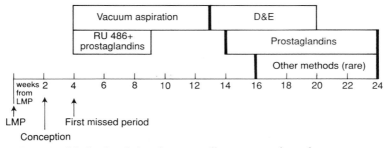

Fig. 4.1 Methods of abortion according to gestation of pregnancy.

It is also thought to increase production of prostaglandins. RU 486 has potential as a post-coital contraceptive, to enhance the effects of prostaglandins in second trimester abortions, and to induce abortion in early pregnancy. It is likely to be licensed by 1992 and its main use will be for early medical abortions.

Given to women in early pregnancy (up to 9 weeks), mifepristone on its own produces abortion in 40 per cent of pregnancies. A recent UK trial (Templeton and Urquhart 1990) found that when combined with prostaglandin pessaries, it produced abortion in 94 per cent of pregnancies up to the 63rd day with only 6 per cent needing surgical evacuation. None of the women at less than 43 days gestation needed this. The main complications were pain (with 28 per cent needing opiate analgesia, this being more common in primips) and bleeding (24 per cent of women complained, but it was severe enough to need intervention in less than 13 per cent). At a recent conference organized by the Birth Control Trust (Williams 1990) it was estimated that 5 per cent of women would need curettage and that the complication rate (pain or bleeding) would be about 3 per cent, that is, similar to conventional methods.

600 mg of mifepristone in the form of tablets is taken initially at an approved clinic or hospital. The abortion process starts slowly and the woman is often sent home at this stage. She may experience some pain and bleeding in the next 48 hours and in up to 2 per cent of women the abortion is complete after mifepristone alone. The woman returns after 48 hours and if necessary is given a prostaglandin pessary (currently Gemeprost is most commonly used). Contractions are induced, with some women (see above) needing pain relief; but most women will be ready to go home after four to six hours. There may be further pain and bleeding for the next few days. As there is a small chance (see above) that abortion will not be induced, follow-up is very important.

The law and mifepristone/Gemeprost.   At present both mifepristone and gemeprost must be administered in an NHS hospital or approved premises. The law does not require the woman to stay during the abortion process but it is likely that regulations will insist on a bed being available for some hours after gemeprost administration and that there is immediate access to specialist help and theatre facilities. The 1990 Act allows the Minister of Health to recognize premises for medical abortion and it is possible that GPs may be able to administer mifepristone in the future.

Women's experience of mifepristone.   Medical abortion has been available in France for three years and has been chosen by 25 per cent of women having first trimester abortions. Most women have found it uncomfortable but acceptable, and most would choose it again if necessary. Although abortion with mifepristone/Gemeprost takes up more time than the suction procedure, some women prefer it because it avoids the need for anaesthetic.

For mifepristone to become part of abortion provision in this country an organized early abortion service will have to be implemented. Speedy referral by GPs and speedy hospital appointments will be a vital part of this provision.

Other methods of first trimester abortion

Menstrual aspiration.   This is the name given to very early abortion per-formed, usually without anaesthetic, using a fine cannula and vacuum source (large syringe) to evacuate the uterus without dilating the cervix. Before very early pregnancy tests were introduced, this method was sometimes used to evacuate the contents of the uterus at or just after menstruation (Savage and Paterson 1982). With the advent of early testing, menstrual aspiration has a role in the development of a service for very early abor-tions. There is a small risk at this stage that the fetus will be missed because of its small size, so follow-up is vital. Unfortunately this method is not widely available today.

Vacuum aspiration.   This has been used successfully for some years and can be performed safely until 13 weeks gestation. The cervix is dilated if necessary and the contents of the uterus are evacuated by suction. Early in pregnancy (up to six weeks) this can be done with minimal dilation, and even without anaesthetic if the setting is supportive and the woman wishes it. A vacuum aspiration can be carried out under local anaesthetic up to 13 weeks but traditionally most are performed under general anaesthetic. (It is easier for the operator and there is less need to select women carefully.) The procedure is safe and with appropriate arrangements it can be carried out as a day case on women at low risk of complications. When referring women for day care, it is important to know the protocol of the local service to avoid the possibility of refusal. NHS gynaecologists, unfortun-ately, have not generally accepted day care. Despite being cheaper, and very acceptable to women, day care is still more widely available in the private/charitable sector. GPs should indicate their willingness, if appropriate, to provide after-care for women undergoing day-care abortions. It may be worth approaching individual gynaecologists on a woman's behalf.

Second trimester abortion

Dilatation and evacuation.   From 13 to 16 weeks, dilatation and evacuation is the safest method of abortion but is still more widely used in the private sector than in the NHS. It can be unpleasant for staff and is time-consuming to teach. Vaginally administered prostaglandins have recently been introduced to aid cervical dilatation, and RU 486 has also been used experimentally. This technique in skilled hands is recommended up to 18–20 weeks gestation (Savage 1990).

Prostaglandins.   The commonest second trimester method of abortion used in Britain today entails the use of prostaglandins. These are used either extra-amniotically, by instillation through the cervix, or more recently by inserting prostaglandin pessaries into the vagina; or intra-amniotically via the abdominal wall. RU 486 is now being used in conjunction with prostaglandin pessaries and appears to shorten the induction/delivery interval and lessen pain and discomfort, as a smaller dose of prostaglandin can be used. In abortions using intra-amniotic prostaglandins, urea is sometimes used in conjunction with prostaglandins for the same reason. In most medical abortions the uterus starts to contract within a few hours and the fetus is expelled within 8–18 hours. In about 50 per cent of cases the abortion is not complete and evacuation of the uterus under anaesthetic is required. Some centres perform this routinely to avoid the danger of retained product.

Other methods.   Methods such as hysterotomy are now very rarely used as the side-effects are too great.

Risks of abortion

There is an enormous literature on this subject, much of it difficult to interpret. Research into the long-term consequences of abortion is particularly fraught with difficulties (Savage and Paterson 1982). However, there is agreement on certain matters.

The risks of abortion depend above all on the gestation of pregnancy when the abortion is performed (RCGP/RCOG 1985); and at any gestation the risks also depend on the method used, the age, health, and parity of the woman, and the experience, skill, and attitude of the operator. Thus the incidence of complications will vary from one gynaecological unit to another.

In the RCGP/RCOG Attitudes to Pregnancy Study (1985) of over 6000 women undergoing induced abortion, some morbidity relating to the abortion occurred in 10 per cent of women but in only 2 per cent was this considered to be major. When the requirement of blood transfusion was used to define severe blood loss, major morbidity was reduced to 0.7 per cent, which corresponds closely to figures of 0.7 per cent from two large studies in the United States.

The impact of abortion on subsequent fertility has been extensively studied, and a review of the literature (Hogue 1986) reveals that women whose first pregnancy is terminated have no increased risk of subsequent infertility unless their abortion is complicated by pelvic infection. This also applies to risk of ectopic pregnancy. *Chlamydia trachomatis* has been found to have a prevalence of 8–10 per cent in young women in inner-city general practice (Southgate 1983; Longhurst 1987), and GPs should bear this in mind. Other long-term risks (e.g. recurrent spontaneous abortion or premature delivery due to cervical incompetence) are rare and are less likely with first trimester abortion. Long-term risks may increase with recurrent abortions and this should be discussed if appropriate.

First trimester abortion

First trimester abortion by vacuum aspiration is safe (Potts *et al.* 1977). Major early complications (e.g. perforation of the uterus, haemorrhage, and infection) are uncommon (RCGP/RCOG 1985) and the mortality is very low indeed (one per 100 000 compared to a maternal mortality of eight per 100 000). Retained products can cause bleeding and pain some days after the procedure and this may necessitate readmission to hospital and re-evacuation of the uterus. If a woman has not been screened for sexually transmitted diseases the possibility of pelvic infection should also be considered.

Second trimester abortion

There is no doubt that immediate complications of abortion (trauma, haemorrhage, infection, retained products) are more common as gestation of pregnancy increases. With more widespread use of prostaglandins the complication rate has decreased, but it could probably be reduced still further by more use of D and E in skilled hands (Savage 1990). There is no large study of pregnancy outcome in women subsequent to late vaginal terminations but MacKenzie and Fry (1988) found that 104 out of 105 women who had had a previous second trimester prostaglandin abortion succeeded in conceiving.

The lessons for GPs are that women should be referred as soon as possible, that the service should provide minimal delay, and that GPs should get to know which local gynaecologists and agencies can provide a skilled and caring service for their patients.

Psychological risks

The psychological risk of abortion is small (Gibbons 1984). Many women experience feelings of guilt and sadness immediately after an abortion but these feelings are usually transient and are often accompanied by a marked feeling of relief. Although women having late abortions are more likely to find the procedure distressing, they do not seem to be at greater risk of severe psychological consequences (Brewer 1978). However, women who have been advised to have an abortion for medical reasons are more likely to experience long-term depression (Donnai *et al.* 1981). Those who are psychiatrically disturbed before the abortion are also more likely to suffer serious psychological effects, but this is a likely result whatever the outcome of pregnancy (*British Medical Journal* 1976). Overall, severe psychological disturbance is much less common after abortion than after childbirth (Brewer 1977*a*).

Interpreting the 1967 Abortion Act (amended 1990)

The 1967 Abortion Act requires two doctors to decide whether a woman has grounds for abortion. However, doctors vary enormously in their interpretation of the Act and this has been a cause of much controversy. We offer here a liberal view as a basis for discussion.

A doctor who has a conscientious objection to abortion may opt out of referring a woman for abortion 'though he has a duty to assist the patient to obtain alternative medical advice . . . if she wants' (BMA *Handbook of medical ethics* 1984). Any doctor who does not have a conscientious objection to abortion is required by the Abortion Act to make a *clinical* decision concerning, in most cases, the comparative risks of having an abortion or continuing the pregnancy. This decision should not be concerned with whether the woman 'deserves' an abortion or not (Aitken-Swan 1977).

From Table 4.5 it can be seen that most abortions are performed under (pre-1991) Grounds 2 or 3, which require the doctor to make a clinical decision concerning the risk to physical or mental health of continuing the pregnancy compared to having the pregnancy terminated. If the woman has children already, how will their physical or mental health be affected if this pregnancy continues? What risks would be entailed for *her* if she continues this pregnancy? Here it is important to consider the psychological risk to the woman of having to continue with a pregnancy that is unwanted (Gibbons 1984). How will the risks be affected by her circumstances, both 'actual' and 'reasonably foreseeable'?

Having assessed the risks of continuing the pregnancy, these must be compared to the risks of having an abortion. This will depend, above all, on the stage at which abortion is performed. Nine out of ten women who request an abortion consult their GP by nine weeks of pregnancy (Cartwright and Lucas 1974); thus nearly all women who request an abortion will be within the first trimester. As discussed earlier, the physical and psychological risks of an abortion performed during the first trimester are very small. Taking into account the risk entailed in having a general

Table 4.5   *Grounds for abortion 1989*

Statutory grounds	Mention of each of grounds as percentage of all grounds mentioned
1. Risk of life of woman	0.2
2. Risk of injury to physical or mental health of woman	88.5
3. Risk of injury to physical or mental health of existing child(ren)	10.2
4. Substantial risk of child being born abnormal	1.0
(All grounds = 170458 (100%))	

Source: OPCS Abortion Statistics 1989.

anaesthetic, one can say that, for any woman in good health, the risk to her physical and mental health of an abortion during the first trimester is less than the risk of continuing with an unwanted pregnancy. Thus it might be argued that most women requesting an abortion would have grounds under the law (BMA 1984). This argument has not been ventilated in court but as Kennedy comments, 'there is no logical answer to it' (Kennedy and Grubb 1989).

However, a few women do not consult their doctor until the second trimester. As pregnancy advances the psychological risks of abortion do not increase but by 16–18 weeks the physical risks probably outweigh those of continuing the pregnancy (see 'Risks of abortion' above). This will vary from unit to unit.

Later in pregnancy the decision is more difficult. However, very few women request an abortion after 20 weeks and there are usually serious reasons for the delay. The law does not make special reference to late abortions but in deciding whether or not to refer a woman for an abortion after 20 weeks, it is worth noting the BMA ethical guidelines on this matter:

The doctor should recommend or perform termination after 20 weeks only if he is convinced that the health of the woman is seriously threatened, or if there is good reason to believe that the child will be seriously handicapped (BMA 1984).

THE ROLE OF THE GENERAL PRACTITIONER TODAY

When a woman consults about an unwanted pregnancy, the emotions felt on both sides sometimes make it difficult for the doctor to offer the help that would be appropriate.

The woman may be upset and full of self-blame; her distress may make communication difficult. Or she may appear to be irritatingly over-casual and off-hand. She may try to convince the doctor of her case for abortion or she may talk unrealistically of her plans to care for the child. The doctor may feel annoyed that the woman has conceived so unwisely, perhaps in spite of the contraceptive advice that the doctor has given.

If the emotions on both sides can be accommodated, there is a great deal that the doctor can do to help by:

(1) confirming the pregnancy;

(2) helping the woman to make a decision about the future of her pregnancy;

(3) carrying out the decision;

(4) follow-up.

Each of these will be dealt with in turn.

Confirming the pregnancy

Many women who consult about an unwanted pregnancy are already certain that they are pregnant; some are not. All need to have the pregnancy confirmed and the gestation assessed but this should not be a cause of delay.

It is now possible, using radio-immunoassay techniques, to detect beta-subunit human chorionic gonadotrophin (HCG) in the serum or urine within a few days of conception. Tests detecting β-HCG are now available both for home tests and for use in GP's surgeries. Most will confirm pregnancy within a few days of a missed period. GP tests are inexpensive and can be useful if a woman consults early and is anxious to know if she is pregnant. One of these may be particularly appropriate if she wants the pregnancy terminated and there is a service for very early abortion in the area.

Most doctors have access to hospital pregnancy testing. Hospital labs often perform latex agglutination inhibition to detect HCG in urine at six weeks or more amenorrhoea, which is cheaper than the new β-HCG tests. Commonly-used tests only take minutes to perform and there is no reason for delay in producing a result. The same tests are available for surgery use and are very reliable.

However, β-HCG tests are widely available and it is increasingly likely that women will consult having done their own test.

Although a positive pregnancy test is reliable and false positives are uncommon, a pelvic examination is worthwhile to check gestation. Examination is also worthwhile if the test is negative, as tests can remain negative for some time in a few women, and in some cases can become negative in the second trimester of pregnancy. Examination also helps to exclude other causes of amenorrhoea.

If the test is negative but there is a possibility of pregnancy, the woman should be asked to return for a repeat test after one week (bringing an early-morning urine sample), rather than waiting for the next period to be missed. Hormonal preparations designed to induce a withdrawal bleed should never be used. They often produce a withdrawal bleed even if the woman is pregnant, and they may cause congenital abnormalities.

One pitfall for the unwary is the danger of making assumptions. It should not be assumed that a happily married woman will be pleased or that an unmarried teenager will be unhappy to be pregnant. Even before the pregnancy is confirmed it may be worthwhile to ask, 'How would you feel if you were pregnant?'

Helping the woman to make a decision

Once the pregnancy is confirmed, a decision must be made about the future of the pregnancy. Any woman who is pregnant has three possible courses of action: she may continue the pregnancy and keep the baby, she may continue the pregnancy and have the baby adopted, or she may request an abortion. Who should make the decision? This is a controversial area where the needs of the woman, the views of the doctor, and the intention of the law often become confused.

It is possible to untangle these three sometimes conflicting strands by dealing with the decision-making process in two stages. Whatever the views of the doctor and whether or not the law will allow her to carry out the decisions she has made, it is important for the woman to make a realistic decision for herself about what she wants. A woman will gain more self-understanding from making such a decision even when it cannot be carried out than if her decision is dictated by the views of her doctor or by the law. Once the decision has been made, she and her doctor can explore the possibility of carrying out this decision within the limits of the law or the resources available.

In practice some women seem unwilling to make this decision but seem to want it made for them. They may need positive encouragement to take responsibility for their future. The doctor may be tempted to make a decision for the woman but this should be resisted.

Despite possible initial relief, people feel ultimately demeaned if responsibility is taken from them; they also have a way of undermining decisions that they feel have been imposed on them (Cheetham 1977).

A woman persuaded to have an abortion or to give up her baby for adoption may seem to comply readily with the arrangements made for her but then she may become pregnant again very soon afterwards. A woman who is apparently easily persuaded that she must continue with a pregnancy that she does not want may seek and obtain an abortion elsewhere.

It should be possible for any doctor to help a woman to decide the future of her pregnancy, even if the doctor's views make it difficult to pursue certain courses of action once the decision is made.

In order to decide the future of her pregnancy a woman needs:

(1) information about the alternatives available, what they entail and their risks, if any;

(2) an opportunity to explore the implications of these alternatives in the light of her own feelings and attitudes.

In practice, most women have made a decision, sometimes with great difficulty and often with regret, before they consult their GP. Although they may need only information and support, they may also welcome the opportunity to discuss their situation further. Others consult when they are still undecided or they may feel they are being pressured into a decision by someone else. Or there may be other problems that have been brought to light by this pregnancy. Thus, although all women will need information, they will vary greatly in how much other help they need.

Helping a woman in this way is often described as 'pregnancy counselling' (as opposed to 'abortion counselling' which implies that only women requesting an abortion need this help). The need for such counselling was emphasized by the Lane Committee in its Report in 1974 and was confirmed by the Department of Health and Social Security in a circular to all health authorities in 1977 (DHSS 1977), where counselling is described as follows:

Counselling should aim to ensure that the pregnant woman has a full opportunity to make a reasoned assessment of her own wishes and circumstances, to obtain any advice she may need in reaching her own decision and to secure that any after-care facilities including social work help which she may need can be made available. In helping the woman to understand the implications of termination or the continuation of pregnancy, it is essential that counselling should be both non-judgemental and non-directional. It is in no sense a way of putting pressure on the woman either for or against abortion.

The *aims* of pregnancy counselling are:

(1) to enable the woman to reach an informed decision that she won't regret;

(2) to lessen the risk of emotional disturbance whatever decision is reached;

(3) to lessen the risk of a further unwanted pregnancy.

However, counselling can sometimes achieve far more than this. The situation of crisis may help the woman to come to a better understanding of herself and her behaviour, not only about her use of contraception but also about her attitudes to her own sexuality and about difficulties she may have had with relationships. This understanding may help her to learn something from her experience and gain for the future. She may find herself not only better able to avoid a repetition of the circumstances that led to the unwanted pregnancy but also better able to plan and control other aspects of her life. Thus an unwanted pregnancy can be the trigger which leads to positive change and personal growth. Although such gains may rarely be achieved, the potential of such counselling makes it very worthwhile.

Too often pregnancy counselling is seen as a barrier that a woman must pass through before she can have an abortion. To see counselling in this way is to diminish its purpose and worth.

Discussing the alternatives

However certain a woman seems of her decision, it is important to consider the alternatives with her as this may be the only opportunity that she will have to do this. Most women will have discussed their situation with one or more other people before consulting the doctor and their opinions may be strongly influencing how the woman feels about her pregnancy. Perhaps the most useful role the doctor can play is to offer information and support in an atmosphere free of pressure and free of the constraints that may have limited the woman's ability to think clearly and decide for herself.

Although this chapter is concerned mainly with abortion, we shall deal briefly with some of the factors that will need to be considered by those who wish to continue the pregnancy or at least wish to consider this option.

Keeping the baby.   Many women who consult the general practitioner about unwanted pregnancy are married or partnered and already have children; they may have little need of factual information about pregnancy itself but may require information about childcare, child benefits or housing.

A single woman may have more questions to consider. Is she in a relationship? Is there mutual agreement about a future together? Is there pressure from outside to make it work (to 'get married')? Is this pregnancy a bid to hold a relationship together? Are her parents her main form of support? What form does this take? Perhaps her parents are offering to adopt the child. How would this feel? Can she see it working in the long term?

She will need factual information about finance, housing, and childcare. This is a complicated and specialized area but the doctor may wish to become acquainted with the basic information, especially as it relates to the local situation. The rules concerning benefits change rapidly and up-to-date information is best obtained from leaflets published by the DSS, obtainable from benefit offices, social services departments, or Citizens Advice Bureaux. Information about housing is best obtained from the local housing department, social services department, or from a Shelter Housing Aid Centre. The availability of childcare varies from area to area; there may be day nurseries, private nurseries, or child-minders. A health visitor attached to the practice may have much of this information or it is usually obtainable from the social services department.

The National Council for One Parent Families and its Scottish counterpart, the Scottish Council for Single Parents, are excellent sources of information, support, and sometimes practical help. Gingerbread is a national self-help organization for one-parent families which has many local groups operating day care projects or drop-in information centres. In some areas there are other voluntary organizations which may have some help to offer.

It may be appropriate for the GP to share antenatal care with the hospital so that contact with the woman can be maintained throughout pregnancy; the health visitor should also be involved at an early stage.

It is perhaps worth emphasizing the difficulties that still face single mothers today, two-thirds of whom will remain dependent on income support (DSS 1989).

Adoption. In recent years there has been a move away from adoption and, for most women, the choice now lies between abortion and caring for the child themselves. However, some women will choose adoption; often they are women who are morally opposed to abortion but are unable to care for the child themselves, or occasionally they are those who have opted for abortion but this has been refused. Women who wish to have their child adopted should be referred to the local social services department or to an adoption agency. Information about these agencies can be obtained from the British Agencies for Adoption and Fostering. Under the terms of the Child Care Act 1980, adoptions can only be arranged by registered adoption societies, including social services departments, except when the proposed adopter is a relative of the child.

Some women, especially young women, who are forced to leave home may need temporary accommodation during the last few months of pregnancy and for a few weeks after the baby is born. Although they are declining in number, mother-and-baby homes still exist. For example, the Life Care and Housing Trust (set up in 1977 by the anti-abortion organization, Life) offers accommodation to young pregnant women in over 40 areas of the country. However, this accommodation is only temporary and there may be little or no continuing support for the mother even if she decides to keep the baby.

When a woman is considering adoption it is important to remember the risk of depression after the birth. The doctor may feel it appropriate to warn her of this risk and should be aware that she is likely to need support at this time and may not ask for it.

Abortion. A woman who is considering an abortion should be offered information about what the operation involves and the risks entailed (see pp. 129–31); using models or diagrams, it should be possible to do this in a few minutes. When discussing the risks, it is important to discuss their implications.

The woman should be told how long she will need to be in hospital and what kind of anaesthetic she will have (if this is known). It is helpful to mention the possibility that she may feel sad and weepy or even full of regrets after the abortion and that it will be worthwhile to arrange for someone close to her to be available to offer support at this time.

Exploring feelings and attitudes

Up this point the doctor has had to concentrate on asking questions and giving information to the pregnant woman. Now a change is needed. The woman needs the opportunity to explore her feelings and attitudes and to discuss any problems that this pregnancy may have brought to light. The purpose is not to offer advice nor to try to make her change her mind but to listen and interpret.

When counselling a pregnant woman, it may help for the doctor to have a checklist of points to cover. Although the majority of women will have few problems, and the discussion may be quite brief, some women may have worries that they find difficult to express and a checklist may help to reveal these.

These are the main points to cover:

(1) *Why is this pregnancy unwanted?* If this question is not asked, the wrong assumption may be made. There may be practical difficulties that need to be resolved. Or the woman may have unrealistic fears—about fetal abnormalities or about pain in labour, for example. She may even be seeking reassurance about these worries so that she can continue the pregnancy.

(2) *Has she been able to talk to others about her predicament?* Some women may welcome help in discussing their situation with others. For example, a young woman may wish her parents to know but may find it difficult to tell them herself; she may wish the doctor to broach the subject with them. Other women will remain unable to talk to anyone else and they need extra support in tackling whatever they decide to do.

(3) *When she first suspected that she might be pregnant, what was her attitude to the pregnancy?* Here one is concerned about the woman's own view of this pregnancy. She may reveal a degree of ambivalence about being pregnant and may need help in understanding this to avoid the danger that whatever decision she makes, she may subsequently feel that it was wrong. If the pregnancy was motivated by a need to change her environment in some way (e.g. by a need for attention or a desire to leave home) she may need help in understanding this and help to deal with her difficulties in other ways.

(4) *If she has talked to others, how did they react and what did they suggest she might do?* It is important to check that she isn't being pressured into a decision by others. Although she may be influenced by the views of those close to her, ultimately she will need to make her own decision independently of them.

(5) *Before she found herself pregnant, what was her view of abortion, of illegitimacy, of adoption, of single parenthood—both in general and for herself?* If she finds herself having to make a decision which does not fit in with her previous views, she may need extra help in coming to terms with her decision. For example, a woman may have strong feelings against abortion, even believing it to be murder, and yet may still request an abortion.

(6) *What is the nature of the relationship she is in, if any?* When an unwanted pregnancy occurs in a stable relationship, there may be support available from the partner. However, even the most stable relationship can be threatened by an unwanted pregnancy. Sometimes the pregnancy is used to test the relationship, which is then found to be wanting. If a relationship that was previously seen to be secure has suffered as a result of the crisis, the woman may need help in coming to terms with this.

(7) *What is the worst aspect of her present situation?* It is useful to ask this at some stage. She may have worries or fears about her situation that she finds difficult to express. For a young woman it may be fear of her parents' reaction. Or she may have decided on a course of action but may have some remaining doubts. For example, she may want an abortion but may be worried about the operation or the risk of sterility afterwards. If such doubts and worries can be expressed and dealt with at this stage, they may be less likely to trouble her later.

(8) *Has this crisis come out of the blue or does she have other problems with which she needs help?* For many women an unwanted pregnancy is a crisis which upsets an otherwise settled existence; once the crisis has been resolved she may need no further help. For other women an unwanted pregnancy may be just one more disaster in a life full of difficulties of an emotional or practical kind. Such women need on-going practical help and support after the present crisis is over.

(9) *How did this pregnancy happen and how can a further unwanted pregnancy be avoided?* Was this pregnancy the result of contraceptive failure, risk-taking ambivalence, or possibly even a desire to be pregnant? Sometimes her motives will not be clear to the woman herself and she may need help in understanding them. Can she learn from this self-understanding for the future so that she is less likely to find herself in this situation again? Does she need to reconsider her method of contraception or her reasons for not using any? Although these questions need to be tackled at some

stage, it may not be appropriate to do so in detail until the immediate crisis has been resolved; this will depend on the woman's feelings and immediate needs. For example, she may find it difficult to consider her need for future contraception if she is not in a relationship. She should not be pressured into making a decision at this stage, particularly not a decision about sterilization (see p. 147).

Who else should be seen?   If the woman agrees to this, it is often appropriate to see others who are involved, such as the woman's husband, boyfriend, or parents. This may be helpful to the woman as it may enable her to express feelings to them which she found difficult to do on her own; it may allow her to understand more clearly how these others view her situation. It may also help the others to work through their own distress about the situation or to accept the woman's decision when it is in conflict with their own wishes. Thus it may be useful to see the other(s) both alone and with the woman, but it is always essential to spend some time with the woman alone so that her own views can be aired rather than being overridden by others.

Difficulties with counselling

Although the general practitioner is ideally placed to counsel a woman with an unwanted pregnancy, such counselling is not without difficulties.

Time.   On average a GP will see five or six women with an unwanted pregnancy in a year. For the majority of women a discussion of the alternatives is unlikely to take longer than 20–30 minutes. But sometimes this discussion reveals the need for further help which may need to be extended over two or three sessions. It is worthwhile making time for such extended counselling for the few who need it, as it may help them to cope more easily with the decision they make, as well as in the future. But a busy doctor may not be able to make time for this and referral elsewhere may be necessary.

The doctor's attitude.   It is difficult to offer help to a woman in reaching her own decision if one hopes to persuade her of one course of action rather than another. Not only can factual information be presented in a misleading way but it is also difficult to encourage a woman to explore her feelings if the doctor cannot accept them. Doctors are usually aware of their attitudes: they may be against abortion in all circumstances or they may feel it is wrong for a young girl to have a baby and care for it herself. Sometimes, however, such attitudes are less easy to recognize as they may not apply in all circumstances. One particular woman may induce a response in the doctor who may then find it difficult to offer her help. For example, a doctor may be irritated by a woman who seems very casual about her request for abortion. In fact, a casual manner often conceals considerable distress; women do not often request an abortion lightly.

Although such negative feelings cannot be avoided altogether, it is important to be aware of the extent to which they affect one's ability to help. It may be helpful to discuss such cases with colleagues.

The woman's response to the doctor's role.   Some difficulties with counselling arise from the doctor's role and how the woman perceives this. When the pregnancy is confirmed the woman may feel angry with herself for what has happened and sometimes this anger will be directed at the doctor—the messenger bringing the bad news. The doctor must establish how the pregnancy occurred, an enquiry that may be perceived as criticism, and then must give factual information about the options open and their risks. The next stage is quite different. The doctor will try to create an atmosphere in which the woman can talk freely. But sometimes the woman's anger and the atmosphere created during the early stages of the consultation may make this difficult. It is important to make a clear change from the didactic approach involved in giving information. It may sometimes be appropriate to break off after giving the necessary information and arrange another appointment to discuss things further. This will also give the woman time to absorb the information and to talk to others who may be involved.

Another problem stems from the fact that the doctor is the final arbiter as to whether a woman may have an abortion or not and the woman usually knows this. She may feel that she needs to convince the doctor of her case and this may make it difficult for her to express any doubts that she may have (Allan 1981). If the woman is requesting an abortion, it may be appropriate to make a hospital appointment at an early stage. Once an appointment has been made 'a woman will probably be more able to look at her situation calmly, and to acknowledge any doubts she may have, without fearing that the expression of ambivalence will lead to the doctor's refusal to consider abortion any further' (Cheetham 1977). Some women may be so preoccupied with the question of whether they can *get* an abortion that they are quite unable to consider whether they *want* an abortion until the first question has been resolved.

If, in spite of these precautions, a woman still finds it difficult to talk freely to the doctor yet would welcome the opportunity for further discussion, it may be appropriate to refer her elsewhere for help, especially to someone who is not required by law to make the decision.

Special groups
Teenagers.   Counselling a teenager with an unwanted pregnancy may present special difficulties.

1. Teenagers often present late having denied the possibility of pregnancy to themselves or because they fear the reaction of their parents or the doctor (Bury 1984).

2. Abortions, especially late abortions, in young teenagers have an

increased risk of causing cervical damage and thus difficulties in future pregnancies (Bury 1984). But pregnancy and childbirth in this age group also carry substantial risks, quite apart from the difficulty that a young woman may have in coping with a child (Huntingford 1981).

3. A young woman may be quite unable to assess realistically her ability to cope with a child and she may even look forward to having a baby whom she believes will offer her the unconditional love that she may have lacked herself.

4. She may wish to have an abortion but without her parents' knowledge. This is always a difficult situation but especially if she is under 16 years. As the legality of performing a termination without parental consent is uncertain, such consent is always advisable and in practice few gynaecologists will perform an abortion on an under-16-year-old without such consent. Conversely 'a termination should never be carried out in opposition to the girl's wishes even if the parents demand it' (Medical Defence Union 1974).

5. If a teenager comes with her mother it is essential to spend some time with the young woman alone to find out what *she* wants to do; she may have no opportunity to express this while her mother is there. In practice the young woman, her boyfriend, and her parents are often in agreement about the best course of action. But even here it is important that the young woman should be able to feel that she has made this decision for herself. Being given the responsibiity for determining her future can then be a stage in her developing maturity rather than a confirmation of her immaturity and dependence.

6. A young woman may have difficulty in accepting her need for contraception even if she is in a stable relationship. This may be partly due to fear of parental disapproval and this should be explored.

Repeat abortion.   Women who have had a previous abortion often cause considerable concern. In fact repeat abortions account for 21 out of every 100 abortions performed (OPCS 1989). In some instances it will be found that the woman has been particularly careless in her use of contraception or that she is particularly ambivalent about pregnancy and she may need help in coming to terms with this. However, such women often differ from other women with an unwanted pregnancy only in that they have more difficulties with contraception—they are often just unlucky (Brewer 1977*b*). The decision about whether a woman has grounds for abortion should depend on her present circumstances and not on whether she has already had an abortion. Although some studies have shown a slightly greater risk of long-term complications after repeat abortions, the significance of this is doubtful (Savage and Paterson 1982).

Some doctors express concern that the increased availability of legal abortion has encouraged women to rely on abortion as an alternative to using contraception but there is no evidence for this.

Abortion for fetal abnormality. Abortions performed because of a risk of handicap (Ground E of the amended 1967 Act) account for only 1.5 per cent of all abortions. They present quite separate problems: the pregnancy is usually planned and wanted; the woman has often undergone an amniocentesis which is, in itself, often associated with anxiety; and the abortion is often performed late in pregnancy, after fetal movements have been felt. It is not surprising therefore, that the risk of long-term depression is greater after such abortions (Donnai *et al.* 1981).

Such women need careful counselling, including full information before the abortion and support afterwards. Unfortunately, the general practitioner is not always involved in the decision to abort, nor in the immediate follow-up. However, the GP is in an ideal position to offer long-term support, particularly around the time that the baby would have been born and during a subsequent pregnancy.

Other counselling services

If the doctor does not feel able to counsel the woman, who else can do this? An attached health visitor may be willing to undertake it. She may need some training and, like the doctor, she would need to be aware of her attitudes, but her role in health education and her contact with mothers and young children in the community may make her a very good counsellor. Alternatively, a social worker attached to the practice, at the local gynaecology unit or social services department may be willing to offer counselling to pregnant women.

In some areas there are other sources of counselling help available; the charitable pregnancy advisory services (BPAS and PAS) have over 30 agencies throughout the country. They offer counselling for a small charge (which for women in some areas is met by the local health authority). There are also Brook Advisory Centres in some areas where pregnancy counselling may be available free of charge. Other voluntary agencies such as Relate, although not specializing in this field, may offer counselling to pregnant women. However, some organizations (e.g. Lifeline) offer 'counselling' which may seek to persuade women to continue with their pregnancy. It is therefore essential to find out what kind of help is offered before referring a woman.

Carrying out the decision

We have already referred to the support that is available for those women who decide to continue their pregnancy. Here we shall be concerned with those women who, after counselling, decide on abortion.

Whom to refer

If a woman wants an abortion it is necessary to consider whether she has grounds within the law. This has already been discussed in the section on interpreting the 1967 Abortion Act (see p. 121, above).

If the doctor considers that the woman does not have grounds for abortion, this should be explained to her, together with the reasons for this decision. If she is still adamant that she wants an abortion, the doctor may decide to refer her to a gynaecologist for a second opinion. Such a referral should not be used as a means to delay her and she should be warned if the gynaecologist is unlikely to accept her request. Alternatively, the doctor may offer her information about other services where she can seek advice. If, on the other hand, she accepts the doctor's opinion and decides to continue the pregnancy, she may need extra help and support.

Where to refer

If the woman has grounds for an abortion, referral should be made to a gynaecologist who will consider her request sympathetically, and ideally this referral will be to an NHS gynaecologist in a local hospital. So it is essential to know the views of the local gynaecologists. One way to ascertain this on moving to a new area is to telephone the gynaecologist about a woman who is being referred.

The likelihood of a successful NHS referral will vary very much from one region to another (see above, Table 4.3), and in any region will depend on the gestation of pregnancy. For example, some gynaecologists who adopt a fairly liberal policy during the first trimester, will perform no abortions after 12 weeks. Where an NHS referral is unlikely to be successful, the general practitioner may feel it appropriate to refer the woman elsewhere; indeed, the woman herself may prefer this. Few NHS gynaecologists accept referrals from women outside their catchment area, so a referral to the private sector may be necessary.

Within the private sector, the non-profit-making pregnancy advisory services, BPAS and PAS, have clinics in a number of areas and between them they perform approximately 47 000 abortions each year, that is, approximately half of all abortions outside the NHS. Both organizations operate a loan and grant scheme for those who find it impossible to pay and in some areas the cost of an abortion may be met by the local health authority. Where there is no charitable clinic nearby, it is necessary to investigate the profit-making services available. Before making a referral to a private clinic, doctors should satisfy themselves about the standard of care offered. In some cases it may be preferable to travel further to obtain a better service.

For women who can afford to pay, referral to the private sector may be speedier (see 'Delays', below), as well as safer. In the recent RCGP/ RCOG study (1985) women having terminations in the private sector encountered a lower morbidity from the operation than women having NHS terminations. This applied particularly to women having an abortion at 13–16 weeks gestation.

How to refer

Some areas (e.g. Newcastle) operate a central referral system (Lawson *et al.* 1976) but in most areas appointments have to be made with individual consultants. Time can be saved by making an appointment by telephone; when a woman is close to 12 weeks or is late in pregnancy, direct contact with a consultant by telephone may be helpful. Appointments should always be made with a named consultant whose views are known. (The consultant with the shortest waiting list for appointments may not do abortions).

The referral letter should indicate the woman's circumstances, the grounds for abortion, the gestation of pregnancy, and how far counselling has been pursued. If the referring doctor is supporting the request, an abortion certificate (blue form in England and Wales, Certificate A in Scotland) should be signed and enclosed. If the request is not being supported, the doctor should say so. While the woman is waiting for her appointment or is awaiting admission to hospital she may welcome further support and this should always be offered.

If the request for abortion is refused, the desirability of another referral should be discussed with the woman; this will often be to the private sector. At any stage some women will change their minds and they may need help in coming to terms with their new decision.

Delays

In general, the earlier an abortion is performed the safer it is; even when a woman consults at six weeks, a delay will increase the risks (Roe 1988). Yet women requesting an abortion are often delayed unnecessarily by the medical services (Allan 1981). Cartwright and Lucas (1974) found evidence of general practitioners who delayed deliberately 'in the hope that the pregnancy would be accepted or that it would be too late to get an abortion.' This still happens (Pro Choice Alliance 1991).

Most delays are not deliberate and there are many ways in which they can be avoided, while still allowing ample time for the woman to make a decision. In the RCGP/RCOG study (1985) of over 6000 women under-going induced abortion, 27 per cent of women having an NHS abortion had to wait at least three weeks from first consulting their general practitioner to their operation, compared to 14 per cent of those having their operation in the private sector. The main cause of delay in the NHS was in the wait for an appointment with the gynaecologist, rather than in waiting for the operation.

An existing example of what can be achieved where a co-ordinated approach is used is in the North Devon Health District where McGarry provides a rapid service and GPs have direct access to him. Here the proportion of abortions done before nine weeks (79 per cent) is twice the England and Wales average (34.1 per cent).

Follow-up

Careful follow-up is important whatever the outcome of the pregnancy. If a woman is continuing with a problem pregnancy or has had an abortion she may welcome the opportunity to talk further about her feelings. After an abortion or after giving up a child for adoption there may be a period of acute distress when much support will be needed and may not be provided by friends and family.

Although some hospitals and clinics see the woman again for a post-abortion check, some do not. It is advisable that the woman be examined between two and four weeks after the abortion to confirm that the abortion has been successful and that she does not have retained products or an infection.

Most women do not experience pain after an abortion. Bleeding usually becomes no more than a pink or brown loss within 1–2 weeks of the abortion, although this loss may continue until the first menstrual period. If the woman has previously had a regular cycle, this period usually comes within 4–5 weeks of the abortion.

Further bright red bleeding with or without clots, approximately one week after an abortion and especially if associated with pain and fever, is suggestive of retained products and infection. If the uterus is enlarged, re-admission to hospital for re-evacuation is advisable; alternatively a course of antibiotics may suffice.

The pregnancy test sometimes remains positive for a few days after an abortion but should always be negative by two weeks afterwards.

At follow-up it is important to consolidate the gains made during counselling. Has this crisis given the woman any insights into her behaviour? Does she need to make any changes in her life to avoid repetition of the circumstances? This may be no more than a need for more efficient contraception but it may involve a more profound exploration of her attitudes and behaviour, requiring several consultations.

The follow-up appointment is often an appropriate time to establish a woman on contraception and most women will be highly motivated to consider contraception at this time. However, some women may not accept their need for contraception and they will require particularly careful follow-up.

It is sometimes appropriate to start contraception earlier than this, at the time of the abortion. An IUD can be inserted immediately after the procedure. Insertion at this time is associated with an increased risk of infection and of expulsion but these risks may be acceptable to the woman if she is anxious to avoid any further risk of pregnancy. Alternatively, the contraceptive pill can be started on the day of the abortion or the following day and many women prefer to do this rather than wait until the first menstrual period. The time to start contraception will often depend on the woman's ability to make a firm decision about her future contraception before the abortion; she may prefer to consider this after the procedure is over. However, it is important to remember—and to emphasize to the woman— that she could conceive within a few days of having an abortion; ovulation may occur as early as 10 days afterwards.

A general practitioner may find it difficult to offer after-care to a woman who has referred herself for an abortion. In fact, it is quite likely that she went elsewhere for help because she did not know how the doctor would respond to her request or, for a young woman, because she feared her parents would find out. Thus the decision to bypass the doctor may reflect the woman's uncertainty and lack of confidence rather than any criticism of the doctor.

Sterilization

Some women who have completed their family and others who do not wish to have children may wish to consider sterilization. Although the unwanted pregnancy may have provoked the need to consider this option, the decision should be made quite independently of the decision about the pregnancy. They involve quite different considerations, and decisions about the long-term future are not easy to make when in a crisis.

It has been suggested that some gynaecologists have on occasion agreed to perform an abortion only on condition that the woman agrees to be sterilized at the same time (Savage 1981). This is clearly unethical. Sterilization performed at the same time as abortion is far more likely to be regretted than when it is performed as an interval procedure; combining sterilization with abortion may also increase the mortality from abortion (Savage 1981; RCGP/RCOG 1985). There are circumstances when it may be appropriate to consider sterilization at the same time as abortion (e.g. when a woman conceives while awaiting a sterilization operation) but she should be told the risks and offered the option of having the sterilization at a later date.

Prevention of unwanted pregnancy

The general practitioner has an important role to play in the prevention of unwanted pregnancy. This requires an understanding of the causes of unwanted pregnancy as well as knowledge of contraceptive practice. These subjects are dealt with in Chapter 3.

CONCLUSION

The general practitioner is ideally placed to help a woman with an unwanted pregnancy. This can be a demanding and time-consuming task but the potential gains for the woman—and for her relationship with the doctor make it very worthwhile.

ACKNOWLEDGEMENTS

Katy Gardner and Lis Davidson would like to thank Judith Bury, who originally wrote this chapter, and Wendy Savage, for their help in updating it.

USEFUL ADDRESSES

Pregnancy testing

Ortho Diagnostics, Denmark House, Denmark Street, High Wycombe, Bucks HP11 2ER (makers of GRAVINDEX).

Organon Laboratories, Crown House, London Road, Morden, Surrey SM4 5DZ (makers of PREGNOSTICON).

Unipath Ltd, Norse Rd, Bedford MK41 0QG (makers of CLEARVIEW).

Pregnancy counselling

Brook Advisory Centres, 153a East Street, London SE17 2SD. Tel: 071 708 1234.

Pregnancy counselling and abortion

British Pregnancy Advisory Service, Austy Manor, Wootton Wawen, Solihull, West Midlands B95 6DA. Tel: Henley in Arden 3225.

Pregnancy Advisory Service, 11–13 Charlotte Street, London W1P 1HD. Tel: 071 637 8962.

Single parents

National Council for One Parent Families, 255 Kentish Town Road, London NW5 2LX. Tel: 071 267 1361.

Scottish Council for Single Parents, 13 Gayfield Square, Edinburgh EH1 3NX. Tel: 031 556 3899.

Gingerbread, 35 Wellington Street, London WC2E 7BN. Tel: 071 240 0953.

Shelter Housing Aid Centre, 189a Old Brompton Road, London SW5 0AR. Tel: 071 373 7276.

Adoption

British Agencies for Adoption and Fostering, 11 Southwark Street, London SE1 1RQ. Tel: 071 407 8800.

REFERENCES AND FURTHER READING

Aitken-Swan, J. (1977). *Fertility control and the medical profession*. Croom Helm, London.
Allan, I. (1981). *Family planning, sterilisation and abortion services*. Policy Studies Institute, London.
Ashton, J. (1983). Trends in induced abortion in England and Wales. *British Medical Journal*, **287**, 1001–2.
Birth Control Trust (1980). *Abortion counselling*. Proceedings of a meeting held at the Royal College of Obstetricians and Gynaecologists in 1978. (Obtainable from BCT, 27–35 Mortimer Street, London W1N 7RJ, price 75p.)
Bone, M. (1982). The 'pill scare' in England and Wales. *IPPF Medical Bulletin*, **16**, 2–4.
Brewer, C. (1977*a*). Incidence of post abortion psychosis: a prospective study. *British Medical Journal*, **i**, 476–7.
Brewer, C. (1977*b*). Third time unlucky: a study of women who have had three or more legal abortions. *Journal of Biosocial Science*, **9**, 99–105.
Brewer, C. (1978). Induced abortion after feeling foetal movements: its causes and emotional consequences. *Journal of Biosocial Science*, **10**, 203–8.
BMA (British Medical Association) (1984). *The handbook of medical ethics*. British Medical Association, London.
British Medical Journal (1966). Report by the BMA Special Committee on Therapeutic Abortion. *British Medical Journal*, **2**, 40.
British Medical Journal (1976). Psychological sequelae of therapeutic abortion. *British Medical Journal*, **i**, 1564–5.
Bury, J. (1984). *Teenage pregnancy in Britain*. Birth Control Trust, London. (Obtainable from BCT, 27–35 Mortimer Street, London W1N 7RJ, price £3.50.)
Cartwright, A. (1987). Trends in family intentions and the use of contraception among recent mothers 1967–81. *Population Trends*, **49**, 31–4.
Cartwright, A. and Lucas, S. (1974). *Survey of abortion patients for the Committee on the Working of the Abortion Act*, Vol. III of the Lane Report. HMSO, London.
Cheetham, J. (1977). *Unwanted pregnancy and counselling*. Routledge & Kegan Paul, London.
DHSS (Department of Health and Social Security) (1977). *Arrangements for counselling of patients seeking abortion*. Health Circular. HC (77) 26.
DSS (Department of Social Security) (1989). DSS Statistics. HMSO, London.
Diggory, P. (1991). *Abortion: an introduction. Guidance on technique, complications and the provision of services*. Birth Control Trust (in press).
Donnai, P., Charles, N., and Harris, R. (1981). Attitudes of patients after 'genetic' termination of pregnancy. *British Medical Journal*, **i**, 621–2.
Gibbons, M. (1984). Psychiatric sequelae of induced abortion. *Journal of the Royal College of General Practitioners*, **34**, 146–50.

Hall, M. H. (1990). Changes in the law on abortion. *British Medical Journal*, **301**, 1109–10.

Henshaw, S. K. (1990). *Induced abortion: a world review*. Allan Guttmacher Institute, New York.

Hogue, C. J. (1986). Impact of abortion on subsequent fecundity. *Clinical Obstetrics and Gynaecology*, **13**,(1), 95–103.

Huntingford, P. (1981). The medical and emotional consequences of teenage pregnancy. In *The consequences of teenage sexual activity*. Brook Advisory Centres, London.

International Planned Parenthood Federation (1976). *Abortion counselling: a European view*. IPPF, London.

Kennedy, I. and Grubb, A. (1989). *Medical law: text and materials*. Butterworth, London.

Lafitte, F. (1975). *The abortion hurdle race*. BPAS, England. (Obtainable from BPAS, Austy Manor, Wootton Wawen, Solihull, West Midlands B95 6DA.)

Lane, Lord Justice (1974). *Report of the Committee on the Working of the Abortion Act*. HMSO, London.

Lawson, J. B., Yare, D., Barron, S. L., *et al.* (1976). Management of the abortion problem in an English city. *Lancet*, **ii**, 1288–91.

Longhurst, H. J., *et al.* (1987). A simple method for the detection of *Chlamydia trachomatis* infections in general practice. *Journal of the Royal College of General Practitioners*, **37**, 255–6.

MacKenzie, I. Z. and Fry, A. (1988). A prospective self-controlled study of fertility after second trimester prostaglandin-induced abortion. *American Journal of Obstetrics and Gynecology*, **158**,(5), 1137–40.

Maresh, M. (1979). Regional variation in the provision of NHS gynaecological and abortion services. *Fertility and Contraception*, **3**, 41.

Roe, J. (ed.) (1988). *Reducing late abortions: access to NHS services in early pregnancy*. Birth Control Trust, London.

RCGP/RCOG (1985). *Induced abortion operations and their early sequelae*. Joint study of the Royal College of General Practitioners and the Royal College of Obstetricians and Gynaecologists. *Journal of the Royal College of General Practitioners*, **35**, 175–80.

Medical Defence Union (1974). *Consent to treatment*. MDU, London.

OPCS Abortion Statistics Series. AB 1–11, 1974–90.

Potts, M., Diggory, P., and Peel, J. (1977). *Abortion*. Cambridge University Press.

Pro Choice Alliance (1991). *Abortion: who decides*. (Obtainable from Pro Choice Alliance, 54 Grange Road, Lewes, Sussex BN71 1TU.)

Savage, W. (1981). Abortion and sterilisation—should the operation be combined? *British Journal of Family Planning*, **7**, 8–12.

Savage, W. (1990). Late induced abortion. *Contemporary Review of Obstetrics and Gynaecology*, **2**, 163–70.

Savage, W. and Paterson, I. (1982). Abortion: methods and sequelae. *British Journal of Hospital Medicine*, **28**, 364–84.

Scottish Health Statistics 1969–90. HMSO, Edinburgh.

Simms, M. (1977). *Report on non-medical abortion counselling*. Birth Control Trust, London. (Obtainable from BCT, 25–37 Mortimer Street, London W1N 7RJ, price 50p.)

Southgate, L. J., Treharne, J. D., and Forsey, T. (1983). *Chlamydia trachomatis* and *Neisseria gonorrhoeae* infections in women attending inner city general practices. *British Medical Journal,* **287,** 879–81.

Templeton, A. A. and Urquart, D. R. (1990). The efficiency and tolerance of mifepristone and prostaglandin in first trimester termination of pregnancy. UK multicentre trial. *British Journal of Obstetrics and Gynaecology,* **97,** 480–6.

Wililams, C. (1990). *The abortion pill (mifepristone/RU 486): widening the choice for women.* Birth Control Trust, London. (Obtainable from BCT, 27–35 Mortimer Street, London W1N 7RJ, price £4.95.)

Further reading for doctors and patients

Davies, V. (1991). *Abortion and afterwards.* Ashgrove Press, Bath.

Frater, A. and Wright, C. (1986). *Coping with abortion.* Chambers, Edinburgh.

Neustatter, A. with Newson, G. (1986). *Mixed feelings: the experience of abortion.* Pluto, London.

5. Premenstrual syndrome

Katy Gardner and Diana Sanders

Premenstrual syndrome (PMS) has received much publicity, in both the lay and medical press. Although there is still much debate over the syndrome's definition, aetiology, and treatment, nowadays there is a greater understanding of PMS and a range of ways of managing the problem. It is a complex and fascinating topic which raises many questions about the interactions between hormones and physiological changes and life events and stress; and it is no wonder that many women, and their general practitioners, feel bewildered over how to deal with it. The primary health care team are increasingly meeting women with PMS, and facing the task of gearing the management of problems to each individual woman. Women are taking an active and positive role in acquiring knowledge and information about health issues and many women today recognize that PMS is a problem for them and are taking steps to try to deal with it. With information, patience, and encouragement, women can work out ways of helping themselves, but may also come to seek medical advice from their GP.

DEFINITION

Many women notice changes in their emotional and physical feelings during the menstrual cycle. While for the majority such changes are acceptable, for others they are distressing. These distressing premenstrual changes have recently been described as 'Premenstrual syndrome' rather than as 'Premenstrual tension', in recognition of the variable nature of the symptoms which may not always include tension. The definition of PMS has been fraught with problems, since the type of symptoms and their severity can vary enormously, both between women and between cycles for individual women; and because the symptoms can be experienced at times other than during the luteal phase of the cycle. There are a number of definitions of PMS available, including Magos's (1990): '. . . distressing physical, psychological and behavioural symptoms not caused by organic disease which regularly recur during the same phase of the menstrual cycle and which significantly regress or disappear during the remainder of the cycle'; and O'Brien's (1990): '. . . a disorder of non-specific somatic, psychological or behavioural symptoms recurring in the premenstrual phase of the menstrual cycle. Symptoms must resolve completely by the end of menstruation leaving a symptom free week. The symptoms should be of sufficient severity to produce social, family or occupational disruption. Symptoms must have occurred in at least four of the six previous menstrual cycles.' Over 150 symptoms have been described; common features are shown in Table 5.1. Some women notice only mood changes, others only physical symptoms, but it is more common for both to be experienced together. Although different sub-types of PMS have been defined (Abraham 1983), the distinction between types of PMS remains arbitrary and based on clinical observations, and in general individual women tend to report their own unique combination of symptoms.

Distressing changes may start up to 14 days before menstruation, although it is more common for the symptoms to last for up to a week, and disappear at or shortly after the start of menstrual bleeding. Many women say that the severity varies from cycle to cycle, depending on general life events or stresses. The most important defining feature of PMS is the appearance of symptoms in the luteal phase and disappearance at menstruation; until the timing in relation to menstruation is established, PMS

Table 5.1 *Features of premenstrual syndrome*

General
1. Symptoms occur 1 to 14 days before menstruation begins.
2. Symptoms disappear at, or shortly after, the onset of menstrual bleeding.
3. The woman feels well for the rest of the cycle.
4. Symptoms occur regularly, for most menstrual cycles.
5. PMS causes distress and possibly other problems, such as with relationships.

Symptoms

Physical changes	*Psychological changes*
Breast tenderness	Depression or feeling low
Swelling or bloated feelings, possibly with swollen face, abdomen, or fingers	Feeling upset
	Tiredness, lethargy, or fatigue
	Tension or unease
Headaches	Anxiety
Appetite changes	Irritability
Carbohydrate cravings	Clumsiness or poor co-ordination
Acne or skin rashes	Difficulty concentrating
Constipation or diarrhoea	Changes in sexual interest
Palpitations	
Changes in sleep	
Muscular stiffness or aches and pains	
Abdominal pains or cramps	
Backache	
Exacerbation of epilepsy, migraines, asthma, rhinitis, urticaria	

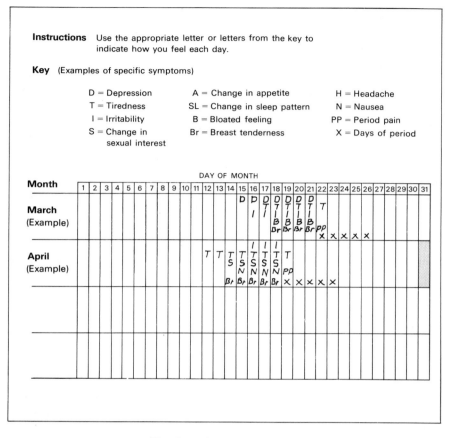

Fig. 5.1 A menstrual diary.

can be confused with more general problems such as anxiety or depression, and may be mis-diagnosed or mistreated. Hence, the first step in diagnosis is careful and regular symptom recording to establish the nature and timing of the problems. Women should be asked to complete menstrual charts, recording their moods, feelings, and symptoms for at least two cycles. Various menstrual diaries are available (Fig. 5.1), or a simple practical alternative is the self-assessment disc, the PMT-cator (Magos and Studd 1988).

INCIDENCE

It is hard to evaluate how many women experience PMS since the distinction between PMS and more common but less severe cyclical changes is not always clear. Epidemiological studies indicate that between 75 and 90 per cent of ovulating women experience cyclical changes at least some time in their lives. For many these are in no way a problem. They can indeed be a positive part of their lives and could be regarded as normal 'physiological' aspects of the menstrual cycle. Logue and Moos (1988) found that between 5 and 15 per cent of women actually feel better in the premenstrual phase, experiencing increased well-being, energy, and activities before menstruation. For other women, however, premenstrual changes are upsetting but not devastating, and Sampson (1989) refers to such changes as 'premenstrual vulnerability' rather than PMS. Severe and distressing PMS leading a woman to seek advice is less common. Johnson (1987) estimates that while about 20 to 30 per cent of women experience PMS as a problem for which they have sought various kinds of self-help and may have tried treatment from their general practitioner, for about 10 per cent PMS is severe and disabling. This leads to a significant number of consultations for PMS in the surgery. It is likely that what brings a woman to seek medical help is the effect of PMS on her life. Women seek help when symptoms interfere with personal, home, or working life, and in particular with relationships with family, children, partner, friends, or colleagues.

EFFECTS OF PMS

PMS is undoubtedly distressing for many women, not only for themselves but also for those around them. Women with small children too young to understand PMS may feel extra stress and be worried about the effect their feelings are having on their children. Cyclical mood changes, particularly if seemingly unpredictable, may be a problem in relationships with a partner, unless PMS is discussed, understood, and accepted. Women whose colleagues at work are unsympathetic and dismiss suggestions or complaints on their part as 'it's that time of the month again' will obviously find PMS hard to bear. Women often worry that their performance at work may be impaired before menstruation but studies have shown that this is largely not the case (Johnson 1987), and that many women who suffer with PMS organize their work and home life so that they avoid stressful events premenstrually. Evidence suggests, however, that women who are admitted to psychiatric hospital, attempt suicide, or commit crimes are more likely to be in the luteal phase of their cycle. This is not to say that all premenstrual women are at risk of these events, but women who are likely to require psychiatric admission or commit crimes, and who experience PMS, may be more vulnerable in the premenstrual phase.

PMS may well influence women's sexuality, and there is no doubt that mood changes interact with sexual feelings. A woman who experiences severe premenstrual tiredness or breast tenderness may find this reduces her interest in sexual activities before menstruation, although sexual interest may well increase after menstruation once she feels an improvement in well-being. However, some women feel more sexually interested in the premenstrual phase. Fluctuations in sexual interest may cause worry to women, and possible problems in relationships unless links to the menstrual cycle are understood. Problems of varying sexual interest, linked to PMS, may be one reason for consulting the general practitioner.

WHO EXPERIENCES PMS?

There appears to be no distinctive 'type' of woman likely to experience PMS, although in general it appears to be more common in women in their thirties and forties and in women who have children. Certain events may be linked to the onset of PMS, such as stopping the oral contraceptive pill, the birth of a child, or sterilization. The observation that PMS may often occur for the first time after the birth of a child raises the question of whether the stress of having a child precipitates or exacerbates PMS or whether there is some hormonal connection (Brush 1985). PMS can still be experienced following hysterectomy if the ovaries remain (Backstrom *et al.* 1981). Women who are experiencing severe period problems, such as menorrhagia or dysmenorrhoea, may also experience PMS in anticipation of bad times to come. Once the menstrual problems are treated, the premenstrual difficulties may reduce. PMS seems to be common across all social classes although it seems that women who seek medical help specifically for PMS are more likely to be in social classes I and II. Therefore the primary health care team should be alert to the possibility of PMS in women consulting for other problems, such as anxiety or depression. There also appears to be a general link between adverse life events and PMS. Women tend to experience PMS as more of a problem during times of stress, such as when there are problems at home or at work, or during examinations or moving house, than during holidays or when life is generally going well.

Despite some views that PMS is a complaint of 'neurotic' women, there is no consistent relationship between women's personalities and PMS. There do, however, appear to be links between PMS and general psychological health. Women who are psychiatrically ill may experience more, and more severe, premenstrual psychological symptoms than psychologically healthy women (Clare 1983). Recently, interest has focused on PMS in premenopausal women. During the time leading up to the menopause, PMS can become more severe and blur into the menopause. It is possible that some women are more vulnerable than others to hormonal fluctuations, and are therefore at risk of problems with PMS, the menopause, and a mild form of postnatal depression, and so require extra support at these times.

PMS AND THE PRIMARY CARE TEAM

Increasing numbers of women are seeking medical help for PMS. This is partly due to a genuine increase in premenstrual problems, partly reflects the greater openness about menstrual problems and PMS, and is partly because more help is available. The general practitioner is often the first point of contact, although premenstrual difficulties may be discussed with health visitors, practice nurses, or social workers attached to the surgery.

Now that many practices have well woman and family planning clinics the 'best person' to deal with PMS may be any member of the team. It is probably helpful to have someone with some expertise in PMS in the practice because it is such a common and complex problem. Health visitors, counsellors, and nurses, as well as GPs, should be aware of PMS and how it may be affecting their clients. Groups for women with PMS—run in the surgery or in a local community centre as part of the practice's health promotion sessions—are very valuable for women with PMS and their partners or families. Some women may be helped by a discussion about PMS as part of a series of meetings on women's health issues where they can obtain information and discuss their problems. Specific PMS groups have been run by general practitioners and psychologists, giving women a chance to air their feelings, try out self-help techniques such as relaxation, and discuss medical treatments.

CAUSES OF PMS

There has been no shortage of hypotheses to explain PMS, the most plausible including variations in ovarian steroid production, abnormal tissue responses to normal levels of ovarian hormones, endorphin changes, abnormalities of other neurotransmitters, and abnormalities in prostaglandin pathways. To these can be added nutritional theories, including deficiencies of pyridoxine and essential fatty acids, hypoglycemia, low magnesium levels, and various psychological and social theories. Although researchers have attempted to come up with the definitive explanation, it is most likely that different aetiological factors apply to different women, given that symptoms vary so widely between, and even within, individuals.

PMS most probably results from a combination of physiological, psychological, and social factors interacting with life events. Various causes of PMS have been extensively reviewed in the literature (O'Brien 1987; Backstrom 1988; Brush 1988; Sampson 1989), and will be mentioned as relevant to treatment.

MANAGEMENT

PMS is a common problem which deserves sympathetic attention and appropriate management. Many women find that with support and encouragement they can work out solutions for themselves; and if problems persist, then various medical treatments can be tried. General approaches to management are summarized in Table 5.2.

Self-help

Women coming to the surgery with PMS need time to work out what the problems and solutions are, and so a number of appointments may be

Table 5.2   *Approaches to management of premenstrual syndrome*

General PMS:	
MILD	Discussion
	Self help
	Groups
	Attention to general health and lifestyle
	Make allowances for PMS
MODERATE	As above but also:
	Pyridoxine
	Evening primrose oil
	Danazol
SEVERE	Danazol
	Oral contraceptives
	Oestrogens in older women (as in HRT)
For particular symptoms:	
DEPRESSION	Pyridoxine
TIREDNESS	
HEADACHES	Antiprostaglandins
MIGRAINES	
BLOATING	Diuretics
MASTALGIA	Evening primrose oil
	Danazol if severe
ANXIETY	Relaxation
TENSION	Consider diazepam for occasional emergency use
MENORRHAGIA	Antiprostaglandins
DYSMENORRHOEA	Progestogens
	Oral contraceptive

Note: Any drug treatment **must** be accompanied by attention to lifestyle and self-help.

necessary. The woman and her adviser can both gain a great deal from a *menstrual chart* in defining and managing the problem (Fig. 5.1). A chart is also very valuable in determining whether remedies or treatments are helping, and the woman should be encouraged to keep the chart for several months. Knowing in some detail how she may feel at any time of the month helps a woman to deal with her feelings, since this introduces some predictability into cyclical changes and allows her to plan for the difficult times. It is very helpful to make allowances for PMS, and many women have benefited from fairly simple rearrangements to their schedules of work and activities to reduce the stress during the premenstrual days.

Talking to her GP, health visitor, or practice nurse may open the door for a woman to talk to others, such as her partner, family, friends, or colleagues. This means that problems are brought out into the open, rather than the woman feeling isolated or 'going round the bend'. Talking to others can also reveal a wealth of remedies and strategies for dealing with PMS. These include yoga, swimming, relaxation techniques (those learnt in preparation for childbirth may be very useful), vigorous exercise, beating up cushions or having a supply of old plates to smash if she feels very angry, having a premenstrual sauna or steam bath, having a good cry, or reading a gripping novel. Many women spend their time looking after others and an important part of the strategy to combat PMS is for the woman to look at *her* needs and to nurture herself. Local women's health groups will also have information and leaflets on self-help strategies.

A check on general health is vital. It is generally believed that a person will be fitter and deal better with stress if eating a balanced 'healthy' diet. There is some evidence that eating less fat will reduce breast pain in women with cyclical mastalgia (Goodwin *et al.* 1988). While this has a bearing on treatment for premenstrual breast pain, it seems reasonable for women with PMS to look at their dietary fat intake. It is possible that women are more sensitive to changes in bood sugar levels in the premenstrual days, resulting in feelings of weakness, fatigue, and carbohydrate cravings. Careful attention to diet can help, eating frequent, small, protein-rich meals, particularly if the woman tends to skip meals or eat sugary snacks. It is well worth looking at caffeine intake, since caffeine can increase levels of anxiety and irritability. Many people drink more tea and coffee than they realize, and cutting down or cutting these drinks out completely can be very helpful. The following case history illustrates the importance of diet:

Sandra is a 29-year-old youth worker who came to the Well Woman Clinic defining herself as having PMS and having tried vitamin B_6 and evening primrose oil with no benefits. She was interested in the nutritional theories of PMS and had heard that hypoglycemia was a possible cause. Breast tenderness and irritability were her main symptoms and she brought along her chart showing cyclical changes. Discussion revealed that she tended to eat junk food at work, regularly drank seven or eight cups of tea and coffee each day, and that premenstrually she craved chocolate. Life in general was fine and she described herself as happy although recent promotion at work meant more stress. Although initially she asked about vitamins and mineral supplements, talking about her diet helped her to see that it might be better to concentrate on her nutrition and cutting down on caffeine rather than buying expensive supplements. We wondered if her premenstrual treats could be, for example, a luxurious soak in the bath, rather than chocolate bars. She went away to try these strategies and report back in two months.

There may be links between *smoking* and premenstrual symptoms, so cutting down or stopping smoking is obviously part of the general health advice. Exercise can help many of the physical and emotional symptoms of PMS, including tiredness, anxiety, irritability, or bloating. Learning simple relaxation techniques or meditation can help too (Goodale *et al.* 1990). Premenstrual tiredness may be exacerbated by women making allowances for needing more sleep premenstrually. If breast tenderness is a problem, a well-fitting sports bra helps. General bloating and fluid retention may be helped by cutting down on fluids and salt, and avoiding salty foods and those that contain 'hidden' salt.

One of the most distressing symptoms of PMS is aggressive irritability which women say affects their activities and relationships. Although in our culture women are generally brought up to be more passive and nurturing than men, it is possible that PMS may bring out real anger about real problems in an otherwise docile woman. She and those around her may perceive this as irritability, and dismiss the underlying problems which need to be explored. The premenstrual days may not be the best time to tackle problems which are making her angry, but this is not a reason for ignoring them. Another case history follows:

A woman was brought to the Well Woman Clinic by her husband who said she was very ill with PMS. After discussion it was clear that the woman did experience moderate symptoms before her periods, particularly anger and aggression, but that there were significant and stressful events in her life. When seen alone, she said that for many years her husband had been drinking regularly, returning home aggressive and sometimes violent. She had decided to stay with him while their two children were growing up, but now that they had left home she was debating whether and when to leave. She was able to tolerate his drinking most of the time, but felt angry and upset about it during her premenstrual days. After several sessions with both of them, the husband came to see that he had a severe problem, and that his wife was not ill with PMS but understandably angry with the problems at home. The couple were referred to Relate.

Many *books* on PMS and self-help remedies are available, with sections on diet, relaxation, and exercise. (See Sanders 1985; Harrison 1991; Duckworth 1990.) More information can be obtained from the Women's Health and Reproductive Rights Information Centre (WHRRIC) or from PREMSOC, the society supporting research, education, and care on PMS. (See 'Useful addresses', below.) If no groups about PMS or women's health are run in the surgery, there are usually local groups or courses which women can be referred to.

Finally, many women have successfully sought help for PMS from various *'complementary'* or *'alternative'* medical practitioners, including acupuncturists, homoeopaths, and herbalists. Although alternative medicine is private, most practitioners operate sliding scales of fees according to the individual's ability to pay, and so are reasonably accessible these days. It is valuable for the surgery or health centre to keep lists of local registered practitioners, and notes of recommendations.

Medical treatments

There are many different medical approaches for PMS although, as for self-help remedies, there is a scarcity of well-conducted clinical trials. One problem in evaluating the efficacy of treatments is that most trials conducted show a very large placebo effect, particularly in the first month of treatment: in one study (Magos *et al.* 1986), 94 per cent of the women in the placebo group showed a significant improvement. Hence any drug trial or monitoring should be accurately controlled and continue for at least three months.

The general approach to medical management should be to start with those treatments known to be least toxic and with the least side-effects, such as pyridoxine or evening primrose oil, and if these are not effective, to try other treatments. A symptomatic approach may be helpful, since the research is indicating that different treatments work for individual symptoms; however, careful attention must be paid to adverse side-effects. A final approach is to look at abolishing ovulation or suppressing cyclical changes using drugs such as the oral contraceptive pil, danazol, LHRH analogues, or HRT. All treatments should be monitored for at least three months using a chart or diary. If the treatment is helpful, it should be continued for another six months and then stopped and the effects monitored. Some treatments can be combined; for example, pyridoxine and progestogens, but this makes it difficult to know which treatment is working and why (Magos 1990). Any treatment used for PMS must be thought about in terms of its possible hazards in pregnancy, and women should be warned about these, particularly with endocrine treatments. The authors' point of view is that no drug can be regarded as absolutely safe in early pregnancy, although Brush (1985) states that pyridoxine and evening primrose oil can be safely taken at this time. Women should also be reminded that no treatment, except the Pill, can be regarded as contraceptively effective.

A number of hospitals run out-patients PMS clinics, and referral to a specialist clinic can be useful for very severe PMS, or when considering one of the more sophisticated treatments discussed below. Menopause clinics may also see women with PMS; it is useful to check what facilities are available locally. Simply referring women to a gynaecologist may be unhelpful unless s/he has an interest in PMS and is sympathetic to the problem.

Pyridoxine—vitamin B_6

Pyridoxal phosphate is a co-factor in the synthesis of neurotransmitters including dopamine and tryptophan. Researchers have postulated that pyridoxine might be relatively deficient in premenstrual depression in some women, possibly related to cyclical changes in levels of steroid hormones (Brush 1988). However, results of controlled studies of women taking pyridoxine for PMS have been unclear (Williams *et al.* 1985; Magos 1990; Kleijnen *et al.* 1990). A recent study in general practice suggested a significant improvement in depression, irritability, and tiredness in women taking 50 mg per day of pyridoxine compared with those on placebo, although this trial involved only small numbers of women (Doll *et al.* 1989). The consensus is that more work needs to be done on the effectiveness of B_6. There is also some concern about the toxicity (peripheral neuropathy) of pyridoxine at doses over 500 mg daily; and occasionally women suffer from indigestion and gastritis at doses over 100 mg daily.

Our recommendation if a woman wanted to try pyridoxine would be to start with 50 mg twice a day and not to exceed 200 mg a day. It should be started three days before the expected onset of symptoms or may be taken continuously if cycles are irregular.

Gamma-linolenic acid—evening primrose oil

Supplements of gamma-linolenic acid in the form of evening primrose oil (EPO) have been given to women to correct a theoretical disorder of prostaglandin E_1 and essential fatty acids in women with PMS which possibly affects the binding of progesterone in tissues and hence the effects of progesterone (Brush and Goudsmit 1988). This theory is still under investigation. Double-blind controlled trials have been contradictory. A randomized trial of EPO in cyclical mastalgia (Pye *et al.* 1985) found that it was effective in 45 per cent of 291 women but less effective than danazol or bromocryptine—although EPO caused fewer side-effects. EPO has recently been licensed for prescription in women with premenstrual breast tenderness. The recommended prescription dose is three to four capsules of 40 mg twice daily after food, from three days before the expected onset of symptoms, tailoring to a lower dose if relief is obtained.

Diuretics and aldosterone antagonists

Most women who experience a feeling of bloating and weight gain premenstrually do not in fact gain weight and probably the feeling is due to weight redistribution. Some trials have shown that spironolactone may be beneficial for this symptom (O'Brien 1987), at a dose of 25 mg twice daily from days 18 to 26, or 10 days premenstrually. Care is needed in the use of diuretics, particularly non-potassium-sparing preparations; it is important not to prescribe them continuously since they can cause dangerously low potassium levels even if taken intermittently for PMS. Continuous use of diuretics can cause or exacerbate fluid retention, leaving a woman more symptomatic.

Prostaglandin inhibitors

Prostaglandin levels fluctuate in response to changing levels of oestradiol and progesterone. Although it is not known how prostaglandins may actually be involved in PMS, a double-blind controlled trial of mefenamic acid (Mira *et al.* 1986) showed it to be significantly better than placebo for physical and mood symptoms, particularly fatigue, general aches and pains, and headaches. A similar result was found in a study of naproxen, 550 mg twice daily from seven days before menstruation until day 4 (Facchinetti *et al.* 1989). Prostaglandin inhibitors may be especially useful for women prone to premenstrual headaches and migraine, and are also worth considering if a woman is suffering from dysmenorrhoea and/or menorrhagia as well as PMS. Treatment should probably start 10–14 days before expected menstruation, but side-effects such as gastrointestinal disturbances must be carefully monitored as these can potentially be severe. Gastrointestinal effects can be reduced if the drug is taken with food.

Endocrine therapies

These attempt to either abolish the menstrual cycle or ablate some of the hormonal fluctuations in it. It must be emphasized that we still know very little about what makes one woman suffer PMS and another not, and about the precise role of hormones in causing symptoms. There has been much publicity of the idea that women with PMS are suffering a hormone imbalance, and so informed patients sometimes ask for hormone measurements. Unless the GP feels the woman may be menopausal or suffering from some other complaint such as thyroid problems, hormone assessments are usually inappropriate.

Bromocryptine and danazol

Bromocryptine and danazol have been shown to be of significant help in premenstrual breast tenderness, although both are associated with unpleasant side-effects (O'Brien 1987). Bromocryptine acts by lowering prolactin levels, even though women with PMS and breast tenderness do not usually have raised prolactin levels. A dose of 2.5 mg daily is effective in mastalgia, although unfortunately even with this low dose many women have side-effects. It is therefore recommended that the starting dose should be a quarter of this, gradually increasing until the symptom is relieved, and it is advisable to take the drug with meals.

Danazol appears to have a direct effect on premenstrual mastalgia, and in addition has been shown to be beneficial in other PMS symptoms apart from bloating. Danazol is an antigonadotrophin and in large doses (400–800 mg daily) inhibits ovulation, thus presumably preventing PMS by abolishing the cycle. Many women find this dose intolerable because of side-effects, such as weight gain, acne, bloating, and hirsutism (Watts *et al.* 1987). However, danazol appears to alleviate PMS and mastalgia in some women at smaller doses of 200 mg daily and side-effects are reduced considerably.

Progesterone and progestogens

The initial rationale for the use of these was to replace some deficiency of progesterone in the luteal phase. We now know that no such deficiency exists in women with PMS. Katharina Dalton has advocated the use of progesterone and her books make interesting reading. She has also done much to publicize the plight of women with PMS in this country and given women and their GPs much to think about. However, results of controlled trials of progesterone are disappointing. Pure progesterone usually has to be given by pessary or suppository which some women find difficult. The results of a trial of oral micronized progesterone appeared to show a benefit for progesterone over placebo (Dennerstein *et al.* 1985), but the trial's analysis has been disputed and oral progesterone is not available in the UK.

Dydrogesterone is the progestogen so far more widely evaluated in women with PMS. Initial uncontrolled trials were hopeful but positive results have not been borne out in controlled trials (Sampson *et al.* 1988). Another trial (Williams *et al.* 1983) found PMS improved more in the progestogen group than in the placebo group only in the third month of treatment. The authors have seen individual women who clearly responded to progesterone or progestogens and these are still being used in general practice. It may be reasonable to try progestogens in a woman who is requesting them, though PMS treatment in the 1990s should be moving towards a rational approach. Progestogens themselves can *cause* PMS-type symptoms in some women and this should be borne in mind.

Medroxyprogesterone acetate (MPA)

One of the benefits mentioned by women using this for contraception is relief of PMS-type symptoms although, like progestogens, occasionally MPA can itself cause those symptoms. A recent study looked at norethisterone and MPA given orally 15 mg daily for 21 days; both drugs relieved PMS compared to placebo (West 1990). Clearly more work needs to be done here.

Oestrogen therapy

Studd and Magos (1986) realized the potential of oestradiol implants in abolishing ovulation. They conducted a double-blind trial in 68 women using implants plus cyclical oral norethisterone versus placebo. There was a significant improvement in six symptoms including concentration, mood changes, fluid retention, and breast pain. Several gynaecologists are now using oestradiol patches to suppress ovulation in women with PMS approaching the menopause, and a study of women aged 30–45 showed that these were more effective than placebo in relieving most PMS symptoms (Garnett *et al.* 1989). Although a large dose may be needed initially, such as two 100 μg patches twice weekly plus cyclical progestogen, the dose may possibly be lowered after a few weeks. Given that many women approaching the menopause may experience an exacerbation in PMS, this treatment can be useful. In the future it may be possible to combine the progestogen vaginal ring with oestradiol patches to produce a safe contraceptive effect as well as relief for PMS.

While oestrogen therapy is now known to have many benefits for women in terms of bone preservation and prevention of heart disease (see Chapter 7 on the menopause), we must not consider this a panacea. Oestrogen patches may cause skin irritation and fall off, progestogens may exacerbate PMS, and there are still some question marks over long-term oestrogen use and breast cancer. In addition, as doses used for PMS have tended to be very high, it might be worth consulting with a local interested gynaecologist before embarking on this treatment.

Gail is 44 and has suffered with PMS all her life. She is a single mother, working full time in a bookshop, with two children, the youngest of whom, aged 10, is deaf. Gail's PMS appeared to worsen after each pregnancy. Her main problems were feeling bloated, severe irritability, and often severe migraines lasting several days; and she felt she treated her children unfairly premenstrually. PMS usually incapacitated her for up to a week each month, which was very difficult both at work and at home. She had tried all kinds of self-help, including yoga and relaxation techniques, and most of the remedies available from the chemist including pyridoxine. These helped somewhat but the irritability and migraine were still hard to cope with. Five years ago her PMS became intolerable and she decided to seek medical help. Her diaries showed that although she was leading a stressful life, she definitely had PMS. She had already cut down on caffeine and because of the migraines was very careful with her diet. After discussion she decided to try progesterone pessaries.

Initially, the progesterone did seem to help the migraines but not the other symptoms, and after nine months the migraines started to reappear and we started her on danazol, having discussed its side-effects. She took 200 mg daily for over a year with relief from both migraines and irritability. Even the bloating decreased to a tolerable level. Eighteen months ago, however, her symptoms gradually started to reappear and in consultation with a sympathetic local woman gynaecologist, we changed treatment to oestrogen patches (100 μg twice weekly) and progesterone pessaries (200 mg twice daily for 12 days out of 28) to provide progestogen coverage.

To begin with, she had some severe breast tenderness with this regime but this soon settled and she is now doing a degree as well as working and looking after her children. She says she feels like a new woman and much more energetic in general.

LHRH analogues

These work by producing a 'medical oophorectomy' (Muse *et al.* 1984) and have been shown to be more effective than placebo in several trials. However, they produce low oestradiol levels and this makes them unsuitable for long-term use because of the risks of osteoporosis. They are also expensive, but they have the advantage of having very few immediate side-effects. Researchers are working on low-dose LHRH analogue treatments and are looking to see if treatment over a short period produces lasting benefits.

Oral contraceptives

While some women experience PMS symptoms, or even an exacerbation of PMS-like symptoms while taking the oral contraceptive pill, particularly the older higher dose pills, some women have reported relief (Magos 1989). In addition, women whose PMS is exacerbated by the thought of terrible periods, heavy bleeding, or dysmenorrhoea will experience relief on oral contraceptives, which can be taken continuously for several months (RCGP 1974). With the advent of new lower dose pills, particularly with different progestogens such as gestodene or desogestrel, the benefits of oral contraceptives for women with PMS urgently need to be reviewed.

Other treatments

Opiate antagonists

Some recent research has questioned whether endorphin production may explain why so many women feel better after exercise premenstrually. A study of the opiate antagonist naltrexone showed possible benefits for PMS, but its side-effects were intolerably severe (Chuong *et al.* 1988).

Benzodiazepines

If a woman is severely stressed and irritable premenstrually, and all causes and exacerbating factors have been eliminated, careful occasional use of a low-dose benzodiazepine may be helpful, as long as the woman understands the dangers of addiction (Harrison *et al.* 1990). Recent studies have looked at the new benzodiazepines but the authors feel that it is much safer to use occasional low doses of well-known and cheaper drugs such as diazepam.

Antidepressants

Psychiatrists are looking at the use of antidepressants in PMS (Harrison *et al.* 1989). More controlled trials need to be done and caution is needed; as in the past many women have complained to us that 'the doctor didn't listen . . . he just gave me these tablets.' GPs should, however, be aware that women who do suffer from PMS may have a lowered threshold for clinical depression if severe life events occur and may benefit from earlier intervention with antidepressants. This may also apply to PMS sufferers in the post-natal period.

Oophorectomy and hysterectomy

For very severe PMS sufferers who are in their forties, particularly those who may also have menstrual problems, oophorectomy and hysterectomy and provision of HRT will result in a cure for PMS. However, women and their GPs must make an informed decision about this as it is a major step; and GPs may be mediators between women and gynaecologists to ensure that the best decision is made for a particular woman (Casper and Hearn 1990).

CONCLUSION

Premenstrual syndrome includes a wide range of physical and emotional changes which vary in severity, duration, and effects on a woman's life. It is unlikely that there is a single or simple cause, and any consideration of the aetiology of PMS must take into account psychological, physiological, and social factors. Management of PMS is not simple, but it is certainly aided by a greater understanding and acceptance of the problem, and the development of a range of approaches and remedies. Women need to devote time to experiment to find an appropriate solution, and may require help from the primary health care team to evaluate how they can help themselves and, if necessary, what medical treatments might be useful. In any individual woman it is essential to determine whether or not she has PMS, what her main problems are, and the circumstances which led her to seek medical help. The first steps are sympathetic discussion of the problems and reorganization of aspects of her life to cope with times of feeling low. Attention to general health and lifestyle is the key to dealing with PMS. Following this a woman may try a variety of self-help approaches; and for those women severely affected by PMS, medical treatment may also be necessary. The approach is to start with less toxic treatments with few side-effects, to consider specific treatments for specific symptoms, and finally to consider cycle suppression in severely affected women. Women who are not helped may be referred to a PMS clinic or to one of the increasing numbers of gynaecologists who are interested in PMS and menopausal problems.

USEFUL ADDRESSES

Women's Health and Reproductive Rights Information Centre (WHRRIC), 52 Featherstone Street, London EC1Y 8RT. Tel: 071 251 6580.
PREMSOC, PO Box 102, London SE1 7ES.

REFERENCES AND FURTHER READING

Abraham, G. E. (1983). Nutritional factors in the aetiology of the premenstrual tension syndromes. *Journal of Reproductive Medicine*, **28**, 446–64.

Bäckström, T. (1988). Endocrine factors in the aetiology of premenstrual syndrome. In *Functional disorders of the menstrual cycle* (ed. M. G. Brush and E. M. Goudsmit), pp. 87–96. Wiley, Chichester.

Bäckström, T., Boyle, H., and Baird, D. T. (1981). Persistence of symptoms of premenstrual tension in hysterectomised women. *British Journal of Obstetrics and Gynaecology*, **88**, 530–6.

Brush, M. G. (1985). The premenstrual syndrome before and after pregnancy. *Maternal and Child Health*, **10**, (1), 19–25.

Brush, M. G. (1988). Vitamins, essential fatty acids and minerals in relation to the aetiology and management of premenstrual syndrome. In *Functional disorders of the menstrual cycle* (ed. M. G. Brush and E. M. Goudsmit), pp. 69–86. Wiley, Chichester.

Brush, M. G. and Goudsmit, E. M. (1988). *Functional disorders of the menstrual cycle*. Wiley, Chichester.

Casper, R. F. and Hearn, M. T. (1990). Effect of hysterectomy and bilateral oophorectomy in women with severe premenstrual syndrome. *American Journal of Obstetrics and Gynecology*, **162**, 105–9.

Chuong, C. J., Coularm, C. B., Bergstralh, E. J., *et al.* (1988). Clinical trial of naltrexone in premenstrual syndrome. *Obstetrics and Gynaecology*, **72**, 332–9.

Clare, A. W. (1983). Psychiatric and social aspects of premenstrual complaint. *Psychological Medicine Monographs Supplement*, **4**, 1–58.

Dennerstein, L., Spencer-Gardner, C., Gotts, G., *et al.* (1985). Progesterone and the premenstrual syndrome: a double-blind crossover trial. *British Medical Journal*, **290**, 1617–21.

Doll, H., Brown, S., Thurston, A., *et al.* (1989). Pyridoxine and the premenstrual syndrome: a randomized crossover trial. *Journal of the Royal College of General Practitioners*, **39**, 364–8.

Duckworth, H. (1990). *Premenstrual syndrome: your options*. Attic Press, Dublin.

Facchinetti, F., Fioroni, L., Sances, G., *et al.* (1989). Naproxen sodium in the treatment of premenstrual symptoms: a placebo controlled study. *Gynaecological and Obstetric Investigations*, **28**, 205–8.

Garnett, I., Savvas, M., Watson, N. R., *et al.* (1989). Treatment of severe premenstrual syndrome with oestradiol patches and cyclical norethisterone. *Lancet,* **8665,** 730–2.

Goodale, I. L., Domar, A. D., and Benson, H. (1990). Alleviation of premenstrual syndrome symptoms with the relaxation response. *Obstetrics and Gynaecology,* **75,** 649–55.

Goodwin, P. J., Neelam, M., and Boyd, N. F. (1988). Cyclical mastopathy: a critical review of therapy. *British Journal of Surgery,* **75,** 837–44.

Harrison, M. (1991). *Self help with PMS.* Macdonald Optima, London.

Harrison, W. M., Endicott, J., and Nee, J. (1989). Treatment of premenstrual depression with nortriptyline: a pilot study. *Journal of Clinical Psychiatry,* **50,** 136–9.

Harrison, W. M., Endicott, J., and Nee, J. (1990). Treatment of premenstrual dysphoria with alprazolam: a controlled study. *Archives of General Psychiatry,* **47,** 270–5.

Johnson, S. R. (1987). The epidemiology and social impact of premenstrual syndrome. *Clinical Obstetrics and Gynaecology,* **30,** 367–76.

Kleijnen, J., Riet, G. T., and Knipschild, P. (1990). Vitamin B_6 in the treatment of the premenstrual syndrome—a review. *British Journal of Obstetrics and Gynaecology,* **97,** 847–52.

Logue, C. M. and Moos, R. H. (1986). Perimenstrual symptoms: prevalence and risk factors. *Psychosomatic Medicine,* **48,** 388–414.

Logue, C. M. and Moos, R. H. (1988). Positive perimenstrual changes: towards a new perspective on the menstrual cycle. *Journal of Psychosomatic Research,* **32,** 31–40.

Magos, A. L. (1989). Premenstrual syndrome. *Contemporary Review of Obstetrics and Gynaecology,* **1,** 80–92.

Magos, A. L. (1990). Advances in the treatment of the premenstrual syndrome. *British Journal of Obstetrics and Gynaecology,* **97,** 7–10.

Magos, A. L., Brincat, M., and Studd, J. W. W. (1986). Treatment of premenstrual syndrome by subcutaneous oestradiol implants and cyclical oral norethisterone: placebo controlled study. *British Medical Journal,* **292,** 1629–33.

Magos, A. L. and Studd, J. W. W. (1988). A simple method for the diagnosis of premenstrual syndrome by use of a self-assessment disk. *American Journal of Obstetrics and Gynecology,* **158,** 1024–8.

Mira, M., McNeil, D., Fraser, I. S., *et al.* (1986). Mefenamic acid in the treatment of premenstrual syndrome. *Obstetrics and Gynaecology,* **68,** 395–8.

Muse, K., Cetel, N., Futterman, L., *et al.* (1984). The premenstrual syndrome: effects of medical ovariectomy. *New England Journal of Medicine,* **311,** 1345–9.

O'Brien, P. M. S. (1987). *Premenstrual syndrome.* Blackwell, Oxford.

O'Brien, P. M. S. (1990). The premenstrual syndrome. *British Journal of Family Planning,* **15,** (suppl.) 13–18.

Pye, J. K., Mansel, R. E., and Hughes, L. E. (1985). Clinical experience of drug treatments for mastalgia. *Lancet,* **ii,** 373–7.

RCGP (Royal College of General Practitioners) (1974). *Oral contraceptives and health.* Pitman Medical, London.

Sampson, G. A. (1989). Premenstrual syndrome. *Baillières Clinical Obstetrics and Gynaecology,* **3,** 687–704.

Sampson, G. A. (1990). The boundaries of premenstrual syndrome—who defines them and how do they affect clinical practice. *British Journal of Family Planning,* **15,** (suppl.) 19–22.

Sampson, G. A., Heathcote, P. R. M., Worsworth, J., *et al.* (1988). Premenstrual syndrome: a double-blind crossover study of treatment with dydrogesterone and placebo. *British Journal of Psychiatry,* **153,** 232–5.

Sanders, D. (1985). *Coping with periods.* Chambers, Edinburgh.

Studd, J. W. W. and Magos, A. L. (1986). Hormone manipulation in the management of premenstrual syndrome. In *Hormones and behaviour* (ed. L. Dennerstein and I. Fraser), pp. 147–59. Elsevier, Holland.

Watts, J. F., Butt, W. R., and Logan-Edwards, R. (1987). A clinical trial using danazol for the treatment of premenstrual tension. *British Journal of Obstetrics and Gynaecology,* **94,** 30–4.

West, C. P. (1990). Inhibition of ovulation with oral progestins: effectiveness in premenstrual syndrome. *European Journal of Obstetrics, Gynecology and Reproductive Biology,* **34,** 119–28.

Williams, J. G. C., Martin, A. J., and Hulkensberg-Tromp, T. (1983). PMS in four European countries. Part 2: a double-blind placebo controlled study of dydrogesterone. *British Journal of Sexual Medicine,* **10,** 8–18.

Williams, M. J., Harris, R. I., and Dean, B. C. (1985). Controlled trial of pyridoxine in the premenstrual syndrome. *Journal of International Medical Research,* **13,** 174–9.

6. Menstrual problems

Margaret C. P. Rees

INTRODUCTION

Disorders of menstruation, 'the curse', 'the devil's gateway', or whatever one likes to call them, form a significant part of the general practitioner's work. This is not surprising since women will each experience about 400 menstruations. In a national community survey, 1069 women aged 16–45 were interviewed in their homes (MORI 1990): 31 per cent reported heavy periods and 38 per cent painful periods. Of these, one-third had consulted a doctor within the past four months. Menstrual disorders are clearly very common and furthermore there is an increasing tendency for women to seek professional help. The Second National Morbidity Survey in General Practice (1981–82) showed that of the commonest specific conditions most often seen in practice, menstrual problems are in the top ten. The consultation rate seems to be increasing; for instance, that for menorrhagia increased by 73 per cent between 1971/72 and 1981/82, and a preliminary survey shows a further increase of 30 per cent by 1990 (Rees 1991, unpublished data).

When it comes to hospital referral, menstrual disorders are the second most common cause for all ages, and both sexes, which would apear to be a disproportionate representation of a quarter of the population (Coulter *et al.* 1989). Menorrhagia is the main presenting complaint in one-third of all women referred to gynaecologists. Ultimately hysterectomy may be required, and up to 40 000 such procedures are performed each year in England and Wales for menstrual disorders. Again, menstrual disorders are the commonest indication for hysterectomy.

Since ancient times the idea of menstruation has had magical and mythical connotations. Pliny noted that while menstrual blood cured epilepsy, gout, malaria, and boils, it also caused iron to rust and copper to turn green. Menstruation has been considered to be a taboo subject. The word *'tabu'* comes from the Polynesian, where it means menstruation as well as things which are both sacred and unclean. In various cultures women have been prohibited from making food, tending plants, and having any contact with men; and have been banished to menstrual huts. In our own society, mothers may still tell their daughters not to bath, wash their hair, or undertake physical exercise during menstruation. These attitudes have no doubt contributed to relatively recent development of effective sanitary protection, with commercial tampons only being introduced in the 1920s.

Furthermore, the UK is one of the few countries where advertisement of sanitary protection on television is restricted.

As a result of these myths it is not surprising that it can be difficult for women to distinguish between normal and abnormal menstruation. The purpose of this chapter is to try and suggest which symptomatology, as usually presented to the general practitioner, might indicate the need for further appropriate investigation and treatment either at a primary care level or by the specialist.

At any one time women might complain that their periods are:

too short
too long
too frequent
too infrequent
too light
too heavy
too painful
too irregular
too early (menarche)
too late (menarche)
too early (menopause)
too late (menopause)
too awful!

This is excluding the complaint that it is unfair that they should have them at all and men are remarkably lucky.

It is probably best when discussing menstrual disorders with patients to use simple descriptive English terms, such as heavy or painful periods, rather than take refuge behind schoolboy classical Greek. For instance, polymenometrorrhagia, literally means 'frequent month womb rushing out' rather than 'frequent heavy, irregular periods'.

This chapter will first discuss the physiology of menstruation and then its problems whether excessive, painful, or absent.

PHYSIOLOGY OF MENSTRUATION

Endocrine changes

The sequence of hormone events occurring in the menstrual cycle during which ovulation takes place is shown in Fig. 6.1. At menstruation, plasma levels of the anterior pituitary hormone, follicle stimulating hormone (FSH), are already rising, stimulating the growth of several Graafian follicles within the ovary. In general, the end result of this follicular development is (usually) one mature follicle and ovum. The developing

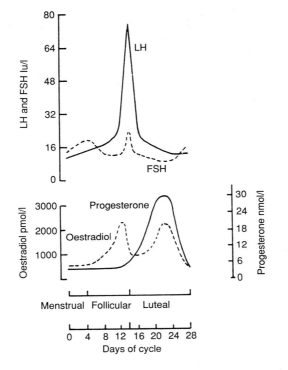

Fig. 6.1 Hormone changes during the menstrual cycle, showing fluctuating levels of the pituitary hormones, luteinizing hormone (LH), and follicle-stimulating hormone (FSH), and of the ovarian hormones, oestradol and progesterone.

follicle produces increasing amounts of oestrogens, notably oestradiol. As levels of oestradiol begin to rise early in the follicular phase of the cycle, production of FSH is suppressed by negative feedback, but oestradiol levels continue to increase over the next few days until a critical level is reached. Here, by positive feedback it triggers the anterior pituitary to release about 24 hours later a surge of luteinizing hormone (LH) with levels up to 50 IU/litre and to a lesser extent FSH with levels up to 15 IU/ litre; such levels only occur for one day. Ovulation follows the onset of the LH surge within about 34–36 hours, and the ruptured ovarian follicle develops into the corpus luteum which secretes both oestradiol and progesterone in the second half or luteal phase of the cycle. Levels of both oestradiol and progesterone therefore rise after ovulation, reaching peak levels between days 18 and 22 of a 28-day cycle. In the last few days of the cycle, if pregnancy has not occurred, the corpus luteum degenerates and oestradiol and progesterone levels fall before menstruation ensues. Plasma levels of progesterone can be measured to assess ovulation and levels greater than 16 nmol/litre on days 18–22 are indicatory. The time period from the LH surge to menses is consistently close to 14 days but may vary normally from 12 to 17 days. However, variability in cycle length among women is principally due to the varying number of days required for follicular growth and development in the follicular phase. Menstrual bleeding can occur in both ovulatory and anovulatory cycles. In the latter the ovary produces enough oestrogen to stimulate endometrial growth and bleeding occurs when oestrogen levels fall. Bleeding in anovulatory cycles tends to be irregular, painless, and heavy. In the past decade it has been found that ovarian follicles also produce peptide hormones such as inhibin and activin which inhibit and stimulate FSH production respectively. While these peptides are not measured routinely, they may be in specialized centres.

Endometrial events

The process of menstruation is poorly understood and it is not really known why women should bleed at all since it does not seem to fulfil any biological function. It only occurs in a restricted number of species: humans and most sub-human primates. Consequently, scientific understanding of the physiological mechanisms involved in the process of menstruation is based on animal as well as human data. Endometrium undergoes growth, degeneration, and regression prior to menstruation and bleeding occurs from endometrial blood vessels especially spiral arterioles. In most species that menstruate, endometrial arterioles are unusual in that they are profusely coiled as they run through the endometrium and they also change throughout the menstrual cycle. These arterioles undergo profound vasoconstriction which starts 4–24 hours before menstruation and lasts until the end of menstrual bleeding. Bleeding results from relaxation of individual blood vessels and then ceases as they constrict. If constriction did not occur, it could not unreasonably be expected that women would bleed to death at the menarche.

Another phenomenon that occurs during menstruation is myometrial contraction. The myometrium contracts throughout the menstrual cycle and there is increased activity during menstruation, especially in women with primary dysmenorrhoea.

Of the pathways thought to play a major role in menstruation, the evidence for altered prostaglandin biosynthesis is the most compelling. Prostaglandins have the capacity to affect both haemostasis and myometrial contractility. Very high levels of prostaglandins are found in uterine tissues and menstrual blood; and, furthermore, administration of prostaglandin $F_{2\alpha}$ during the luteal phase of the cycle results in menstrual bleeding. Prostaglandin levels are further increased in women with menorrhagia and dysmenorrhoea, and clinically inhibitors of prostaglandin biosynthesis are effective in these disorders. In menorrhagia there is also additional evidence of an altered responsiveness to the vasodilator prostaglandin E_2. Increased concentrations of prostaglandin E_2 receptors are present in myometrium collected from women with excessive bleeding. In dysmenorrhoea the leukotriene pathway allied to prostaglandins has also been implicated, in that higher levels of leukotrienes are present in endometrium of dysmenorrhoeic women. Finally, increased endometrial fibrinolysis has been implicated in menorrhagia leading to the use of antifibrinolytic agents.

Variation in menstrual blood loss (MBL)

The amount of blood loss at each menstruation has been measured in several population studies. In several hundred women not complaining of any menstrual problems objective measurement of menstrual blood loss (MBL) shows a skewed distribution with the mean of about 35 ml and the 90th percentile of 80 ml. MBL is considered excessive if greater than 80 ml: without treatment such a loss leads to iron deficiency anaemia and constitutes objective menorrhagia (see Fig. 6.2). Blood losses up to 1600 ml have been measured in some women. Despite variation in the total amount of blood lost, 90 per cent is lost within the first three days, fitting in with patients' description of a tap being turned on and off.

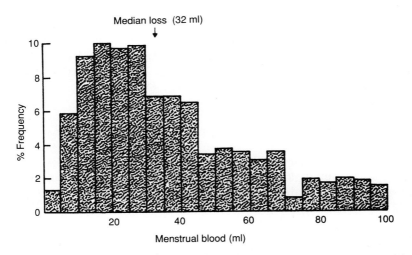

Fig. 6.2 Frequency distribution (%) of menstrual blood loss in several hundred women in Oxford before insertion of a intra-uterine device. Mean menstrual loss is 33 ml; median loss is 32 ml. (From unpublished data of J. Guillebaud, with permission.)

Variation in cycle length

Cyclical vaginal bleeding is known to occur at well-defined intervals from
the menarche to the menopause. Since ancient times, it has been shown
that the length of the menstrual cycle (i.e. from day 1 of one period to day
1 of the next) approximated to the phases of the moon. The Greek 'men'
means month. Women in many cultures refer to their periods as 'the moon'
and some women believe they are actually caused by the moon! As recently
as 1938 a textbook for American medical students stated that the majority
of women menstruated with the moon. Not surprisingly, the 28-day cycle
has become the symbol of health and normality in relation to reproductive
function and women begin to worry that something is wrong if their
menstrual cycle deviates from this 28-day 'norm'. Furthermore, medications to induce artificial cycles, such as the oral contraceptive and hormone
replacement, are also geared to producing 28-day 'ideal' cycles. This therefore leads women to seek medical treatment to regulate periods if cycles
become either short or long.

It is important that women should be informed that there is a large
degree of variability in cycle length that is compatible with good health.
Variability in cycle length was best evaluated in the classic study of Vollman
(1977). The famous 28-day cycle happens to be the commonest cycle length
recorded (see Fig. 6.3) but only just, and then in only 12.4 per cent of
cycles documented. Cycle length changes with age forming a U-shaped
curve from the menarche to the menopause. Mean cycle length drops from
35 days at age 12 to a minimum of 27 days at age 43, rising to 52 days at age
55, with an enormous range of cycle length. Clearly, there is a wide
variation in normal cycle length especially in the first few years after
menarche and in the years preceding the menopause. It is important that
normal biological variation be recognized by both women and their doctors
so that they do not become crippled by the 28-day ideal.

THE ABNORMAL MENSTRUAL CYCLE

Menstrual cycle problems and ways of dealing with them in general practice
are now presented, and things important for a general practitioner to
recognize and treat are discussed in detail.

Menorrhagia (heavy blood loss)

Menorrhagia comes from the Greek 'men' month and 'rhegynai' to rush out.
It is a complaint of excessive menstrual bleeding, but in objective terms is a
blood loss greater than 80 ml per period. While various pathologies have
been implicated in menorrhagia, in 50 per cent of cases of objective

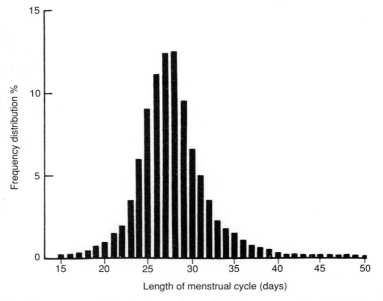

Length of menstrual cycle (days)

Fig. 6.3 Frequency distribution (%) of length of the menstrual cycle in days from menarche to the menopause. 31 645 menstrual cycle lengths recorded by 656 women aged 11–58 years. (Redrawn from Fig. 33, p. 54, in Vollman 1977.)

menorrhagia no pathology is found at hysterectomy. Although 'unexplained' menorrhagia is a very appropriate term, this state is often labelled less clearly as dysfunctional uterine bleeding which implies endocrine abnormalities. It must be emphasized that most cases of menorrhagia are associated with regular ovulatory cycles; anovular cycles tend mainly to occur soon after the menarche or close to the menopause. In ovulatory cycles excessive menstrual loss has been ascribed to abnormal uterine levels of prostaglandins with increased concentrations of receptors to the vaso-dilator prostaglandin E_2, and elevated levels of the fibrinolytic enzyme plasminogen activator.

Assessment of menstrual blood loss

A common presentation of a patient with menorrhagia is a complaint of increased menstrual loss requiring more sanitary protection and including the passage of clots and flooding. While soaking of bed sheets and staining of clothes is suggestive of a heavy period, women find it very difficult to assess accurately the amount of blood loss. Thus some women who are losing several hundred millilitres consider their flow to be normal while others losing only a few millilitres complain bitterly of menorrhagia. Furthermore, numbers of pads and tampons used, as well as degree of staining— parameters often used by doctors—do not give reliable estimates. Women with true menorrhagia may not necessarily drop their haemoglobin concentration; losses of 800–1000 ml can occur without anaemia. Conversely the presence of a hypochromic microcytic anaemia in a woman who menstruates should alert the GP to the possibility that she might have menorrhagia. At present it has been estimated in hospital practice that only 40 per cent of women complaining of menorrhagia have measured losses greater than 80 ml. The percentage could be even higher in general practice!

Although not available routinely, objective measurement of MBL could therefore be considered to be a vital assessment. MBL can be easily measured using the non-invasive alkaline haematin method, which involves soaking sanitary devices in 5 per cent sodium hydroxide to convert the blood to alkaline haematin whose optical density can be measured.

Causes and diagnosis

A diagnosis of unexplained menorrhagia depends on exclusion of pathology. Menorrhagia may be due to systemic or pelvic pathology, or iatrogenic causes. However, this widespread view perpetrated by many gynaecological textbooks is based on clinical impression without essential objective MBL measurement. Disorders of haemostasis such as von Willebrand's disease and deficiencies of factors V, VII, and X, and idiopathic thrombocytopenic purpura, are thought to increase menstrual loss, but blood loss was not objectively measured in the cases originally reported. When it has been measured, platelet disorders (thrombocytopenia) rather than coagulation disorders have been implicated in menorrhagia. With regard to pelvic pathology, fibroids (leiomyomas), endometriosis, pelvic inflammatory disease, and endometrial polyps are thought to cause menorrhagia; but again there is a paucity of data with objective MBL measurement. The few studies where it has been measured show that these lesions are associated with objective menorrhagia in only about half to two-thirds of cases. While iatrogenic causes, such as intra-uterine contraceptive devices, have been shown objectively to increase MBL there is no such data for anticoagulants.

History-taking and general physical and pelvic examination should allow the GP to reach a diagnosis and decide whether hospital referral is necessary. The length and interval of periods and duration of excessive bleeding, as well as any intermenstrual or post-coital bleeding, should be ascertained. The method of contraception should also be noted since intra-uterine contraceptive devices are associated with increased MBL. General examination, including bimanual and pelvic examination, should be performed and a cervical smear obtained. A particular search should be made for polyps protruding through the cervical os and for enlargement or tenderness of the uterus or adnexae. A routine full blood count should be performed to check for anaemia.

The next step is to decide whether an endometrial biopsy need be performed. Since the incidence of endometrial hyperplasia and carcinoma increases significantly after the age of 40, a prudent guideline is that biopsy is mandatory in women over that age but may be deferred in younger women unless the bleeding is severe, does not respond to treatment, or is associated with intermenstrual bleeding. However, in a woman aged over 40 with regular periods and no intermenstrual bleeding, a trial of a prostaglandin synthetase inhibitor or an antifibrinolytic agent could be used first since blood loss reduction tends not to occur in the presence of pathology.

The reasons for referral can therefore be for management of pelvic pathology, endometrial biopsy, or help with assessment of clinical findings if these are uncertain.

Endometrial biopsy

Traditionally endometrium has been obtained for histological examination by dilation and curettage or 'D&C' under general anaesthesia. Although for many years it has been considered a therapeutic procedure curing all menstrual disorders, it is only diagnostic. The reason for this erroneous concept is that traditionally follow-up after any gynaecological procedure is at six weeks when most women will have had only one post-operative period. Objective menstrual blood loss measurement has shown that while the first period after D&C is lighter than previous ones, they are subsequently no different.

In the past decade there has been an increasing trend to perform minor procedures in outpatient departments without general anaesthesia. Here endometrium is obtained either with a suction curette (Rockett) or biopsy loop (Gynocheck). Suction may be achieved with either a small hand pump or with a disposable piston cannula (Pipelle). The technical skills required for the Gynocheck and Pipelle are similar to those needed to fit an intrauterine contraceptive device and could be used in general practice after suitable training. Patients should be warned that they may experience some discomfort as the curette is passed and the biopsy taken (usually 10–15 seconds). For the majority the transient, usually mild, discomfort is outweighed by the advantages of avoiding hospitalization and having the test over with at the time of the initial consultation. The minority of cases who are either difficult to examine, or have a relatively tight cervix, or who decline outpatient testing will still need biopsy under anaesthesia.

Whichever way endometrial biopsy is performed, endometrial polyps and submucous fibroids will tend to be missed. These can only be accurately diagnosed by direct vision with hysteroscopy. Hysteroscopy can be performed either as an inpatient or an outpatient procedure, but is available only in specialized centres.

Whom the general practitioner should treat and how

Women under the age of 40 with otherwise uncomplicated regular heavy periods are extremely unlikely to have endometrial cancer or hyperplasia, and referral for specialist opinion in the absence of clinically detectable pathology seems unnecessary. If there are no worrying signs such as blood-stained vaginal discharge, intermenstrual or post-coital bleeding, the GP can use medical therapy to try and reduce blood loss if this is what the woman wishes. The aim of therapy is to reduce blood loss to a socially convenient level and where the woman is not at risk of anaemia. In the absence of objective MBL measurements it must be remembered that there are two sorts of treatment failures: (1) those with extremely heavy periods, and (2) those with a normal loss where therapy is only effective if the patient is rendered amenorrhoeic. Some women are prepared to put up with their heavy loss if it is not too debilitating or socially inconvenient, and fear the side-effects of drug therapy in the long term; though anaemia should be looked for and corrected. Women over the age of 40 with menorrhagia should probably be referred to a gynaecologist. Not all women over 40 will need referral. The GP may try medical therapy first in women whose loss has been gradually increasing over the years. A sudden change in loss is suggestive of pathology and needs earlier referral.

Young girls with heavy periods in the years after the menarche are very unlikely indeed to have any pelvic pathology. Probably all that is required is for the GP to give reassurance by explaining to the girl (and her mother) that this type of menstrual upset usually settles with time. It is probably part of the maturation of the hypothalamic–pituitary–ovarian axis. General practitioners should be cautious about giving young girls hormonal treatment in the early years after the menarche because of possible long-term consequences. There are a very few young girls with persistent heavy irregular periods associated with anovular cycles. Sustained unopposed oestrogen levels lead to endometrial hyperplasia which may ultimately progress in later years to carcinoma. Specialist investigation is required in these young girls who may then need cyclical progestogens.

Drug therapy

Medical treatment is indicated when there is no obvious pelvic abnormality and the woman wishes to retain her fertility. There is a wide range of preparations which can be divided into either non-hormonal or hormonal (Table 6.1). The former need only be taken during menstruation and have the added advantage that the women are treated only when they are not unknowingly pregnant.

Non-hormonal. The implication of excessive prostaglandin levels in menorrhagia has led to the use of prostaglandin synthetase inhibitors in the treatment of this disorder. The effectiveness of these agents was first demonstrated by Anderson *et al.* (1976). In this study, it was observed that mefenamic acid reduced menstrual blood loss by an average of 50 per cent, and furthermore need only be taken during menstruation. These findings

Table 6.1   *Drug therapy for menorrhagia*

Preparation	Dose
Non-hormonal	
Prostaglandin synthetase inhibitors	
Mefenamic acid	500 mg q.i.d. during menstruation only
Antifibrinolytics	
Tranexamic acid	1–1.5 g 6–8 hourly during menstruation
Ethamsylate	500 mg 4–6 hourly during menstruation
Hormonal	
Norethisterone	5 mg b.d. or t.i.d. days 19 (or earlier) to 26
Danazol	200–400 mg daily continuously
Gestrinone	2.5 mg twice weekly

have since been confirmed. Follow-up 12 to 15 months after commencing treatment shows that mefenamic acid continues to be effective in reducing MBL. Mefenamic acid is contraindicated in women with a history of peptic ulceration, but seems to have few side-effects if taken for only a few days each cycle. Other prostaglandin synthetase inhibitors, for example ibuprofen, also reduce MBL.

Recently a dual mode of action has been demonstrated for fenamates. As well as reducing prostaglandin synthesis, they inhibit binding of prostaglandin E to its receptor and this additional effect may contribute to their efficacy in the treatment of menorrhagia.

The suggestion that fibrinolytic activity may be abnormal in menorrhagia has led to use of antifibrinolytic agents such as tranexamic acid. Taken during menstruation they also have been found to be effective in reducing MBL. Although there have been worries about thrombo-embolic risks these drugs seem safe in normal healthy women. It would be prudent, however, not to give them to women with a previous history of thrombosis or other risk factors such as a low anti-thrombin III level.

Ethamsylate is a drug which is said to increase capillary wall strength and it can reduce MBL, but there are few studies of its efficacy.

Hormonal.   Although progestogens are the most popular therapy for menorrhagia, the available evidence with objective measurement of menstrual blood loss does not show a significant reduction in flow. Their use is based on the idea that women with menorrhagia have anovular cycles but, as stated earlier, most women with menorrhagia and regular cycles are ovulating. Progestogens are probably more useful to regularize menstrual cycles since their effect on blood loss is limited. It is interesting that dose

ranging studies have never been performed. Very large doses of progestogens can be given to arrest torrential vaginal bleeding. Norethisterone up
to 30 mg daily will usually stop the bleeding in 24–48 hours. The dose can
then be reduced and finally stopped over the next few days, when another,
usually lighter, bleed will occur. Bleeding of this magnitude needs specialist
assessment but may require emergency measures by the GP.

Oral contraceptives are particularly useful in women who also require
contraception. Danazol taken continuously will either reduce MBL or produce amenorrhoea depending on the dose used. It is an isoxazol derivative
of 17α-ethinyl-testosterone which acts on the hypothalamic pituitary
ovarian axis as well as having a direct effect on the endometrium resulting
in atrophy. While it inhibits ovulation it cannot be relied on as a contraceptive. Side-effects are weight gain, muscle pains, acne, and headaches.
These combined with its expense limit long-term therapy except in special
cases.

Gestrinone is a synthetic tri-enic 19-norsteroid with antigonadotrophic
and antiprogesterone activity which has recently been licensed. It is also
effective in menorrhagia, but again is expensive. LHRH analogues, by
inducing a medical menopause, may be useful in some cases (see section
below on fibroids). Cyclical oestrogen/progestogen hormone replacement
therapy may be used in women at the perimenopause. Although clinically
it seems to work, again there has been no study to date with objective MBL
measurements. However, measurements of withdrawal bleeds on one
preparation show that they are not heavier than normal periods. It must
always be remembered that menorrhagia tends to cause iron deficiency
anaemia, which requires treatment.

Surgical treatment
Surgical treatment may be necessary to deal with pelvic abnormalities such
as polyps, fibroids, chronic pelvic inflammatory disease, or endometriotic
masses. Operations should be as conservative as possible in women who
wish to retain their fertility. Surgical treatment is also indicated when
medical treatment has failed, and includes removal of cervical or endometrial polyps, myomectomy, and ultimately hysterectomy.

Hysterectomy is offered more often now to younger women whose
families are complete because many are reluctant to take treatment for
several years until the menopause. Although 100 per cent effective, hysterectomy is accompanied by significant morbidity (pyrexia, haemorrhage,
infection) but fortunately a low mortality rate of 6 in 10 000. A new final
solution to reduce MBL or cause amenorrhoea is removal of the endometrium, again under hysteroscopic control, either by resection (TCRE
transcervical endometrial resection) or laser ablation. Hospital stay and
recovery after transcervical resection of the endometrium are much shorter
than after hysterectomy and it is being promoted as a cheaper alternative.

It should provide a useful option to women who wish to avoid hyster-ectomy, but there has not been time to evaluate the efficacy or long-term risks of transcervical procedures.

Treatment of fibroids

Uterine fibroids are common benign tumours which arise in the myomet-rium. They are dealt with here in a separate section because they are the commonest form of pathology in women complaining of regular heavy periods. Fibroids are composed predominantly of smooth muscle with a variable amount of connective tissue. Three sub-types are recognized de-pending on their situation in relation to the uterine wall, namely sub-mucous, subserous, and intramural. They are commonly multiple and may result in considerable uterine enlargement. Between 20 and 25 per cent of women over the age of 35 have fibroids.

Fibroids are thought to be oestrogen dependent since they do not occur prior to puberty and become smaller after the menopause. It is currently believed that oestrogen exerts an effect on fibroid growth via other factors such as growth factors which have been detected in the uterus. Fibroids are frequently asymptomatic but may cause menorrhagia, although the pro-portion associated with objective excessive menstrual loss is not well docu-mented. The mechanism by which fibroids cause excessive blood loss is uncertain but could be related to vasodilator prostaglandin release by these tumours. Uterine fibroids are usually diagnosed clinically but they may be difficult to differentiate from ovarian masses. Ultrasound is useful in this situation, but again there may be difficulty in distinguishing between pedunculated subserous fibroids and solid ovarian tumours. If any doubt remains, patients need referral and laparoscopy or laparotomy may be considered.

The management of a woman with uterine fibroids depends on their size, any associated symptoms, as well as her age and reproductive wishes. Small asymptomatic fibroids rarely require treatment but need to be moni-tored regularly. One concern is sarcomatous changes in fibroids, but this is now thought to be very low being less than 0.2 per cent. Women with fibroids and menorrhagia are usually treated by hysterectomy. For those wishing to conserve their fertility myomectomy may be offered. The ad-vent of new endoscopic techniques means that it is possible to remove subserous and intramural fibroids by laparoscopy, and submucous fibroids by hysteroscopy, thus avoiding laparotomy.

There is considerable demand for an alternative to surgery in the man-agement of fibroids. Protaglandin synthetase inhibitors are probably of limited effect in reducing heavy menstrual bleeding. The 19-norsteroid danazol and gestrinone may be effective and may indeed shrink uterine volume. A therapeutic innovation is the use of LHRH analogues to induce a temporary and reversible menopausal state. These analogues produce amenorrhoea and fibroid shrinkage. Unfortunately, shrinkage is rarely complete and not sustained after cessation of therapy. Another concern is the bone mineral loss associated with a prolonged hypo-oestrogenic state. Nevertheless LHRH analogues should be considered in women where surgery is contraindicated and as pre-operative treatment, since shrinkage of fibroids makes surgery technically easier.

Financial implications of menorrhagia
The theme of the White Paper now makes costings of investigation and treatment a very important consideration. The White Paper defines a medical audit as the systematic critical analysis of the quality of medical care, including procedures used for diagnosis and treatment, use of re-sources, and resulting outcome and quality of life for the patient. It is difficult to give precise figures for medical treatments since they depend on the dose and duration employed, and therefore average costs are pre-sented. Hospital costs are based on charges made to private patients which include hospital and theatre charges as well as surgeons' and anaesthetists' fees (Table 6.2). The costs do not include consultations to general prac-titioners and hospital doctors. It must not be forgotten that the patient and her employer will also have to bear costs in terms of loss of earnings during absence from work. In this light, hysterectomy could easily be costed in the region of £5000.

Throughout this section is has been suggested that among women receiv-ing medication or surgery for a complaint of heavy menstrual bleeding, about half do not require such treatment because they do not have object-ively heavy menstruation. These women can only be correctly identified by

Table 6.2 *Costs of treatment of menorrhagia*

	Cost per menstrual cycle (£)
Medical treatment	
Mefenamic acid	2
Tranexamic acid	4
Norethisterone	3
Danazol	31
Gestrinone	56
Surgical treatment	Cost £
Dilation and curettage	700
Hysterectomy	2700
Endometrial resection	2500
Menstrual blood loss measurement per menstruation	5

objective measurement of their menstrual blood loss. It could therefore be argued that objective measurement should be available in primary care so that informed decisions are made about whom to treat.

Dysmenorrhoea (painful menstruation)

Derived from the Greek meaning 'difficult monthly flow', the word dysmenorrhoea has come to mean painful menstruation. Dysmenorrhoea can be classified as either primary or secondary. In the former type there is no pelvic pathology, while the latter implies there might be.

Primary dysmenorrhoea

In general, primary dysmenorrhoea appears 6 to 12 months after the menarche when ovulatory cycles have become established. (The early cycles after the menarche are usually anovular and tend to be painless.) The pain usually consists of lower abdominal cramps and backache and there may be associated gastrointestinal disturbances such as diarrhoea and vomiting. Symptoms occur predominantly during the first two days of menstruation. Primary dysmenorrhoea tends not to be associated with excessive menstrual bleeding: it is rare for women to have both dysmenorrhoea and menorrhagia.

It is only in the past two decades that intra-uterine pressure measurements have been performed which demonstrate for the first time that women complaining of dysmenorrhoea are not neurotic! Primary dysmenorrhoea is associated with uterine hypercontractility characterized by excessive amplitude and frequency of contractions and a high 'resting' tone in between. During contractions endometrial blood flow is reduced and there seems to be a good correlation between minimal blood flow and maximal colicky pain, favouring the concept that ischaemia due to hypercontractility causes primary dysmenorrhoea.

It is now generally agreed that the myometrial hypercontractility pattern found in primary dysmenorrhoea is associated with increased prostaglandin production. More recently elevated levels of leukotriene C_4, D_4, and E_4 (substances allied to prostaglandins) have been found in endometrium collected from dysmenorrhoeic women. Increased vasopressin levels have also been implicated.

Although excessive levels of prostaglandins, leukotrienes and vasopressin have been found in primary dysmenorrhoea, the primary stimulus for their production remains unknown.

Secondary dysmenorrhoea

Secondary dysmenorrhoea is associated with pelvic pathology such as endometriosis, adenomyosis, pelvic inflammatory disease, submucous leiomyomas, and endometrial polyps. The use of an intra-uterine contraceptive device may also lead to dysmenorrhoea. Secondary dysmenorrhoea tends to appear several years after the menarche and the patient may complain of a change in the intensity and timing of her pain. The pain may last for the whole of the menstrual period and may be associated with discomfort before the onset of menstruation. The mechanism by which various pathologies cause pain is uncertain and again prostaglandins may be involved though the evidence is less clear.

Assessment

A full gynaecological history is an essential part of investigation. The onset of dysmenorrhoea and its relation to menstruation usually differentiates between primary and secondary dysmenorrhoea. The presence of an intra-uterine contraceptive device or a history of infertility should also be noted. In young girls one can usually assume a diagnosis of primary dysmenorrhoea and it is probably unnecessary to examine them. If the history is suggestive of secondary dysmenorrhoea, a bimanual pelvic and speculum examination should be performed. A particular search should be made for polyps protruding through the cervical os and for enlargement, tenderness, or fixity of the uterus or adnexae.

Referral to a gynaecologist may be necessary if pathology is suspected; and laparoscopy and, in specialized centres, hysteroscopy may be recommended to make a diagnosis.

Treatment

The clear involvement of prostaglandins in primary dysmenorrhoea has led to the use of prostaglandin synthetase inhibitors such as mefenamic acid, naproxen, and ibuprofen to treat the disorder; and they are effective in reducing menstrual pain in 80–90 per cent of patients. Commencing treatment before the onset of menstruation appears to have no demonstrable advantage over starting treatment when bleeding starts. This observation is compatible with the short plasma half-life of prostaglandin synthetase inhibitors. The advantage of starting treatment at the onset of menstruation is that it prevents the patient treating herself when she is unknowingly pregnant; thus potential teratogenic effects at this stage can be avoided.

The presence of elevated leukotriene and vasopressin levels may explain why not all women respond to prostaglandin synthetase inhibitors. The role of the various agents which affect the leukotriene pathway has not yet been fully evaluated in the treatment of primary dysmenorrhoea. Vasopressin antagonists have been examined but are not available for routine use at present. It must not be forgotten that the combined oestrogen–progestogen oral contraceptive pill is a useful agent for the treatment of primary dysmenorrhoea especially when contraception is required. In fact young girls using the pretext of dysmenorrhoea may really be seeking contraception. The Pill is effective in 80–90 per cent of women and probably acts by reducing the capacity of the endometrium to produce prostaglandins.

Concern remains about the 10–20 per cent of patients with primary dysmenorrhoea who fail to respond either to prostaglandin synthetase inhibitors or to oral contraceptives. Some of these women may really be suffering from secondary dysmenorrhoea with pelvic pathology, requiring appropriate investigation, but the concern has led to the examination of new agents such as leukotriene and vasopressin antagonists.

Effective treatment of secondary dysmenorrhoea must be based on a correct diagnosis since different pathologies require different therapies. In addition, the type of treatment offered must take into account the patient's age, her desire for conception, the severity of the symptoms, and the extent of the disease.

Amenorrhoea (absent menstruation)

The absence of periods disturbs women just as much as other disturbances of menstruation especially since it has implications of loss of a normal bodily function related to fertility. While some women may be concerned about loss of femininity others will worry about an unwanted pregnancy. It seems relatively clear that women wish to menstruate regularly, not too much nor too little, but not to be without periods altogether.

To menstruate women require a functioning hypothalamic pituitary ovarian axis with a responding endometrium and genital outflow tract in the absence of endocrine or systemic disease or drug therapy, and in the presence of a normal chromosome complement. In the vast majority of women presenting in general practice the cause of amenorrhoea will be hormonal. There has been a preoccupation in the past over distinguishing between primary and secondary amenorrhoea, but this should probably be defused since there is so much overlap between the two. Instead the differential diagnoses should be based on the pathological categories (Table 6.3).

Assessment

The initial step in the work-up of the amenorrhoeic patient is exclusion of the possibility of pregnancy, even in a woman with primary amenorrhoea. It is important that the GP should warn women with primary or secondary amenorrhoea of hormonal aetiology that they are not necessarily infertile and are at risk of pregnancy should a sporadic ovulation occur.

History-taking and examination should elicit the following information and physical characteristics in all cases of amenorrhoea:

(1) age at menarche

(2) development of secondary sex characteristics–pubic and axillary hair, breasts, menstrual history before amenorrhoea;

Table 6.3   *Main causes of amenorrhoea*

Hypothalamic—pituitary disorders:
   Prolactin hypersecretion ± prolactin-secreting pituitary adenoma
   Tumours
   Weight loss—anorexia nervosa
   Obesity
   Psychogenic
   Post-oral contraception
   Isolated gonadotrophin deficiency (Kallman's syndrome)
Ovarian, uterine, or vaginal disorders
   Polycystic ovarian disease
   Ovarian failure (premature menopause)
   Gonadal dysgenesis (e.g. Turner's syndrome)
   Absence of uterus (e.g. testicular feminization) or vagina
   Haematocolpos
Other diseases
   Thyroid hormone deficiency or excess
   Adrenal disorders (e.g. Cushing's disease, congenital adrenal hyperplasia)
   Severe general disease (e.g. leukaemia or Hodgkin's disease treated with
   chemotherapy)

---

 (3) galactorrhoea;

 (4) recent changes in body height and weight; height and weight;

 (5) medication: oral contraception, chemotherapy;

 (6) family history of genetic anomalies;

 (7) recent emotional upsets;

 (8) hirsutism;

 (9) hot flushes and sweats and dry vagina;

(10) previous surgery: curettage, oophorectomy, other endocrine organs;

(11) symptoms of endocrine disorders: thyroid, pituitary, adrenal;

(12) systemic, abdominal, and pelvic examination with special attention to reproductive tract and inguinal hernias.

Laboratory tests to determine the cause of amenorrhoea involve measurement in serum in all cases of the anterior pituitary hormones FSH and LH, as well as prolactin and thyroid function tests. Testosterone should be measured in women with hirsutism or where testicular feminization is suspected. The karyotype should be checked if there are suspicions of a chromosomal disorder such as testicular feminization and Turner's syndrome (see below). It is important to remember that the presence of a Y chromosome requires surgical removal of the gonadal areas because the presence of testicular components carries a 25 per cent risk of malignant tumour formation. About 30 per cent of patients with a Y chromosome will not develop signs of virilization. Therefore this investigation should be undertaken also in women presenting with primary amenorrhoea and normal secondary sexual characteristics where gonadotrophin levels are high. (See Table 6.4.)

A useful diagnostic test is administration of a progestogen challenge. This will determine if there is sufficient ovarian activity to produce significant amounts of oestrogen to stimulate the endometrium, a responsive endometrium, and a competent genital outflow tract. A suitable progestogen challenge is norethisterone, 10 mg daily for five days, and bleeding usually follows within a few days of ceasing treatment.

If a patient is referred for specialist opinion the following investigations may be undertaken. In cases of hyperprolactinaemia a CT scan is used to evaluate the pituitary fossa. Laparoscopy and examination under anaesthetic are used to evaluate pelvic organs especially in cases of primary amenorrhoea. At surgery ovarian biopsy may be performed. The endometrial cavity can be examined by hysteroscopy when a diagnosis of Ascherman's syndrome is suspected. Assessment of the renal tract may be instigated since abnormalities of this system are associated with developmental defects of the reproductive organs.

Specific causes

Delayed menarche.   How long should a general practitioner wait before investigating the girl who has never menstruated? Since most girls will have menstruated by the age of 16, this could be considered the upper age of the normal menarche. But referral is essential earlier if secondary sex characteristics have not developed, or if there appear to be anatomical disorders of the genital tract, or signs of a chromosome abnormality. Rarer possibilities are testicular feminization syndrome (maturation of breasts with absent axillary and pubic hair, and absent uterus with normal or short vagina; 46XY with testes); or Turner's syndrome (many variants, but with typical short stature, sexual infantilism, webbing of the neck, cubitus valgus, 45XO with streak gonads). Absent development of the lower genital tract resulting in haematocolpos is another rare cause where secondary sexual development will be normal. There may be intermittent lower abdominal pain and a lower abdominal cystic swelling in the vagina palpable per rectum; and a tense blue-coloured membrane may be seen at the introitus. Referral is obviously necessary for incision and drainage.

If secondary sexual development is normal or appears to be progressing satisfactorily, and there is no anatomical problem, then the likely cause is hormonal and can be elucidated with an endocrine screen.

Premature menopause.   This is characterized by high FSH and LH with normal prolactin levels. Other symptoms may be present such as hot

Table 6.4 *Laboratory findings in major causes of amenorrhoea*

	FSH	LH	Prolactin	Testosterone	Karyotype
Hyperprolactinaemia	Normal	Normal	High	Normal	Normal
Premature menopause	Very high	High	Normal	Normal	Normal
Polycystic ovarian disease	Normal	Slightly raised	Normal or slightly raised	Slightly raised	Normal
'Hypothalamic'	Normal	Normal	Normal	Normal	Normal
Turner's syndrome	High	High	Normal	Normal	45XO or mosaics
Testicular feminization	High	High	Normal	High	46XY

flushes and night sweats, as well as atrophic vaginitis. Sadly, premature ovarian failure can occur at any age. If the woman is concerned about fertility, specialist referral is required for laparoscopy and ovarian biopsy. Treatment with cyclical oestrogen/progestogen therapy is indicated in women with premature ovarian failure both to treat symptoms and to protect against premature heart disease and osteoporosis.

In the past these women were considered sterile and counselled that future pregnancy should be impossible. However, in recent years it has become apparent that some may resume normal ovarian function either spontaneously or while taking hormone replacement therapy, and may become pregnant. The picture has also changed with the possibility of fertilized ovum donation in some IVF programmes. Therefore it is important for women with premature ovarian failure to realize that there is a possibility of pregnancy, although it may be remote.

Hyperprolactinaemia. The discovery of human prolactin and the realization of its involvement in reproductive function opened new doors in the management of amenorrhoea and infertility. The incidence of hyperprolactinaemia in amenorrhoeic populations varies with individual clinical practice but averages about one-third of women with no obvious cause for their amenorrhoea. Galactorrhoea is present in 30 per cent of hyperprolactinaemic women but galactorrhoeic women who do not have menstrual disturbance only rarely have hyperprolactinaemia. High prolactin levels cause amenorrhoea by inhibiting the normal pulsatile secretion of GnRH by the hypothalamus.

There are many causes of hyperprolactinaemia, the most important being prolactin secreting tumours of the anterior pituitary. Tumours less than 1 cm in diameter are referred to as microadenomas, and those greater than 1 cm as macroadenomas. The exact incidence of the clinical problem is uncertain with between 9 and 27 per cent of pituitary glands in routine autopsy series having been found to contain adenomas. Women with hyperprolactinaemia should therefore have a visual field assessment and a CT scan of the pituitary gland.

It must be remembered that the commonest cause for a moderately elevated serum prolactin level is stress and therefore it is important to take a repeat blood sample when the patient is more relaxed, if that is possible. Drugs including metaclopromide, phenothiazine, reserpine, methyldopa, and cimetidine may also cause hyperprolactinaemia and therefore an accurate drug history is important.

Menstruation, ovulation, and fertility can be restored in patients with hyperprolactinaemia with the drug bromocriptine, which can be used for macro- as well as microadenomas. The starting dose should be small, taken in bed at night to minimize the side-effects of nausea and faintness due to hypotension. The dose is increased to the levels required to lower prolactin levels and, in the case of macroadenomas, produce tumour regression. If a patient wants her fertility restored then obviously she should be treated with bromocriptine; but there is controversy over patients with micro-adenomas who do not wish to become pregnant. If they are given bromo-criptine they require contraception, preferably with a barrier method. Alternatively, they could be given hormone replacement therapy to counteract the hypo-oestrogenic effects on their bones and cardiovascular system. Approaches over the years have become more conservative with documentation of a benign clinical course leading to spontaneous resolution in many patients.

Hypothalamic amenorrhoea. Hypothalamic problems are usually diagnosed by exclusion of pituitary lesions and are the most common category of hypogonadotrophic amenorrhoea. They usually present as secondary amenorrhoea. The condition should normally be investigated if the woman has been for six months or more without periods. Biochemically it is found that gonadotrophins are normal or low with a normal prolactin.

The clinical picture is usually associated with weight changes, vigorous exercise, stress, and cessation of the oral contraceptive pill. Since weight loss and anorexia nervosa may lead to amenorrhoea it is important for the general practitioner to enquire about recent weight changes and to check weight for height. Where the problem is thought to be weight loss it is better to achieve a return of menstruation via weight gain rather than drug therapy. The ponderal index (weight (kg/height^2 (m))) is valuable in that a target weight can be calculated for the likely return of periods based on a score of 19 or more being the threshold for menstruation. If a response of weight gain is not being achieved then the doctor must consider whether the patient has anorexia nervosa and is thus in need of psychiatric help to prevent the serious consequences of that condition.

Those who take too much exercise have been observed since the first century AD by Soranus to have amenorrhoea. It is currently observed in athletes, some intensive joggers, and ballet dancers. When training starts before the menarche the first menstrual period can be delayed by as much as three years. The mechanism relates to the lowering of body fat mass below a critical threshold for normal hypothalamic pituitary ovarian function. A similar hypothalamic cause is found in association with stress, as in the student who always menstruated regularly until leaving school and home and coming to university or college; menstruation often returns once the final examinations are passed. Post-pill amenorrhoea can also give the biochemical picture of normal FSH, LH, and prolactin, although there is no need to investigate this for six months after stopping the Pill since spontaneous return to menstruation can occur during that time.

For many women despite reassurance that nothing is wrong it is difficult to accept amenorrhoea which is perceived as a loss of femininity. Some may want to know that their endocrine system can be switched on, and clomiphene may be used. But it should be used for only a limited amount of time and reserved for achieving pregnancy.

Recent concerns are the long-term conequences of the hypo-oestrogenic state on bone density and the cardiovascular system. Cyclical oestrogen–progestogen hormone replacement therapy may be used; or the combined contraceptive pill, depending on the woman's contraceptive needs. She should understand that HRT is not contraceptive.

Polycystic ovarian disease (PCOD).   First described by two gynaecologists Stein and Leventhal in the early 1930s, this syndrome was originally ascribed to patients with amenorrhoea, hirsutism, obesity, and bilateral polycystic ovaries. It is clear, however, that any form of menstrual irregularity can occur—oligomenorrhoea, or menorrhagia with regular or irregular cycles—and the term polycystic ovarian disease or syndrome is now preferred. There is still a problem of definition, however, and doctors may disagree as to whether a particular woman with less florid symptoms can be said to have the syndrome. It is generally thought that about 90 per cent of women with oligomenorrhoea and 30 per cent with amenorrhoea have the syndrome; but the extent to which the underlying ovarian dysfunction exists in the general population is more uncertain. It has been suggested that as many as 20 per cent of the normal population have ultrasonically defined polycystic ovarian disease, though further analysis of the data showed that the majority of women for whom the ultrasound diagnosis was made had irregular periods. In women with regular periods it was diagnosed in only 7 per cent.

The condition involves:

(1) the presence of an excessive number of small follicles placed peripherally in the ovaries and a relative failure of follicular selection processes which should produce a dominant follicle;

(2) a continuous background of oestrogen production by the small follicles;

(3) ovarian stromal hyperplasia associated with excessive androgen production.

The increased androgen production and tonic oestrogen feedback, as well as increased inhibin levels, result in increased LH relative to FSH and this accentuates the process in a vicious circle. However, the expression of excessive androgen production depends not simply on blood levels of testosterone and androstenedione but on the peripheral metabolism of testosterone to dihydrotestosterone in the specific androgen-sensitive end organs (the hair follicles). This is the main difference between hirsute and non-hirsute women with PCOD.

Various diagnostic criteria are used by different gynaecologists. Biochemically, LH is elevated with respect to FSH with a ratio of 3:1, and testosterone levels are also increased. On ultrasound the classic picture is a string of small follicles, 2–8 mm in diameter, arranged like a necklace in the periphery of the ovary with a minimum of 10 follicles in each ovary.

Treatment depends on the woman's desire for pregnancy. It must be remembered that the chronic anovulatory state in PCOD increases the risk of endometrial cancer. Cyclical progestogens given for 12 days each month can be used if the patient does not want her fertility restored. Alternatively the excess LH and hence androgen production can be suppressed with a combined oral contraceptive pill. If hirsutism is a problem, one containing the anti-androgen drug cyproterone can be used, e.g. Dianette. In women who wish to become pregnant ovulation induction with clomiphene may prove effective, but progression to gonadotrophin therapy, possibly with pituitary control using LHRH analogues to suppress LH production, is often required. In PCOD gonadotrophin therapy is more often associated with ovarian hyperstimulation. Surgery in the form of bilateral wedge resection used to be a favoured treatment. It probably acted by reducing the mass of stroma and small follicles, thus interfering for a time with the 'vicious circle'. Currently, the favoured surgical approach is laparoscopic laser or diathermy used to pepper the ovarian surface. This is believed to be less likely to cause the adhesions which were a problem after wedge resection.

Oligomenorrhoea (infrequent and scanty menstruation)

A woman with infrequent periods should be investigated in the same way as a woman with amenorrhoea, since the causes in general are the same. Scanty regular menstruation needs no investigation; blood losses as low as 2 ml per month have been found in normal parous women. It may herald the menopause or rarely have an endocrine basis but in general is not a worrying symptom.

Prolonged menstruation

A recent study of 321 women showed that the commonest cycle lengths were 5 and 6 days, found in 49 per cent of women. However, 20 per cent bled for more than 7 days and 1 per cent bled for more than 12 days. As discussed earlier, the number of days of bleeding does not necessarily relate to menstrual blood loss since most of the loss is passed in the first three days of menstruation whether the overall loss is light or heavy. Prolonged menstruation in itself does not require investigation but may go along with other complaints such as menorrhagia. Periods can be prolonged by being preceded or succeeded by spotting in association with an IUD or the progestogen-only pill: reassurance is usually all that is required. Several days of spotting before a period can be a sign of an endometrial or cervical polyp, even malignancy, and visualization of the cervix, a cervical smear, and bimanual pelvic examination should be carried out by the GP with referral to a gynaecologist if there are suspicious findings.

Irregular menstruation and bleeding

Irregular periods

Women often worry if their previously regular periods become irregular but, as discussed earlier, this is most likely to be no more than a variation on the physiological. Irregular menstruation, both long and short cycles, is most common at the extremes of reproductive life, soon after the menarche or before the menopause. These cycles are usually anovulatory. In adolescent girls this does not need investigation unless there are signs of obvious disease, and should not be treated with hormonal therapy to regularize periods. Rather the GP should reassure the girl that it is part of the normal maturation process and her periods will spontaneously become regular. If she requires contraception this will outweigh all other considerations and an oral contraceptive may need to be used. In later life, nearer the menopause, irregularity of periods is so common that not all women could be investigated. If the period becomes heavy as well as irregular, or there are problems such as intermenstrual or post-coital bleeding, referral to a gynaecologist is wise.

Intermenstrual and post-coital bleeding

Investigation and management mainly depend on the age of the patient. In perimenopausal women these symptoms cannot be ignored. Speculum examination is essential to exclude a cervical lesion—malignancy, ectropion, or polyp—and pelvic examination will define any obvious uterine or ovarian problems. Referral to a gynaecologist should be made in older women (over 40) unless, for example, a cervical polyp is present. This can be easily avulsed by the GP using long forceps to twist off the polyp and cauterizing the raw area with a silver nitrate stick. The polyp should be sent for histology but is rarely malignant. If the bleeding settles after removal of a polyp then referral is not necessary. In young women mid-cycle bleeding is often associated with ovulation and does not require investigation. Intermenstrual and post-coital bleeding in young women is rarely associated with malignancy but again it is important that the cervix is visualized, cervical smears taken, and a bimanual pelvic examination carried out. If the bleeding persists over several cycles referral should be considered.

Postmenopausal bleeding

This is defined as bleeding occurring six months after the last period. It always requires examination and urgent referral because of the high incidence of malignancy. While the most common malignancy is endometrial, cancer of the cervix, vulva, or ovary may present in this way. It may however be due to non-malignant causes such as atrophic vaginitis or a polyp.

Variations in colour and smell of menstrual blood

Women may report to their doctor a change in the colour or smell of their menstrual blood which may worry them. There is no known association with pelvic pathology and these symptoms. If anything, these changes are associated with different rates of menstrual flow. Thus patients should be reassured.

HOW TO POSTPONE A PERIOD

Sometimes women ask for 'something' to postpone a period because of, for example, a special event such as a wedding, an examination, or a holiday. Periods can be postponed using either a progestogen such as norethisterone, 5 mg three times daily, starting three days before the anticipated period and used for up to one month; or a combined contraceptive pill taken continuously, if given several months warning.

TOXIC SHOCK SYNDROME

This short piece on toxic shock syndrome (TSS) has been included here as this seems to be the most appropriate place for it. One might be forgiven for thinking that TSS was specific to women who used tampons. In fact, it was first described in children in 1978 as a multisystemic disease characterized by rapid onset of fever, hypotension, hyperaemia of the mucous membranes, and rash followed by desquamation and multisystem involvement. However, descriptions of Staphylococcal scarlet fever suggest that TSS was noted already in 1927. In 1980 an increase in TSS was noted among previously healthy young women with onset during menstruation. Initial studies of menstrual TSS demonstrated that tampon use was a risk factor for disease and a particular brand was implicated which was withdrawn in 1980. Since then non-menstrual cases associated with hospital-acquired infections, parturition, and contraceptive barriers have been increasingly recognized. Some women are subject to recurrences of menstrual TSS even when tampons have not been used.

The association between TSS and *Staphylococcal aureus* infection was firmly established when an exotoxin from isolates of TSS-associated *S-aureus* was isolated in 1981. The exotoxin has since been called toxic shock syndrome toxin 1 (TSST-1) and is generally considered to be the major cause of TSS. Other pathogens such as *E. coli* have more recently been implicated as well.

The exact role of tampons in menstrual TSS is uncertain. Initially it was believed that high absorbency of tampons such as those containing carboxymethylcellulose or polyacrylate was an important factor. Indeed these substances are no longer used. However, the role of absorbency is now being questioned since the original studies did not distinguish the effects of absorbency from the effects of chemical composition or other tampon characteristics that are correlated with absorbency. One persistent problem in understanding the aetiology of TSS is that the vaginal environment is anaerobic but the production of TSST-1 requires the presence of oxygen. Therefore it has been suggested that insertion of a tampon might provide the oxygen necessary for toxin production. Another theory is that highly absorbent tampons bind magnesium ions: in a magnesium deficient environment production of TSST-1 increases dramatically.

It is important to put the risks of developing TSS in perspective. It is a very rare disease with no justification for women to avoid using tampons. On the other hand, if one suspects that a woman has TSS it is important to arrange hospital admission for appropriate antibiotic treatment since the disease has a high mortality.

REFERENCES AND FURTHER READING

Anderson, A. B. M., Haynes, P. J., Guillebaud, J., *et al.* (1976). Reduction of menstrual blood loss by prostaglandin synthetase inhibitors. *Lancet,* **1,** 774–6.

Coulter, A., McPherson, K., and Vessey, M. (1988). Do British women undergo too many or too few hysterectomies? *Social Science Medicine,* **27,** 987–94.

Coulter, A., Noone, A., and Goldacre, M. (1989). General practitioners' referrals to specialist out-patient clinics. *British Medical Journal,* **299,** 304–8.

Rees, M. C. P. (1989). Heavy, painful periods. In *Clinical obstetrics and gynaecology: dysfunctional uterine bleeding and menorrhagia* (ed. J. O. Drife), Vol. 3(2), pp. 341–56. Baillière Tindall, London.

Vollman, R. F. (1977). *The menstrual cycle.* W. B. Saunders, Philadelphia.

7. Menopause

Jean Coope

NATURAL HISTORY

The word menopause is derived from the Greek words '*men*' month and '*pausis*' halt. It means the end of menstruation and the last menstrual period marks the end of reproductive life.

The mean age at menopause is just over 50 and this is remarkably constant throughout the Western world. Moreover, a recent survey of Malaysian women showed a mean age at menopause of 50.7 years, and another of seven Asian countries found that most women reached menopause around 50. These findings relate to cross-sectional studies of large female populations. Recently longitudinal studies have been carried out in Southern England, Norway, Canada, and Massachusetts (Holte 1990). These show similar results and confirm the only important factor to influence age at menopause: cigarette smoking advances it by about two years.

All the sociological studies confirmed the importance of cultural and social factors in determining a woman's attitude to menopause. For example, Rajput women of Northern India perceive the menopause as an end of taboos and social restrictions and do not suffer any symptoms. On the other hand, reports of North American women indicate that over 80 per cent suffer from hot flushes and many suffer from a general decline in health status. In the USA, and in Australia and Western Europe, the concept has emerged of the menopause as a deficiency disease which needs treatment by hormone replacement therapy.

The experience of British women at menopause has been investigated by sociologists (McKinlay and Jefferys 1974) and epidemiologists (Bungay *et al.* 1980). About 80 per cent of women experience flushes but only 20 per cent feel that their symptoms are severe enough to require medical help. Flushing and sweating are the only symptoms to show a sharp peak at or just after the menopause. Minor mental symptoms such as depression and loss of confidence show a smaller rise just before the last menstrual period. Other symptoms, such as headaches, urinary frequency, insomnia, back pain, and irritability are not specifically associated with menopause and major psychiatric illness is not more common at this time. Sexual difficulties and loss of libido increase in frequency with advancing age in both sexes, and vaginal dryness and atrophy are common in postmenopausal women. Osteoporosis does not usually present with symptoms in mid-life but the imperceptible bone loss which begins at menopause may culminate

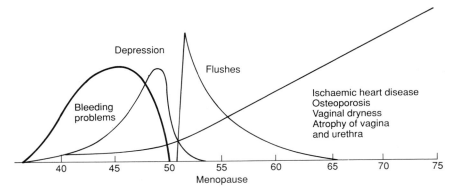

Fig. 7.1 Timing of symptoms related to menopause. (Adapted from many epidemiological studies and Fig. 1 in *Research on the menopause*, World Health Organization, 1981.)

in fractures or spinal pain 20 years later. Ischaemic heart disease is much commoner after menopause and is the most common cause of death in postmenopausal women. (See Fig. 7.1.)

Longitudinal studies by McKinlay *et al.* in Massachusetts (1990) and Hunter in England (1990) have confirmed the importance of previous behaviour patterns and use of medical services in determining whether women actually experience symptoms and seek medical help at menopause. For individual women the experience of a worthwhile career and a satisfactory long-term sexual relationship protects against symptoms.

The menopause itself is merely a date in a woman's life (the date of the last menstrual period) and is diagnosed retrospectively after a year has elapsed without menstrual bleeding. However, the menopause coincides approximately with the *climacteric*, a much more important event.

THE CLIMACTERIC

This is a gradual waning of ovarian function which takes place over a number of years and has a profound effect on bones, blood vessels, and collagen.

HORMONAL CHANGES

The ovary secretes both androgen and oestrogen from puberty to old age. The high oestrogen levels present in young women fall after the menopause and androgen levels rise.

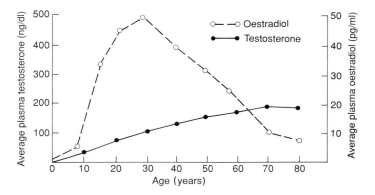

Fig. 7.2 Plasma levels of oestradiol and testosterone in human females according to age. [From: The menopause and aging. In *The menopause: comprehensive management* (ed. B. A. Eskin), Macmillan, New York, 1988. Reproduced with permission of the author and the publisher.]

The effect of increased androgen relative to oestrogen is exaggerated because of postmenopausal reduction in sex hormone binding globulin. This has a greater affinity for testosterone than for oestradiol (Fig. 7.2). Sex hormone binding globulin exaggerates the clinical effect of oestrogen. It is only the unbound portions of the sex hormones that are clinically active and can be attached to receptors on the cells of target organs.

In young women and HRT-users, oestrogen stimulates the liver to produce sex hormone binding globulin which binds selectively to circulating testosterone. Circulating free androgens are reduced thus raising the effect of oestrogen on the target organ. Older women have lower oestrogen production, less sex hormone binding globulin is produced, and free circulating androgens rise. This probably explains the hirsutism and male pattern baldness which occurs in some elderly women.

Oestrogen is secreted in the ovary and is also produced by peripheral conversion of androgens from the ovary and adrenal gland. Even the postmenopausal ovary produces some oestrogen and testosterone.

The premenopausal woman produces 50–500 µg of oestradiol daily, mostly from the ovary. After the menopause 15–100 µg of oestrone are produced, mainly from aromatization of ovarian androgen precursors and conversion of adrenal androstenedione in fatty tissues. FSH and LH levels rise dramatically, and FSH over 20 U/litre is regarded as diagnostic of menopause. In ordinary circumstances it is not necessary to use a laboratory test to confirm menopause; the presence of flushes in a woman over 45 who has amenorrhoea for a year is sufficient. In hysterectomized patients, or those already taking the combined pill or HRT with regular bleeding, it is useful to obtain FSH assay. A high level means that the patient is menopausal. A low level in a patient who is taking HRT or the combined pill does not necessarily exclude menopause as these preparations cause lowering of FSH and LH.

The ovarian follicles may become less sensitive to circulating gonadotrophins with time. The follicular phase shortens and shortening of the cycle to 18–24 days often occurs after the age of 40. After this the cycles lengthen and there are often gaps of amenorrhoea before periods stop altogether. Women may need reassurance that short cycles are a normal pattern.

Fertility falls rapidly in the ten years before the menopause and ovulation often becomes sporadic.

There is evidence that hysterectomy with conservation of the ovaries is associated with earlier ovarian failure (Siddle *et al.* 1987), and this may be due to a reduction in the blood supply to the ovaries following surgical clamping of the uterine arteries. Animal studies have demonstrated that uterine tissue is necessary to ensure the development of ovarian follicles.

CLINICAL PROBLEMS ASSOCIATED WITH THE MENOPAUSE

Dysfunctional bleeding

Irregular and falling production of progesterone means that the endometrium may be exposed to unopposed oestrogen stimulation for many weeks. This causes prolongation of the proliferative phase and perhaps hyperplasia, which may progress to cystic or atypical hyperplasia, a precancerous condition.

Heavy bleeding occurs when oestrogen levels fall and the thick endometrium separates. Very heavy, painful, or irregular bleeding needs investigation to exclude uterine pathology and women need to be educated that this is not simply 'part of the menopause'. Postmenopausal bleeding needs investigation and so does very late menstruation past the age of 54 as there is a higher incidence of malignancy in these patients (see Chapter 6).

Amenorrhoea

If amenorrhoea occurs in women below the age of 45 there may be a problem with diagnosis. The progestogen-only pill or depot injection are possible causes and pregnancy should be excluded. Pelvic examination, height, weight, FSH, LH, and prolactin can be measured.

$$\text{Low body mass index:} \quad \frac{\text{(weight in kg)}}{\text{(height}^2 \text{ in metres)}} \quad \text{below 20}$$

plus recent weight loss and normal LH, FSH, and prolactin levels may indicate anorexia nervosa. Emotional trauma can cause this. Young women who undertake very heavy exercise can also experience amenorrhoea with lowering of oestrogen production (Cann *et al.* 1984). These patients are at high risk of osteoporosis and need HRT. Such young women should be referred to a specialist endocrine unit.

Hyperprolactinaemia results in high prolactin and normal FSH and LH. A positive assay needs referral.

Menopause is indicated by high FSH and LH and probably flushes and night sweats. In women with irregular cycles it is just possible that a high FSH is due to the test being carried out during the ovulatory FSH peak and it should be confirmed after a couple of weeks.

SYMPTOMS AND SIGNS OF THE MENOPAUSE

Menses

Changes in menstrual pattern occur frequently in the last few years before the menopause. It is common for the cycle to shorten and after the age of 40 many women have cycles of 21 or even 18 days, which may lengthen to two or three months before ceasing altogether. Hot flushes often occur during the menstrual periods as this is the time when circulating oestrogen is at its lowest. Women who stop the contraceptive pill at this age often experience flushes which are triggered by falling oestrogen levels, rather than a constant low level of hormone.

Flushes and sweats

These are common and usually peak in the year following the cessation of menses. They may cause embarrassment and interfere with sleep but are otherwise harmless. They are made worse by anxiety and our double-blind placebo/oestrogen study shows the high response to placebo during the first month of treatment.

However, placebo only partially relieved flushing whereas oestrogen eliminated it. Other workers have confirmed these high responses to placebo. Several other treatments, such as clonidine, have failed to produce an improvement which is significantly greater than that due to placebo in the first half of the trial. Our study also shows the high level of rebound flushes in the second half of the study when oestrogen was withdrawn.

Flushes are worse in hot weather and Fig. 7.4 shows the significant correlation between mean number of daily flushes and ambient temperature in a group of twenty-five menopausal patients. Withdrawing oestrogen treatment can be difficult and should be done by reducing the dosage

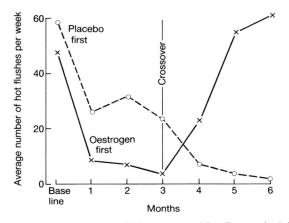

Fig. 7.3 Hot flushes in two groups of 15 women, taking Premarin 1.25 or placebo, in a double-blind crossover trial. (From: Coope *et al.* 1975.)

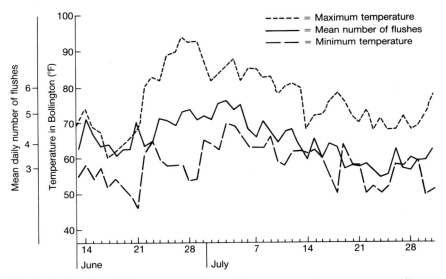

Fig. 7.4 Relationship between number of flushes and daily temperature. (From: Coope *et al.* 1978.)

gradually, keeping the progestogen supplement until the end to ensure safety.

Flushes are associated with a generalized discharge of the sympathetic system with vasodilation of the blood vessels of the face, neck, and hands. The increase in skin temperature coincides with a fall in internal body temperature and occurs in women with an intact hypothalamus following withdrawal of oestrogen. There is a surge of LH secretion and a release of B-endorphins. Flushes have been treated with hypnosis and a recent study of 142 menopausal women in Sweden found that physical exercise reduces their frequency. Nevertheless it is often helpful to give short-term oestrogen treatment for flushes at a time of crisis, for instance during a family wedding or a holiday abroad. Many women who do not wish to embark on long-term therapy because they fear dependence on the drug are grateful for the temporary improved sleep and lowered anxiety levels which accompany the relief of flushes.

Depression

A summary of a population of women in Dundee (Ballinger 1975) found that there was a peak of mild depressive illness and anxiety just before the menopause. However, Jenkins and Clare (1985) in a review of the literature concluded that true depressive illness is not commoner at this time. There is no doubt that depression is commoner in women than in men but this may be largely due to social factors such as the psychological pressures of childbearing, shortage of money, and lack of interesting well-paid work. Careful research on a population of 408 menopausal women in Glasgow (Cooke and Greene 1981) found that psychological stress was directly related to adverse life events, particularly bereavement.

On the other hand, some workers have treated depression successfully with large doses of oestrogen (Klaiber *et al.* 1979) although the safety of very high dosage must remain in doubt. Women who experience depression and loss of libido after surgical castration are enormously helped by oestrogen/androgen implants but they often become dependent on this treatment and much of the effect may be due to testosterone.

Montgomery *et al.* (1987) have attempted to reduce scores of depression measured on Kellner and Sheffield scales, using oestradiol/testosterone implants or placebo. They found that after the menopause women responded better to placebo but perimenopausal patients were significantly improved on oestrogen. This group have also demonstrated the efficacy of anovulatory doses of oestrogen in treating premenstrual depression. My own double-blind study of 55 women in general practice (1981) did not show a significant difference between oestrogen and placebo in the treatment of depressed patients over a period of six months. However, the oestrogen used (piperazine oestrone sulphate) was not as potent as the oestradiol implants.

The conclusion must be that depression at the menopause is caused by many factors and careful assessment of the social and cultural environment is needed. The depth of depression needs to be measured, perhaps using a validated questionnaire such as the Beck Inventory, and suicidal patients need referral. A sympathetic nurse is invaluable in finding the hidden causes such as an unsatisfactory marriage or problems with children. Perimenopausal patients respond better to oestrogen than postmenopausal ones and this may be due to the large swings in hormone levels which occur at this time.

Genito-urinary problems

There is no convincing evidence that oestrogen improves urinary incontinence. However, it increases blood flow and epithelial thickness of the vagina and is useful in patients who use ring pessaries or in the preoperative months for those awaiting vaginal operations. Oral oestrogen should be stopped a month before operation.

Vaginal dryness and atrophy cause painful intercourse and can be particularly troublesome in women who are starting a new relationship after a gap of some years. Oestrogen by any route is of enormous benefit. A lubricant such as KY jelly is also helpful.

However, sexual problems *at* the menopause are not usually caused *by* the menopause (vaginal atrophy is postmenopausal). These depend on the sexual pattern in previous years and on the relationship between the couple; on levels of anxiety and confidence; and whether either partner is taking drugs such as hypotensives which reduce libido or potency (Leiblum and Bachmann 1988).

Cardiovascular disease

Numerous studies have shown an increase in ischaemic heart disease after the menopause, especially in young women who have their ovaries removed surgically (Oliver and Boyd 1959). A recent study from Holland (Witteman *et al.* 1989) showed an increase in atherosclerosis of the aorta which was demonstrated radiologically to be three to five times greater in postmenopausal patients.

Epidemiological studies have confirmed that oestrogen prevents cardiovascular disease. Large population studies from the USA (Stampfer *et al.* 1985; Ross *et al.* 1981) have demonstrated a reduction of about 30–40 per cent in oestrogen-users. A recent British study of 4000 women attending hormone clinics found a significantly reduced risk of death from circulatory disease (risk ratio 0.37) (Hunt *et al.* 1990). The risk of stroke is also reduced by oestrogen medication (Paganini-Hill *et al.* 1988).

All the American studies relate to the use of conjugated oestrogen without progestogen. We do not yet know the clinical effect of oestrogen plus progestogen supplement, although laboratory studies suggest that this is still beneficial. Androgenic progestogens such as norethisterone and d-l-norgestrel have an adverse effect on lipids.

The beneficial effect of oestrogen is thought to be due to a combination of factors:

(1) reduction of total cholesterol levels;

(2) increase in HDL fraction;

(3) lowering LDL fraction;

(4) reduction of atherosclerosis;

(5) vasodilation of the coronary arteries and general vasodilation.

The prevention of cardiovascular deaths and symptoms such as angina is probably the strongest reason for taking HRT as a preventive therapy.

Osteoporosis

The other important preventive use of HRT is to preserve bone density and prevent fracture. Numerous population studies have shown that fractures in women increase sharply after the menopause (Melton and Riggs 1983).

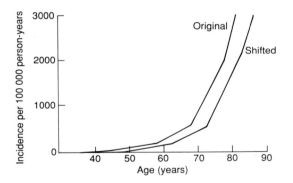

Fig. 7.5 Age-specific incidence of proximal femur fracture among women in Rochester, Minnesota, as originally reported and as it might appear if osteoporosis onset were delayed or progression slowed sufficiently to shift each rate to an age group 5 years older. From: B. L. Riggs, and L. J. Melton (1986). *New England Journal of Medicine*, **314**, 1676. Reproduced by permission of the authors, the editor, and J. C. Stevenson and Parthenon Publishing Group, USA.

Measurement of bone density in men and women has demonstrated that peak bone density is attained around the age of 35. After this age, women lose bone at 1 per cent per annum, accelerating to 3–5 per cent around the menopause, and slowing about 10 years later. Cooper *et al.* (1987) have demonstrated the association between loss of bone density and fractures. The architecture of trabecular bone is damaged and the amount of bony tissue is smaller in osteoporotic patients. Prevention becomes important as new bone can be laid down on the pre-existing trabecular network. Many experimental studies have shown the positive effect of oestrogen in preventing osteoporosis.

Epidemiological studies of large populations (Weiss *et al.* 1980) confirm that oestrogen used for five to six years will halve the risk of subsequent fracture. It halts bone loss through its effect on oestrogen receptors which have been demonstrated in bony tissue. Oestrogen has a positive effect on the collagen matrix and on collagen in skin (Brincat *et al.* 1988).

Thus it is reasonable to assume that treatment of women with oestrogen for six or more years around the time of the menopause will halve the incidence of subsequent fractures and greatly reduce the suffering, loss of earnings, and pressure on hospital beds due to this disease. The Consensus Conference held in Denmark (Smith 1987) recommended that oestrogen treatment given for 10 years would delay the onset of osteoporosis by 10 years and delay the expected peak of femoral fractures until close to the end of the expected span of life (Conference Report 1987).

Patients often ask if it is too late to take hormones if they are past the menopause. It is never too late. If older women with a uterus are willing to accept the resumption of 'periods', the administration of oestrogen effectively stops bone loss during the period of therapy.

Figure 7.6, taken from Christiansen's study of two groups of Danish women given either oestrogen or placebo, shows the effect on bone density.

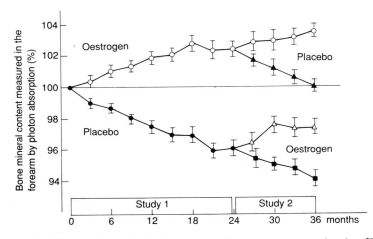

Fig. 7.6 The effect on bone density in women given oestrogen or placebo. [From: C. Christiansen and I. Transdøl (1981). Bone mass in postmenopausal women after withdrawal of oestrogen/gestagen replacement therapy. *Lancet*, **1**, 459–61. Reproduced with permission of the authors and the editors of the *Lancet*.]

Those women who were given oestrogen maintained or increased bone density until therapy stopped. Those on placebo experienced steady loss of bone, which stopped when oestrogen was given instead. Population bone density screening to detect those women who are most at risk is under investigation.

New treatments for osteoporosis which do not necessitate monthly withdrawal bleeding include continuous very small doses of combined oestrogen and progestogen (though this may cause irregular bleeding). A drug related to the anabolic steroids which does not cause endometrial stimulation is being studied. Older women with osteoporosis, who do not wish to take sex hormones, are appropriately treated with anabolic steroids, such as stanozolol, and oral calcium supplements, such as calcium hydroxyapatite. Fluoride supplements are effective but cause unpleasant side-effects. Recently two trials of etidronate given for two weeks followed by calcium supplements for 11 weeks have shown restoration of bone density and reduced incidence of fracture (Watts *et al.* 1990).

It is important that women who have had their ovaries removed or irradiated *before* the menopause should be given adequate oestrogen therapy for a long period in order to prevent the accelerated loss in bone density which sometimes occurs. (This does not apply to women who have a major contraindication such as breast cancer.) Many of these patients need to be told about the reasons for therapy, and that they may need to take HRT for a long period—perhaps as long as 25 years.

There is a consensus that women should be offered the option of HRT as a preventive treatment against heart disease and osteoporosis. This implies that the doctor is adequately informed about risks and benefits and can offer initial screening and supervision during therapy (Coope 1989). Great importance should be attached to non-hormonal remedies such as sufficient dietary calcium (Wickham *et al.* 1989), stopping smoking (Daniell 1976), correct weight for height, aerobic exercise to improve bone density (Chow *et al.* 1987), and exposure to sunlight to improve vitamin D synthesis (Fraser 1983). This implies data collection and education.

Most women do not want to take hormones (Coope and Roberts 1990). However, they do need education about their possible benefits and the other lifestyle factors which affect future health; and this advice needs to be offered at the time when it is most effective—just before or after the menopause.

MANAGEMENT AND TREATMENT OF THE MENOPAUSE

General management of patient before and during hormone therapy

Diagnosis

Symptoms occurring *at* the menopause are not always *due* to the menopause. The doctor needs to ask the following questions and should examine the patient and discuss her needs and attitudes:

1. Are the symptoms due to another condition, medical or social (i.e. not menopausal)?
2. Has the patient positive symptoms of oestrogen deficit? Flushes? Vaginal atrophy or dryness? Urethral syndrome? Osteoporosis?
3. Is there a contraindication to hormone therapy (Table 7.1)?
4. Does the patient wish to take hormones? If she has a uterus she will need combined oestrogen/progestogen and will have withdrawal bleeds.
5. Has she other needs—for instance, contraception? Screening of blood pressure, pelvis, and smear test is appropriate at this stage.

An accurate diagnosis is necessary using history and examination.

During hormone therapy the patient should be seen every few months. With women who have a uterus, enquiry about withdrawal bleeding should be made. Regular withdrawal bleeding is almost certainly associated with a normal endometrium but any unscheduled vaginal bleeding must be investigated and the patient referred to a gynaecologist for endometrial biopsy or further investigation. It is normal for some women not to bleed at all. 'Premenstrual syndrome' is a common complaint and women can experience depression, bloating, and weight gain. It is worth 'shopping around' to find the most acceptable preparation. Blood pressure should be checked at least once after the first few months on therapy. A yearly blood pressure check is useful, and weight measurement too. Weight gain may occur on progestogen therapy and fluid retention may happen in the early days of oestrogen treatment. Yearly pelvic examination to establish the size of the uterus is thought to be necessary as fibroids may grow quickly. Cervical smears are necessary only every three to five years as part of routine preventive care. Women should be encouraged to examine their own breasts and a regular breast examination should be part of the follow-up. Women with a history of previous benign breast disease especially need breast surveillance on hormone therapy.

Practical points

Smoking is dangerous to the heart, increases the risk of hormone therapy, and is now shown to be associated with increased risk of cervical cancer. Patients should be encouraged and helped to give up, or at least reduce to below five cigarettes daily.

A full blood count, dipstick examination of the urine, and possibly T^4 estimation excludes anaemia, kidney disease, diabetes, and thyrotoxicosis which may mimic menopausal symptoms or contraindicate hormone therapy. Abnormal vaginal bleeding such as intermenstrual, post-coital, or post-menopausal must be investigated and hospital referral is essential.

The following is a summary of the main points of management in a woman on hormone therapy who has an intact uterus:

1. The lowest effective maintenance dose should be found for each patient.
2. Oestrogen with cyclical progestogen supplements is necessary.
3. Some preparations (Prempak C, Trisequens, and Estrapak 50) provide continuous oestrogen during the week of withdrawal bleeding. This minimizes the incidence of flushes during that time.
4. Regular withdrawal bleeding is normal, but does not occur in all patients. Irregular, heavy, or painful bleeding, or uterine enlargement, need referral to a gynaecologist for investigation.
5. Coming off therapy may be difficult for both types of patient (those with and without a uterus). Slow withdrawal by halving dosage is helpful and therapy is better withdrawn in cold weather. Withdrawal flushes can be severe and distressing to the patient and she needs reassurance that they are harmless and will eventually cease.

Hormonal measures

Table 7.2 shows the range of HRT drugs available for treatment of menopausal symptoms. As many studies have shown an association between oestrogen therapy and endometrial carcinoma, in Great Britain it is now commonly accepted practice to treat women with an intact uterus with oestrogen/progestogen combinations. Progestogen prevent atypical hyperplasia and carcinoma of the endometrium if given in adequate dosage for a sufficient number of days in each cycle (about 10–13 days). When progestogen is withdrawn each month the patient usually has a withdrawal

Table 7.1 *Hormone replacement therapy*

For patients who have had a hysterectomy:
　Premarin 0.625 mg or 1.25 mg once daily
　Progynova 1 or 2 mg once daily. 2 mg is necessary to prevent bone loss
　Harmogen 1.5 mg once or twice daily
　Estraderm 50 μg–100 μg. 25 μg may not prevent osteoporosis but is useful in patients with poor tolerance

For patients with a uterus:
　Prempak C 0.625 mg or 1.25 mg
　Cyclo-Progynova 1 mg or 2 mg
　Estrapak 50 μg
　Trisequens
　Nuvelle

---

bleed or 'period'. This ensures her safety as the endometrial cells are shed regularly.

Most women do not want 'periods' after the menopause. However, those with severe symptoms will often accept regular withdrawal bleeding as the price they have to pay for effective therapy. The patient will need reassurance that the return of a monthly bleed does not imply a return of fertility.

Hysterectomized women do not have this problem. They can safely take oestrogen alone continuously, briefly, or long term, or in irregular courses as their symptoms require it. There is no definite age at which therapy has to cease. If a contraindication to therapy develops then the treatment is stopped, but if possible it should be tailed off slowly.

Implant preparations

Although there is no reason *per se* why implants should not be inserted by the general practitioner in the appropriate patient, this will usually be done in a hospital setting. As relatively few patients need them, each general practitioner's experience is likely to be limited. 'Pure' oestradiol is available in implant form as a very small hard-packed pellet, 50 or 100 mg, which can be inserted under the skin, usually of the lower abdominal wall, as an out-patient procedure. It can also be left under the rectus sheath following abdominal hysterectomy when the ovaries have been removed. Oestradiol is slowly absorbed from the implant over the course of about a year. Return of menopausal symptoms can therefore be expected within a few months of insertion but the implant can be renewed as often as is necessary to control symptoms. In the main, an oestradiol implant is given only to women who have had a hysterectomy. Some gynaecologists use this form of oestrogen administration in women who have an intact uterus, and give oral progestogens for 10–13 days to induce cyclical bleeding following withdrawal of the progestogens. Removal of an implant may be difficult owing to problems of identification of the exact site and requires a general anaesthetic.

Vaginal creams

Vaginal creams are extremely useful for older women with a uterus who do not wish to have the trouble and embarrassment of monthly bleeding. Menopausal women may have problems with sexual intercourse. If it is painful, trauma to the narrow rigid vagina may cause bleeding. A two-week course of cream, followed by intermittent small doses, usually benefits this problem. Women who are on the waiting list for colporrhaphy and older women who use vaginal rings often find a short course of local oestrogen cream helpful. A particular group who are grateful for vaginal oestrogen are older women embarking on a new relationship. Women who are separated or widowed often have a gap of several years before re-establishing intercourse and may experience painful trauma.

Vaginal creams are used with an applicator, nightly at first, and then once or twice weekly as required. They are absorbed into the bloodstream and should not be used by women who have a serious contraindication, such as breast or endometrial cancer. Often very small doses are effective as the oestrogen, unlike oral preparations, is not immediately conjugated in the liver. A vaginal lubricant such as KY jelly should be used before sexual intercourse.

Oestrogen/progestogen preparations

For women who are still menstruating, or who are postmenopausal but with an intact uterus, the risk of endometrial hyperplasia and possibly of endometrial carcinoma may be reduced by prescribing preparations designed to give women 12 or 13 days of progestogen in each monthly 'cycle'. All these preparations can be classified as a sequential type of therapy with ideally 12 to 13 days of unopposed oestrogen followed by 7 to 13 days of oestrogen combined with progestogen. Some are given on a 'three weeks on treatment, one week off' regimen (e.g. Cyclo-Progynova); others (Prempak C, Estrapak, and Trisequens) give continuous therapy.

Patients find these preparations easy to use as they are in a calendar pack. Postmenopausal patients are warned that they are likely to have a monthly bleed after the progestogen treatment finishes, although some postmenopausal patients do not bleed, particularly if they are taking low-dose therapy. Absence of bleeding is not dangerous but the size of the uterus should be checked ever year by the GP. Heavy, irregular, or painful bleeding needs investigation.

Progestogens alone

Oral progestogens are rarely prescribed. They can relieve the hot flushes and sweats of the menopause but are of no value in atrophic vaginitis. They are usually prescribed where there are contraindications to oestrogens, for example in women with a history of atypical hyperplasia or thrombosis. If given on a cyclical basis, vaginal bleeding is unlikely to occur in postmenopausal women. The two progestogens which can be used are norethisterone 5 mg daily or medroxyprogesterone acetate 10 mg daily. The dose of progestogen in the progestogen-only contraceptive pill is too small to control menopausal symptoms. Progestogen in high dose protects the bones but has an adverse effect on lipids.

Transdermal oestrogen (oestradiol patches)

This therapy provides oestradiol B in an alcohol base contained in an adhesive patch with a permeable covering. The patch is applied to the buttock or a suitable adjacent area, and oestrogen is released slowly over a period of days achieving a steady daily dose of 25, 50, or 100 μg.

Hysterectomized women can safely use the patches without supplement, applying a new patch every three or four days. It is useful to vary the site of application to prevent skin irritation.

Women with a uterus should take a progestogen supplement for 12 days each cycle to prevent endometrial hyperplasia and cancer. This is provided as norethisterone 1 mg in the calendar packs of Estrapak 50. Work is under way to provide progestogen transdermally but suitable preparations have not yet reached the market.

Transdermal oestrogen is highly effective in maintaining bone mass and preventing further fractures (Lufkin *et al.* 1990). It has a beneficial effect on lipids but it is too early to assess its effect on the incidence of mortality of coronary heart disease. Most women feel very well on it. The main side-effects are the usual swelling of breasts, erectile nipples, and occasional nausea. These preparations are much more expensive than oral oestrogen.

Continuous oestrogen/progestogen

Continuous oestrogen/progestogen can be given and this does not cause withdrawal bleeding. However there is a high incidence of spotting in the first few months and D&C is often necessary. Further research is under way.

The low-dose contraceptive pill

The low-dose contraceptive pill provides effective HRT and prevents osteoporosis; although the effect on the cardiovascular system may not be so beneficial. It is now approved for use up to the menopause in selected cases (e.g. non-smokers). Non-androgenic progestogens such as desogestrol are probably safest.

Livial

This is a product with the properties of weak oestrogen, androgen, and progestogen. Experiments have shown that livial prevents osteoporosis but it is not yet officially approved for this use. It is supposed not to cause withdrawal bleeding but my experience shows that this may occur in the form of irregular spotting or actual 'periods', although the bleeding is much lighter than on conventional HRT. Nandrolone decanoate, stanozolol, or calcitonin can also be used in older women with fractures. Weight gain is common with anabolic steroids.

Etidronate

Several trials have shown the effectiveness of cyclical etidronate in preventing further thinning of bone and fractures in women who already have spinal osteoporosis. Bleeding does not occur which is useful for older women. The dose is etidronate 400 mg daily for 14 days followed by calcium supplements 5 mg daily days 15–88 (Watts *et al.* 1990). These should not be given simultaneously. This drug can be used in general practice although it awaits a product licence for use in osteoporosis.

Table 7.2 *Reasons for positively recommending HRT if there are no contraindications*

1. Removal or irradiation of both ovaries before menopause, or natural menopause before 45 years. Bone loss occurs rapidly in these women and oestrogen completely prevents this for the duration of therapy. Give HRT until 55–60 years old or longer. Oophorectomized patients may need HRT for 20–30 years and periodic mammography is important as there is increased breast cancer risk after nine years' treatment.

2. Hysterectomy before the menopause, even if ovaries are conserved. 25 per cent of these women have early ovarian failure. The appearance of hot flushes and FSH >20 μ/litre is confirmation of menopause. Oestrogen can be given without progestogen and is protective against ischaemic heart disease for the duration of therapy. If given for five years, it halves the risk of future fractures.

3. Sexual difficulty due to tight atrophic vagina, which usually occurs in women over 55 but may occur earlier in hysterectomized patients. This responds dramatically to oestrogen.

4. Fractures, particularly if occurring before the menopause and with minimal trauma. The appearance of a second fracture or compression fracture of vertebra indicates the need for immediate treatment with oestrogen to prevent further fractures. HRT is the safest and cheapest form of treatment. If the patient cannot take this, refer her for bone density measurement and if low ask advice of specialist unit. Etidronate is effective. Calcitonin is useful but expensive. Stanozolol is useful in older women.

5. High risk of ischaemic heart disease, e.g. diabetic, patient already suffering from angina, or high cholesterol >6.8 not responding to diet. Severe family history of cardiac or stroke death <60. Oestrogen is the cheapest and most effective lipid lowering drug for women.

6. Flushes and sweats interfering with sleep or work.

7. Increased risk of osteoporosis. Thinness, lack of exercise, rheumatoid arthritis, use of corticosteroids, heavy smoking at perimenopause, low calcium diet, family history of osteoporosis.

8. Depression associated with labile mood at the perimenopause. Careful assessment of psychosocial background is needed. Also assess depth of depression and suicide risk (Beck Inventory is useful). Psychotherapy or antidepressant drugs may be first-line treatment. Refer if suicidal.

RISKS OF HORMONE THERAPY

Endometrial cancer

Over the last 10 years many reports from the USA have suggested an increase in the incidence of endometrial carcinoma which paralleled in the 1960s and early 1970s increasing sale of oestrogens. In addition, case control studies show an apparent association between oestrogen usage in postmenopausal women and endometrial carcinoma. These latter reports claim an average fivefold increase in the likelihood of endometrial cancer developing in postmenopausal oestrogen users. Several studies suggest that the risk is increased the bigger the dose of oestrogen and the longer the duration of use. The frequency of endometrial cancer among postmenopausal women who never use oestrogens is of the order of 0.7 per 1000. Prolonged use of oestrogens may raise this risk to around three per 1000. The risk of dying of the disease is, however, remote—about one woman in 4000 so exposed, since the five-year survival rate exceeds 90 per cent if the disease is localized in the uterus.

A recent report (Shapiro *et al.* 1985) found a significant increase in risk in women who had used conjugated oestrogens for at least a year and then discontinued them, even after oestrogen-free intervals of over ten years. This is an important observation for general practitioners who carry out long-term supervision of current and ex-users of oestrogen therapy.

However, women who use adequate progestogen supplements from the beginning of therapy do not have increased risk of cancer (Persson *et al.* 1989). A Swedish study of 23 000 patients taking oestrogen (Bergkvist *et al.* 1989) found increased risk of endometrial cancer in users of oestrogen without progestogen. If cyclical progestogens were used throughout the entire period there was no increase. And one study has shown a *reduced* rate of endometrial cancer in users of combined preparations. Progestogen is powerfully protective against both hyperplasia and cancer.

It is possible for women with a uterus to take unopposed oestrogen for long periods in order to prevent heart disease and osteoporosis and this regime is widely used in the USA; but the risk of hyperplasia and carcinoma cannot be overlooked, and frequent endometrial biopsy is needed. Constraints of medical time and expense would make this regime impossible to adopt in the NHS and most women would find frequent invasive procedures distasteful. If women find difficulty in tolerating the progestogens in calendar packs it is possible to use continuous low dose oestrogen and to supplement this with one of the following for 12 days in each 28-day cycle:

Norethisterone 0.7–1.05 mg (= Micronor, 2 or 3 tablets)
Provera 10 mg
Duphaston 10 or 20 mg

Breast cancer

In the past, several studies showed no significant association between oestrogen use and breast cancer, and a large study (Kaufman *et al.* 1984) of American women taking menopausal oestrogen preparations also showed no increased risk. More recent studies have not been so reassuring. One suggested that the relative risk increased with follow-up duration progressing to two per 1000 after 15 years. And the general consensus now is that long-term use of oestrogen (more than ten years) does increase the risk of breast cancer.

The Swedish study of 23 000 hormone-users (Bergkvist *et al.* 1989) reported that the incidence of breast cancer compared to that in non-users was not increased in up to six years' use, but after this the risk increased according to duration of therapy. After nine years' treatment the risk ratio was 1.7 per 1000. This confirms the findings of several cohort studies from the USA. The most recently reported is a British study which updated the analysis and follow-up of 5000 women taking HRT and attending menopause clinics (Hunt *et al.* 1990). Breast cancer mortality compared with that in the general population rose from 0.55 per 1000 in the earlier period of follow-up to 1984, to one per 1000 between 1984 and 1988. This confirms previous reports of low mortality increasing with length of hormone use and follow-up. In both the British and Swedish studies no protective effect was observed when progestogen was given.

Women contemplating oestrogen therapy at the menopause should be questioned about their own or family history of breast cancer. Lumps in the breast detected initially or during therapy must be referred for investigation. Although not all breast cancers are oestrogen-dependent we have no way of knowing beforehand whether a particular tumour will prove to be so. Therefore breast cancer is still regarded as an absolute contraindication to oestrogen therapy—although this issue remains unresolved. (See Chapter 2.) Routine screening by mammography is recommended for all women over the age of 50 (Roebuck 1986).

A practical point in prescribing HRT is the need to consider length of therapy because breast cancer is so common and even a small increase may have disastrous effects. Five to six years' use of oestrogen at the menopause has not been shown to increase the risk, however; and this duration of treatment has also been shown to halve the risk of postmenopausal fracture (Weiss *et al.* 1980).

Therefore in the first instance it may be wise to recommend five to six years' HRT beginning at the menopause when bone loss is most rapid. Women who have their ovaries removed at an early age are strongly recommended to take oestrogen for much longer, perhaps 15–20 years, with the safeguard of periodic mammograms. If a patient wishes to go on longer with treatment she may do so but should have regular physical examination and mammography. Recurrence of carcinoma of the ovary is not more likely to occur if a patient is given HRT (Eeles *et al.* 1991).

Thrombosis

Concerns about risks of hypertension and thrombo-embolic disease in postmenopausal women on oestrogen therapy have arisen because of the risks in older women using oral contraceptives. Some studies have suggested that natural oestrogens in low dosage as used at the menopause have some adverse effects on blood-clotting factors and platelet function although these are minimal when compared to larger doses of synthetic oestrogens (Coope *et al.* 1975). Epidemiological evidence is reassuring.

There is no evidence from population studies that HRT in the usual low doses of oestrogen increases thrombo-embolism; high doses given to men are associated with increased deaths from thrombosis. It is prudent to stop oestrogen treatment a month before major operations involving increased risk of thrombosis, e.g. hip replacement. Auricular fibrillation and *present* deep vein thrombosis or embolism or myocardial infarction would contraindicate therapy but HRT could be resumed after a few months when the clinical picture is normal. Oestrogen would be beneficial for women with ischaemic heart disease. Varicose veins do not contraindicate oestrogen treatment. Blood pressure is not raised by oestrogen although a few women retain fluid and this may cause weight gain and possibly LV failure. Diuretics are effective treatment.

Gall bladder disease

There is conflicting evidence about the risk of gall bladder disease in menopausal women treated with oestrogen. One study suggested a 2.5-fold increase in surgically diagnosed gall-bladder disease; another failed to

Table 7.3 *Contraindications to oestrogen treatment*

Absolute contraindications
　　Cancer of breast or endometrium
　　Major thrombo-embolic disease (including atrial fibrillation)
　　Severe liver or kidney disease

Relative contraindications
　　Lump in breast (needs investigation and possibly removal)
　　Lump in pelvis (needs investigation and possibly removal)
　　Intermenstrual, postmenopausal, or heavy bleeding (needs investigation and
　　　　possibly removal of uterus)
　　Gall-bladder disease
　　Previous adverse reaction to hormone replacement or the pill
　　Otosclerosis (may deteriorate on HRT)

---

confirm this finding. In practice, some women taking oestrogen therapy develop upper abdominal pain after several months, which disappears on stopping treatment. Caution is indicated in prescribing oestrogens for women with established gall-bladder disease.

NON-HORMONAL MEASURES

Even in practices which offer education and supervision of HRT, 80 per cent of women do not wish to take it but prefer to use other means of prevention of heart disease and fracture.

Doctors are usually aware of the preventive measures against coronary heart disease (stopping smoking, attention to diet, aerobic exercise, and weight control) but are less well educated in prevention of osteoporosis (sufficient calcium, sunlight, weight-bearing exercise, and stopping smoking).

There has been a great deal of controversy about the level of calcium intake which is 'sufficient' (and it is now widely accepted that oestrogen is much more effective than calcium supplements in preventing bone loss). However, the bones consist of calcium salts laid down on a protein matrix and patients obviously need a certain minimum intake. The recommended dietary allowance in Britain for menopausal women is 500 mg daily, in the USA 800 mg daily. There is evidence that older women benefit from higher levels and Heaney's study (1977) showed that after the menopause women need 1400 mg daily to stay in zero balance; before the menopause 800 mg is sufficient.

The two major risk factors for osteoporosis are loss of ovarian function and low-peak adult bone mass (Stevenson *et al.* 1989). The latter depends on adequate nutrition in childhood (about a pint of milk daily or the equivalent), plenty of exercise and sleep, and avoiding smoking. Women need to know that these simple remedies may avoid problems 30 years later. Doctors need to know about the calcium content of foods (see Appendix 1), as calcium is better absorbed in the diet than as a supplement and expensive time-consuming prescriptions can be avoided. Fluoride in water protects teeth and may protect bones, although it is too toxic and has too many side-effects to use as routine treatment.

A study of a community of 957 women and men in California (Holbrook *et al.* 1988) showed that the risk of hip fracture was inversely correlated with calcium intake. Several controlled studies have demonstrated the effect of exercise in increasing bone density (Chow *et al.* 1987).

DOCTORS' AND WOMEN'S ATTITUDES TO THE MENOPAUSE

A survey of women's reactions to hormone therapy was carried out by Hunt (1988) who sent questionnaires to 300 British women having treatment. Over 90 per cent found therapy helpful. Hot flushes, irritability, and depression all improved on treatment. However, most of the women had obtained information on HRT from the media or from a friend and 20 per cent had exerted pressure on their general practitioner to obtain a prescription. Draper and Roland (1990) questioned 102 women about their attitudes to HRT for prevention of osteoporosis. 75 per cent were interested in taking hormones to prevent this but wanted more information. A standard questionnaire and interview was used to approach women at their place of work in Glasgow (Barlow *et al.* 1989). Only 12 out of 424 women had received long-term HRT over three years, and 9 of these had had an oophorectomy. 11 per cent were dissatisfied with their GP's handling of the matter. A further study by the same authors (Barlow *et al.* 1991) of nine general practices in the Oxford area showed that under 5 per cent of women had had consultations about the menopause. Prescription of HRT was about 2.5 per cent for women aged 40–69.

Because of the problems of education, screening, and supervision of HRT, we started a preventive clinic in our practice in 1988, offering a preventive health package to 40–60-year-olds (Coope and Roberts 1990). The use of hormones is now over 20 per cent in our practice in women aged 40–60, but there is a strong social-class bias (see Fig. 7.7). The clinic protocols are shown as appendices.

The problems of non-attendance at preventive clinics apply to many other practices and other types of prevention. A general practice in Oxfordshire (Waller *et al.* 1990) found that only 44 per cent of patients had attended for a preventive health check and that smokers and heavy drinkers were less likely to attend. This reflects our own experience, although we are finding that a second trawl of non-attenders is yielding some people who are at high risk of disease but would not attend the surgery for advice unless actively contacted.

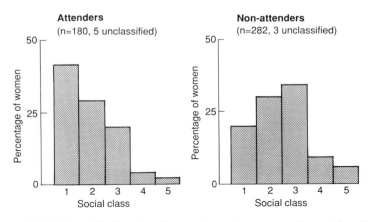

Fig. 7.7 Social class distribution of attenders and non-attenders at the clinic.

Although HRT offers safe prevention against heart disease and fracture it is not a panacea for all the ills of middle-aged women. Doctors and patients need more education and the use of a practice team of doctor, nurse, nutritionist, and physiotherapist in an organized clinic offers a way forward to preventive health.

Appendix 1

PROTOCOL FOR NURSE/DOCTOR WOMEN'S HEALTH CLINIC

A one-off education and screening clinic offered to all women in the practice between the ages of 40 and 60. It educates them about HRT and other preventive strategies against fractures, heart disease, and strokes; and also about nutrition and family health.

Aims: Education and screening of all middle-aged women. This clinic feeds the HRT clinic, enabling women in all social groups to perceive the uses of HRT and attend the HRT clinic.

Manpower: Receptionist/clerk
Practice nurse
Doctor
Physiotherapist
Nutritionist/cook.

Method: Weekly two-hour session using two consultation rooms, a teaching room, a video room.
Appointments Patients are identified from age/sex register and contacted in groups of 15. The secretary sends an invitation to attend on a specific date, at lunch time.
Letter This should be informative, non-threatening, and friendly and explain why we are sending for patients (to educate them, and find out about their lifestyle and any health problems).
Equipment Blackboard or flip chart
    Posters showing high-calcium diet, healthy heart diet
    Leaflets (anti-smoking)
    Diet sheets
    Weighing scales, height measure, cholesterol screening
    Video, TV.

Procedure: (1) Patients come to the receptionist, then sit in a group for a lecture from the doctor. She gives information on the prevention of osteoporosis, the risks and benefits of HRT, etc.

(2) Each patient is seen by the nurse who completes a data sheet recording height, weight, exercise, smoking history, cholesterol level (high risk patients), blood pressure, result of urine dipstick.

(3) Each patient is then seen privately by the doctor who completes LMP, hormone use, calcium intake (calculated from chart overleaf); examines contraindications to therapy; looks at other health problems and alcohol intake; and demonstrates HRT tablets/patches. Together they make a decision (or postpone one) on whether HRT would be acceptable.

(4) Physiotherapist gives monthly exercise class.

(5) Nutritionist/cook gives monthly cookery class.

(6) Videos are used for teaching about osteoporosis.

Prescriptions are issued only after screening breasts and pelvis, and possibly after other tests, such as a mammogram. Patients are followed up in the HRT clinic.

Data sheet for use in Clinic

LMP
....
....
Ovaries
....
....
Calcium
....
Hormones ....
Ultraviolet ....
Smoking ....
Exercise ....
Weight ....
Height ....
Alcohol ....
BP ....
Urine ....
Cholesterol ....
Mammogram ....
Cervical smear ....

TYPICAL CALCIUM CONTENT OF FOOD	
⅓ pint (195 ml) silver top milk	230 mg
⅓ pint (195 ml) semi-skimmed milk	240 mg
⅓ pint (195 ml) skimmed milk	250 mg
1 oz (28 g) Cheddar or other hard cheese	220 mg
5 oz (140 g) pot of yogurt	270 mg
4 oz (112 g) cottage cheese	60 mg
4 oz (112 g) ice-cream	157 mg
2 oz (56 g) sardines (including bones)	220 mg
2 large (60 g) slices white bread	60 mg
2 large (60 g) slices wholemeal bread	14 mg
4 oz (112 g) spring cabbage	30 mg
4 oz (112 g) broccoli	76 mg
4 oz (112 g) baked beans	45 mg
2 oz (56 g) peanuts	34 mg
2 oz (56 g) dried apricots	52 mg

Appendix 2

PROTOCOL FOR DOCTOR/NURSE HRT CLINIC

Aims: To offer
Screening
Prescription and advice
Supervision
for women wishing to use HRT. HRT is viewed as a preventive strategy against osteoporosis and heart disease.

Manpower: Receptionist/clerk
Practice nurse
Doctor.

Method: Weekly two-hour session at surgery, using two consultation rooms and a reception desk. Patients book on their own responsibility or are referred from one of the partners.
Appointments 5–15 minutes depending on problem.
Equipment Usual gynaecological couch, light, etc., wash basin
Computer if generally used in practice
Ordinary records.

Clinical protocol: Patients are advised as to the suitability of HRT for them. *Contraindications* are:

(1) endometrial or breast cancer (current or previous);

(2) otosclerosis (may deteriorate on oestrogen);

(3) *present severe* thrombo-embolism, e.g. myocardial infarction, or risk of DVT as in patient undergoing hip replacement. (Past DVT (especially if due to trauma or obstetrics), or varicose veins are not a contraindication.)

(4) Severe liver or kidney disease. (This prevents efficient metabolism and excretion of oestrogen.)

Ethical considerations:

(1) Patients should be menopausal (periods infrequent or stopped). FSH may be used to diagnose menopause in hysterectomized or doubtful cases; > 20 indicates menopause.

(2) Patients should be informed about the risks and benefits of HRT and *should decide whether they want it*. They should be informed that breast cancer risks do not escalate in under six years' use (Bergkvist *et al.* 1989) and should be

advised that maximum benefit in osteoporosis prevention is obtained *at* the menopause when bone loss is most rapid. Five years' use halves fracture risk and considerably reduces risk of heart disease.

(3) Patients should be offered contraceptive advice and may decide to substitute the combined pill for HRT.

(4) The doctor should be aware of other medical problems and treatments, e.g. corticosteroids, which increase the risk of osteoporosis.

History and examination of patient:

Doctor: Bleeding which is irregular, painful, or very heavy needs investigation. *Vaginal examination* should be carried out by the doctor (unless the nurse has been trained to do this). It is essential for the doctor to exclude pelvic masses. If a mass is found it should be investigated before any decision is taken on treatment. Pelvic ultrasound, D&C, and/or laparscopy may be needed.

Nurse: Breast examination, weight, blood pressure, and urine dipstick can be carried out by the nurse.

Mammography is needed for those with a lump in the breast, discharge from the nipple, or a family history of breast cancer. This is desirable before embarking on long-term therapy.

After discussion with the patient, history, and examination, a decision is made on *whether to offer* HRT. If not, other non-hormonal methods of keeping fit are explained.

Prescribing HRT:

Choice of method: Patches or tablets (continuous) for hysterectomized patients.
Patches and progestogen, or tablets and progestogen for patients with a uterus.

Doctor: Initial prescription.
Follow-up appointment after three months, which should include questions about bleeding pattern. (Pattern may be abnormal in first two months, but bleeding should reappear after progestogen supplement.) Yearly assessment in long-term users.
Trouble-shooting at request of nurse or patient.

Nurse: Weight check, blood pressure throughout.
Follow-up after six months, and after nine months.

Routine questioning of patients should include:
What is the bleeding pattern?
Have you any problems?

Common side-effects include:

(1) oestrogen: fluid retention, breast enlargement, nausea, headaches;
(2) progestogen: premenstrual syndrome, headaches, depression, bloating.

REFERENCES AND FURTHER READING

Ballinger, C. B. (1975). Psychiatric morbidity and the menopause: screening of general population sample. *British Medical Journal*, **3**, 344–6.

Barlow, D. H., Grosset, K. A., Hart, H., *et al.* (1989). A study of the experience of Glasgow women in the climacteric years. *British Journal of Obstetrics and Gynaecology*, **96**, 1192–7.

Barlow, D. H., Brockie, J. A., and Rees, C. M. P. (1991). Study of general practice consultations and menopausal problems. *British Medical Journal*, **302**, 274–6.

Bergkvist, L., Adami, H-O., Persson, I., *et al.* (1989). The risk of breast cancer after estrogen and estrogen-progestin replacement. *New England Journal of Medicine*, **321**, **(5)**, 293–7.

Brincat, E., Versi, T., O'Dowd, C. F., *et al.* (1988). Skin collagen changes in postmenopausal women receiving oestradiol gel. *Maturitas*, **9**, 1–6.

Bungay, G. T., Vessey, M. P., and McPherson, C. K. (1980). Study of symptoms in middle life with special reference to the menopause. *British Medical Journal*, **281**, 181–3.

Cann, C. E., Martin, M. C., Genant, H. K., *et al.* (1984). Decreased spinal mineral content in amenorrhoeic women. *Journal of the American Medical Association*, **251**, **(5)**, 626–9.

Chow, R., Harrison, J. E., and Notarius, C. (1987). Effect of two randomised exercise programmes on bone mass of healthy postmenopausal women. *British Medical Journal*, **295**, 1441–4.

Conference Report (1987). Consensus development conference: prophylaxis and treatment of osteoporosis. *British Medical Journal*, **295**, 914–15.

Cooke, D. J. and Greene, J. G. (1981). Types of life events in relation to symptoms at the climacterium. *Journal of Psychological Research*, **25**, 5–11.

Coope, J. (1981). Is oestrogen therapy effective in the treatment of menopausal depression? *Journal of the Royal College of General Practitioners*, **3**, 134–40.

Coope, J. (1989). *Hormone replacement therapy*. Royal College of General Practitioners, Exeter.

Coope, J., Thomson, J., and Poller, L. (1975). Effects of natural oestrogen replacement therapy on menopausal symptoms and blood clotting. *British Medical Journal*, **4**, 139–43.

Coope, J., Williams, S., and Patterson, J. S. (1978). A study of the effectiveness of propanolol in menopausal hot flushes. *British Journal of Obstetrics and Gynaecology*, **85**, 472–5.

Coope, J. and Roberts, D. (1990). A clinic for the prevention of osteoporosis in general practice. *British Journal of General Practice*, **40**, 295–9.

Cooper, C., Barker, D. J. P., Morris, J., *et al.* (1987). Osteoporosis, falls and age in fracture of the proximal femur. *British Medical Journal*, **295**, 13.

Daniell, H. W. (1976). Osteoporosis of the slender smoker. *Archives of Internal Medicine*, **136**, 289–304.

Draper, J. and Roland, M. (1990). Perimenopausal women's views on taking hormone replacement therapy to prevent osteoporosis. *British Medical Journal*, **300**, 786–8.

Eeles, R. A., Tan, S., Wiltshaw, *et al.* (1991). Hormone replacement therapy and survival after surgery for ovarian cancer. *British Medical Journal*, **302**, 259–62.

Fraser, D. (1983). The physiological economy of vitamin D. *Lancet*, **1**, 969–72.

Heaney, R. P., *et al.* (1977). Calcium balance and calcium requirements in middle-aged women. *American Journal of Clinical Nutrition*, **30**, 1603–11.

Holbrook, T. L., Barrett-Connor, E., and Wingard, D. L. (1988). Dietary calcium and risk of hip fracture: 14-year prospective population study. *Lancet*, **5**, 1046–9.

Holte, A. (1990). *The Norwegian menopause project (NMP)*. Abstract of Sixth International Congress on the Menopause, Bangkok, p. 227. Parthenon Publishing Group, Carnforth.

Hunt, K. (1988). Perceived value of treatment among a group of long term users of hormone replacement therapy. *Journal of the Royal College of General Practitioners*, **38**, 398–401.

Hunt, K., Vessey, M., and McPherson, K. (1990). Mortality in a cohort of long-term users of hormone replacement therapy: an updated analysis. *British Journal of Obstetrics and Gynaecology*, **97**, 1080–6.

Hunter, M. (1990). *Longitudinal studies of the climacteric—the South-East England study*. Abstract of Sixth International Congress on the Menopause, Bangkok, p. 228. Parthenon Publishing Group, Carnforth.

Jenkins, R. and Clare, A. W. (1985). Women and mental illness. *British Medical Journal*, **291**, 1521–2.

Kaufman, D. W., Miller, D. R., Rosenberg, L., *et al.* (1984). Noncontraceptive estrogen use and the risk of breast cancer. *Journal of the American Medical Association*, **252**, (1), 63–7.

Klaiber, E. L., Broverman, D. M., Vogel, W., *et al.* (1979). Estrogen therapy for severe persistent depression in women. *Archives of General Psychiatry*, **36**, 550–4.

Leiblum, S. R. and Bachmann, G. A. (1988). The sexuality of the climacteric woman. In *The menopause: comprehensive management* (ed. Bernard A. Eskin) (2nd edn), pp. 165–80. Macmillan, London.

Lufkin, E. G., Hodgson, S. F., Kotowitz, M. A., *et al.* (1990). Transdermal estrogen treatment of osteoporosis: a randomised placebo controlled double blind study. Abstract of Third International Symposium on Osteoporosis, Copenhagen, p. 197. Department of Clinical Chemistry, Glostrup Hospital, Denmark.

McKinlay, S. M. and Jefferys, M. (1974). The menopausal syndrome. *British Journal of Preventative and Social Medicine*, **28**, 108–15.

McKinlay, S. M., *et al.* (1990). *The Massachusetts women's health study: a prospective study of menopause*. Abstract of Sixth International Congress on the Menopause, Bangkok, p. 229. Parthenon Publishing Group, Carnforth.

Melton, I. J. and Riggs, B. L. (1983). Epidemiology of age-related fractures. In *The osteoporotic syndrome: detection prevention and treatment* (ed. L. V. Avioli), pp. 45–72. Grune and Stratton, New York.

Montgomery, J. C., Brincat, M., Tapp, A., *et al.* (1987). Effect of oestrogen and testosterone implants on psychological disorders in the climacteric. *Lancet*, **i**, 297–9.

Oliver, M. F. and Boyd, G. S. (1959). Effect of bilateral ovariectomy on coronary-artery disease and serum-lipid levels. *Lancet*, **2**, 690–4.

Paganini-Hill, A., Ross, R. K., and Henderson, B. E. (1988). Postmenopausal oestrogen treatment and stroke: a prospective study. *British Medical Journal*, **297**, 519–22.

Persson, I., Adami, H-O., Bergkvist, L., *et al.* (1989). Risk of endometrial cancer after treatment with oestrogens alone or in conjunction with progestogens: results of a prospective study. *British Medical Journal*, **209**, 147.

Roebuck, E. J. (1986). Mammography screening for breast cancer. *British Medical Journal*, **292**, 223.

Ross, R. K., Paganini-Hill, A., Mack, T. M., *et al.* (1981). Menopausal oestrogen therapy and protection from death from ischaemic heart disease. *Lancet*, **i**, 858–60.

Shapiro, S., Kelley, J. P., Rosenberg, *et al.* (1985). Risk of localized and wide-spread endometrial cancer in relation to recent and discontinued use of conjugated estrogens. *New England Journal of Medicine*, **313**, 969–72.

Siddle, N., Sarrel, P., and Whitehead, M. (1987). The effect of hysterectomy on the age of ovarian failure: identification of a subgroup of women with premature loss of ovarian function and literature review. *Fertility and Sterility*, **47**, **(1)**, 94–100.

Smith, T. (1987). Consensus on preventing osteoporosis. *British Medical Journal*, **295**, 872.

Stampfer, M. J., Willett, W. G., Colgitz, G. A., *et al.* (1985). A prospective study of postmenopausal estrogen therapy and coronary heart disease. *New England Journal of Medicine*, **313**, 1044–9.

Stevenson, J. C., *et al.* (1989). Determinants of bone density in normal women: risk factors for future osteoporosis. *British Medical Journal*, **298**, 924–8.

Waller, D., Agass, M., Mant, D., *et al.* (1990). Health checks in general practice: another example of inverse care? *British Medical Journal*, **300**, 1115–18.

Watts, N. B., Harris, S. T., Genant, H. K., *et al.* (1990). Intermittent cyclical etidronate treatment of postmenopausal osteoporosis. *New England Journal of Medicine*, **323**, **(2)**, 73–9.

Weiss, N. S., Ure, C. L., Ballard, J. H., *et al.* (1980). Decreased risk of fractures of the hip and lower forearm with postmenopausal use of estrogen. *New England Journal of Medicine*, **303**, 1195–8.

Wickham, C. A. C., Walsh, K., Cooper, C., *et al.* (1989). Dietary calcium, physical activity, and risk of hip fracture: a prospective study. *British Medical Journal*, **299**, 889–92.

Witteman, J. C. M., Grobbee, D. E., Kok, F. J., *et al.* (1989). Increased risk of atherosclerosis in women after the menopause. *British Medical Journal*, **298**, 642–4.

8. Cervical cytology

Ann McPherson and Joan Austoker

INTRODUCTION

Despite many millions of smears being taken, there has only been a minor reduction in overall mortality from cervical cancer in this country, although the most recent figures are starting to look more promising. It is the purpose of this chapter to look at the epidemiology and natural history of the condition, and the recent organization of the cervical screening programme in primary care. It will examine the continuing controversy over screening, and even whether it is worthwhile. Detailed information on the running of the screening programme, including the taking of smears, is not comprehensively dealt with, as it is in two small booklets (Austoker and McPherson 1992; BSCC 1989). The former was a major source in the preparation of this chapter.

FACTS AND FIGURES

Incidence

In the UK during 1985 (the latest year for which figures are available), 4496 new cases of invasive cervical cancer were registered. This makes it the eighth most common cancer in women, with an incidence rate of 158 new cases per million female population. Eighty-four per cent of new cases of invasive cancer occur in women aged 35 and over. About 9000 women were registered in 1985 with pre-malignant conditions. The vast majority (87 per cent) of *in situ* cases are registered in women under 45.

Nevertheless, trends in the UK between 1971 and 1985 show that there has been a significant increase in the incidence of both carcinoma *in situ* and invasive carcinoma for *young women*. Between 1971 and 1985, in the age group 25–34 years, the rates more than doubled for invasive carcinoma and trebled for carcinoma *in situ*. Carcinoma *in situ* and severe dysplasia are now considered together as cervical intraepithelial neoplasia grade III (CIN III). For carcinoma *in situ* there has been little change in the rates in other age groups, but for invasive carcinoma the rates have decreased in the older age groups, particularly for women aged 45–54 years.

These trends need, however, to be carefully interpreted, because they are influenced by the increase in screening, particularly for younger women. Thus at least part of the trend in age-specific incidence may be the result of the screening programme, not a true increase; although there is certainly a true increase in mortality in younger women.

There is a cohort effect in that women born in the five years around 1921 have higher rates of invasive carcinoma of the cervix and higher mortality rates throughout their lives than for previous birth cohorts this century. For subsequent birth cohorts the rates are lower until 1941. From 1941 the progressively higher incidence and mortality rates for more recent cohorts fits the theory that cervical cancer could be a sexually transmitted disease whose spread has been facilitated by freer sexual relationships.

Mortality

In 1990, 2070 women died of cervical cancer in England and Wales. Ninety-four per cent of these cases were in women aged 35 and over.

Over the last 20 to 30 years there has been a marked decrease in the mortality of women aged 45 and over. However, for younger women there has been a significant increase in mortality despite screening, particularly for women aged 25 to 34. Although this means only approximately 100 women per year, it represents a large number of life-years lost.

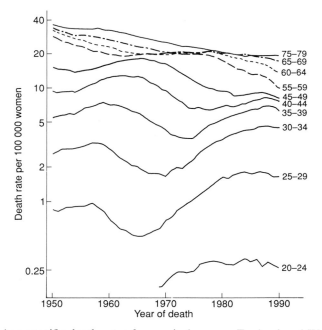

Fig. 8.1 Age-specific death rates for cervical cancer, England and Wales, 1950–90. [Source: P. Sasieni (1991). Trends in cervical cancer mortality. (Letter). *Lancet*, **338**, 818–19.]

There is also a considerable regional variation in cervical cancer mortality in the UK, showing a marked North–South divide. Analysis of the figures for district health authorities (DHAs) show that the 20 DHAs with the highest standardized mortality ratios (SMRs) are all in the northern half of the country.

NATURAL HISTORY

The natural history of invasive cervical cancer and carcinoma *in situ* remains uncertain, a factor which obviously has a profound influence on trying to formulate a screening policy.

The natural history is complicated by the fact that the investigative procedure of performing a biopsy on the cervix may itself in some cases be curative. The questions to which one would theoretically like definite answers *are*:

(1) what number of positive smears progress to invasive carcinoma?

(2) what numbers regress to normal?

(3) how long do these changes take to occur?

(4) what factors influence these changes?

The studies dealing with the first question are conflicting and not made easy to compare by the variation in what has been identified as the different stages of dysplasia as against carcinoma *in situ*. The popular theory is that there is a progression to invasive carcinoma of the cervix through various different phases, as illustrated in Fig. 8.2, although histologically all stages may be present at the same time—a fact that neither refutes nor confirms this hypothesis. Evidence to support this theory comes from several studies.

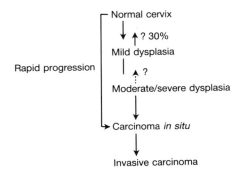

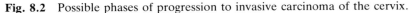

Fig. 8.2 Possible phases of progression to invasive carcinoma of the cervix.

The malignant potential of cervical intraepithelial neoplasia grade III (CIN III, or severe dysplasia/carcinoma *in situ*) is well established. Kinlen and Spriggs (1978) attempted to trace a group of women who had had positive smears with no clinical signs but who for two years had escaped follow-up on treatment, and managed to examine 60 of the original 107. Seven had clinically diagnosed carcinoma of the cervix, and five of these were dying from the disease. Further smears and/or biopsies were carried out on the remaining 53. In 30 per cent of the 60 followed up the smear had become negative or biopsy showed no lesion, suggesting that spontaneous regression had occurred. This regression was confined to women aged less than 40 at the time of the original smear. In 20 cases biopsy showed dysplasia or carcinoma *in situ*; in three microinvasive carcinoma; and in three others invasive carcinoma.

The natural history of minor epithelial atypia (CIN I, or mild dysplasia) remains controversial. Walker *et al.* (1986) followed up 228 women referred to a colposcopy clinic over a 10-year period with mildly atypical cervical cytology who had histological diagnosis established by colposcopically directed biopsy. Sixty-two per cent had CIN II or III and the percentage was greater, 69 per cent, when the smear was dyskaryotic. They concluded that although grossly abnormal cytology correlates well with histological findings, their results did not show such good correlation with lesser grades of cytological abnormality.

The older literature based on cytological and epidemiological evidence suggests that progression from cervical dysplasia to carcinoma *in situ* normally takes over 10 years. Most invasive carcinomas occur in women over 40, most dysplasia in the younger age group. Recently, however, reports have appeared that in a small number of cases progression may be more rapid, and invasive cancer may develop within five years of a normal test (Roberts *et al.* 1985). It is not known what percentage progresses rapidly nor which patients they will be. Obviously an increase in the overall number of rapidly growing cancers could result simply from an overal increase in the incidence of cervical cancer. Some patients with apparently rapidly progressive lesions have had only one previous smear; because of the probability of false-negative results two consecutive satisfactory smears are better evidence that no abnormality is present. It should be stated that in Aberdeen where a large percentage of the population have had a smear, only 2 per cent of women found to have invasive cervical carcinoma had had a negative smear within the preceding five years, while 90 per cent had never had a smear (MacGregor *et al.* 1985).

Further light on the subject comes from the Green 'experiment' in New Zealand. This experiment or trial was set up in 1966 and followed women with minor abnormalities by repeated smears and colposcopy (Coney 1988). Green did not believe that minor abnormalities developed into invasive cancer, and therefore watched the progress of these lesions without giving treatment. Those that did progress were excluded from the trial. The conduct of the trial was seen as a scandal. Unfortunately, because of political sensitivities, a full analysis of the data which could give good information on natural history has not been carried out.

PROGNOSIS

Although this chapter deals primarily with precancerous lesions of the cervix, it is important to know the prognosis once the diagnosis of invasive cancer has been made. It is 'staged', which is a way of describing how far it has spread, and the stages are:

Stage I   Cancer confined to the cervix.
Stage II   Cancer has spread beyond the cervix but not on to the pelvic wall.
Stage III Cancer has spread on to the pelvic wall.
Stage IV Cancer has spread more widely.

The percentages of women who will survive five years after treatment for the different stages are given in Table 8.1.

Table 8.1   *Stage and prognosis of cancer of the cervix*

Stage	Description	5-year survival rate %
	Precancerous lesions	99–100
I	Cancer confined to cervix	79
II	Cancer has spread beyond the cervix but not on to the pelvic wall	47
III	Cancer has spread on to the pelvic wall	22
IV	Cancer has spread more widely	7
All stages		57

Source: CRC Factsheet 12.1.

RISK FACTORS

In order to develop a screening programme it helps to know the risk factors involved in developing carcinoma of the cervix. Factors related to risk either directly or indirectly include:

(1) sexual behaviour;

(2) sexually transmitted factors;

(3) parity and age at first pregnancy;

(4) method of contraception;

(5) occupation and social class;

(6) smoking;

(7) history of dyskaryosis.

One could make up a scoring system, as indicated in Table 8.2, to try and develop a risk table and thus work out a screening policy for each woman.

Table 8.2 *Risk factors in developing carcinoma of the cervix*

Risk factor	Low risk	High risk	Relative risk		
			<2	2–4	4+
Sexual partners	Few	Many			X
Age at first intercourse	Old	Young			X
Social class	Non-manual	Manual	X		
Smoking	No	Yes		X	
STD	Never	Ever			X
OC use	<5 yrs	5 yrs+	X		
Cervical smear	Ever	Never			X
Age	Young	Old			X

Sexual behaviour

Epidemiological studies of risk factors for carcinoma of the cervix have tended, until recently, to pay more attention to the sexual behaviour of women than to that of men. It was not initially realized that not only age at first intercourse, number of sexual partners, and frequency of intercourse of the women may be important, but also the sexual habits of their partners or husbands. Evidence for this comes from a study of two groups of women with and without cervical pathology, all of whom had had only one sexual partner. When these partners were interviewed the number of their sexual contacts was found to be a significant risk factor in the development of cervical pathology (Buckley *et al.* 1981).

Age at first intercourse was always thought to be an important risk factor, but more recently it has been shown that when adjustment is made for the number of sexual partners, there appears to be no clear relationship with age. However, in trying to identify at-risk categories, young age at first intercourse can be included as this group of women are likely to have more partners during their lives than those starting sexual activity later, and will thus be at increased risk. The number of sexual partners is a definite risk factor and there is a linear relationship between the number of partners that a woman has had and the likelihood of her developing cervical changes. Compared to having one partner, two partners increase the age-standardized incidence rate by 3, and three or more partners by 5. What evidence there is does not link increased frequency of intercourse *per se* with increased cervical changes.

Sexually transmitted factors

The most popular theory of the causation of cervical cancer is an infection passed venereally. There is an increasing mass of evidence to implicate certain strains of papilloma or wart virus. In 1976 and 1977 two laboratories working independently reported an association between wart virus infection and cervical cancer. Since then there have been great advances in our knowledge of human papilloma viruses (HPV) and their relationship with cervical neoplasia. Different strains of HPV have been identified. Correlation of virus type with the morphology of the cervical lesion shows that HPV 16 and 18 are present in over 80 per cent of invasive squamous cancers of the cervix, vulva, and penis, and in the higher grades of intraepithelial neoplasia of the cervix and vulva (CIN III and VIN III). In contrast, HPV types 6 and 11 are more often associated with benign warts or mild dysplasia (CIN I or II). It is therefore thought that different HPV strains vary in their oncogenic potential.

A prospective study of 100 women under 30 years old with cytological and colposcopic evidence of mild cervical atypia consistent with CIN I showed that 26 per cent progressed to CIN III; spontaneous regression occurred in only 11 cases, and in four of these CIN recurred. The prevalence of HPV 16 in this group was 39 per cent but in the cases with progressive disease 85 per cent were positive for HPV 16 (Campion *et al.* 1986).

Other theories put forward have included an association with herpes virus type II, a carcinogenic effect of smegma, and that products from sperm may induce malignant change in cervical cells at a particular stage of cell division.

Parity and age of first pregnancy

There appears to be no association between risk and age at menarche. Virgin women have the lowest risk of severe dysplasia and carcinoma *in situ*, and women having a late pregnancy have relative risks lower than those with an early pregnancy. An increased number of pregnancies increases the risk of cervical abnormalities but there appears to be no clear relationship once other confounding factors such as number of sexual partners is allowed for, and it is likely to be an associative rather than a causative factor. Pregnancy outside marriage, termination, and divorce have at some time all been shown to be associated with an increased risk, but it is unlikely that these will all hold up to closer scrutiny once other variables are allowed for.

Method of contraception

Certain methods of contraception may have a direct adverse effect, such as the hormonal influence of the Pill, while others, such as the barrier methods, may actually have a protective effect. Long-term use of oral contraceptives has been shown in several studies to be associated with cervical abnormalities. Some of these findings have been questioned because of inadequate control of confounding factors such as age at first intercourse, number of sexual partners (both men and women), and inclusion of diaphragm users in the control groups. In several studies (Wright *et al.* 1978; Vessey *et al.* 1983; WHO Collaborative Study 1985) in which many of these factors were taken into account, there was still a higher relative risk for people on the contraceptive pill. Another difficulty in trying to evaluate the effect of the Pill is that oral contraceptives may cause eversion of the endocervix making abnormalities easier to detect. Thus, the direct importance of the oral contraceptive in the pathogenesis of cervical dysplasia and invasive carcinoma is still controversial and the issue is unlikely to be resolved until more prospective long-term studies are reported.

On the other hand, diaphragm-users and users of other barrier methods have a decreased risk of cervical abnormalities, as shown in several studies. However, diaphragm-users are less likely to have had coitus at an early age and have usually had fewer sexual partners. Even when these factors and the frequency of intercourse are allowed for, they have a much lower risk; though when looking at barrier methods the possible effect of spermicides should also be considered. But again the difficulties of interpretation are many, for although spermicides may have a direct effect, protective or otherwise, they are not applied by all users of barrier methods.

Occupation and social class

Mortality statistics for cervical cancer show a steep social-class gradient. The disease is five times as common in social class V as it is in the professional classes, which may in part explain the regional variation within England, and it is more common in urban than rural areas. Social class variation may also reflect women's different usage of preventive medical services. It may, of course, not be a direct effect of social class. In one study (Harris *et al.* 1980) that looked at the characteristics of women with dysplasia or carcinoma *in situ*, no social class influence was found once the other risk factors had been taken into account, such as earlier marriage, more pregnancies, more partners, etc.

The wives of men working in certain occupations are more likely to develop cancer of the cervix. For example, wives of miners, quarrymen, fishermen, and glass and ceramic workers have a higher incidence than expected within their socio-economic group. There may well be reasons, sexual or otherwise, to explain this, as some of these jobs involve absence from home, but few epidemiological studies have looked at the social and occupational risks with regard to cancer of the cervix. Nevertheless, the explanation could be a direct one such as dust under the male foreskin (Robinson 1982). Recent data on this are not available.

Until the beginning of the 1970s mortality data for women by their own occupation were only available for single women whose deaths from cervical cancer were few and who were more likely to be sexually inactive than married women. The only occupation that did have a significantly raised cervical cancer rate was textile workers but it is difficult to disentangle the possible effects of husband's occupation and other risk factors until more data are collected which actually look at these possible associations.

Smoking

The emergence in several studies of cigarette smoking as a major risk factor for cervical neoplasia is difficult to understand as at first sight it seems unlikely that the use of tobacco has any direct effect on the cervix. It may be that smoking reflects some important aspect of sexual behaviour or is indirectly linked via other social-class factors. There are no published laboratory findings establishing a direct effect of smoking on cervical cells, although it has been suggested that this is possible as (a) it is known that the carcinogenic products of cigarette smoke are absorbed from the respiratory tract and excreted at distant sites, e.g. breast ducts and in the urine; (b) nicotine and cotinine have been detected in the cervical fluid of smokers; and (c) chemical carcinogens can enhance the *in vitro* carcinogenicity of certain viruses. In many of these studies the sexual habits of the male partner and his occupation have not been allowed for, but where they have, smoking still comes out as a strong independent risk factor.

PRIMARY PREVENTION

Cervical screening is secondary prevention. At present, the exact cause of cervical cancer is not known so that primary prevention is difficult, and from what we do know may not always be socially acceptable. However, from the risk factors already mentioned information can and should be given to women (and men) to allow decisions to be made which may help in primary prevention. Thus available information on primary prevention would include:

(1) fewer partners (for both men and women);
(2) barrier methods of contraception and avoidance of long-term use of the Pill;
(3) avoidance of intercourse with partners with genital or rectal warts, and hence avoidance of the spread of papilloma virus;
(4) advice to heavy smokers to stop or reduce.

GUIDE-LINE FOR SCREENING

The present guide-lines in the UK are that all women aged 20–64 who are or ever have been sexually active should be screened. It is suggested that screening should stop at age 65 if a woman has had regular negative smears, but that there is no upper age limit for having a first smear. It is also suggested that a smear should be taken at least every five years. Women who have never been sexually active do not need to be screened. Different countries and individual doctors operate under different guide-lines. Trying to establish consensus has been extremely difficult.

ORGANIZATION

The vast majority of screening cervical smears are taken in general practice. For the programme to be effective all the participants, i.e. the FHSA, the GP/FHSA interface, and the primary care management team within practices have to be committed and efficient and the screening carried out in a spirit of co-operation. Two major changes have occurred in recent years in the organization of the cervical screening programme. Firstly, there is now a national call and recall system normally based on the FHSAs which have been computerized and can classify which women need smears. The other major change is the method of payment for this service to GPs since the 1990 contract. Payment is dependent on reaching quarterly targets of 50 per cent or 80 per cent coverage of the eligible population with a differential of 3:1 in favour of the latter.

Practice organization

Organization of cervical screening varies from one practice to another and there is no one right way. Smears can be taken at many different times, i.e. in special cervical smear clinics, women's health clinics, family planning clinics, or during normal surgery appointments. The best rates of coverage will be reached by combining a mixture of a call/recall system with opportunistic screening of those who fall through the call/recall net. However it is arranged, it is necessary to have a system and to have *someone* responsible for running it. Whoever takes the smears needs to be adequately trained (increasingly, practice nurses are taking many of them). A sizeable proportion of women would prefer a woman to take their smear, although most women are happy to be examined by their usual doctor.

GPs are now issued with regular FHSA lists of women aged 20–64 who need to be screened. These lists need to be checked before notes are issued. Letters of invitation can be sent via the FHSA or from the practice. The advantage of the latter is that an appointment time can be included, and it has been shown that there is better attendance when this method is used. Explanatory leaflets will also improve the uptake. Patients who do not attend should have their notes flagged so that the opportunistic approach can be used when they next attend the surgery. This is a useful back-up as 75 per cent of women consult their GP in any one year and 90 per cent over a five-year period.

New patients

For *new* patients the registration medical is the ideal time to check on their cervical screening status, and if they have fallen through a previous net or are due for a smear they can be put on the appropriate call/recall system immediately. It is important to do this as there is a time-lag before old notes come through.

Special groups

Temporary and emergency patients are a group who may never get asked about a cervical smear. This does not mean the temporary patient visiting her mother for a few days at Christmas who comes to see the GP because she has a cough. The temporary patients at risk are those who never register permanently, who are frequently on the move, who never get on to an operative call/recall list, and whose lifestyle may put them at increased risk. They are not included in practice targets but even in this money-oriented age they should not be neglected! Other groups that may require special inputs to encourage them to have smears taken are Asian women and travellers. Personal visits and videos have proved effective in increasing the uptake of cervical smear testing among Asian women in Leicester who have never been tested previously.

Fail safe

The general practitioner has certain clearly laid down responsibilities in the fail-safe mechanism:

(1) checking that all smear reports have been received;

(2) informing the woman of the result;

(3) initiating further investigation;

(4) contacting women who do not attend for further investigation;

(5) informing the FHSA if a woman requiring investigation has moved away;

(6) monitoring the 'suspend' and 'repeat advised' lists sent by the FHSA.

Where smears are taken by GP trainees or practice nurses, responsibility lies with the GP principal recorded on the request form.

Where smears are taken outside the primary care setting and the result is sent to the GP, it is important to check who is looking after the follow-up and referral as necessary.

ATTITUDES TO CERVICAL SCREENING

Some women even if invited will not come forward to have a cervical smear. There may be many reasons why women will not have it done, and myths may need to be dispelled. There is, for example, confusion as to what cervical screening is for. Much emphasis is made by health professionals that screening is to pick up precancerous lesions. However, a survey in east London showed that 71 per cent of women thought it was to pick up cancer, and only 12 per cent realized it was to detect disease at the precancerous stage (Savage and Schwartz 1985). The Women's Institute carried out a survey of members in their groups. Common worries expressed by patients include:

'I thought it would hurt.'

'I felt embarrassed about being examined.'

'I didn't want to see a male doctor.'

'I didn't want to bother the doctor.'

'I no longer have sex, so I didn't think I needed one.'

'I'm too old to need one.'

'You can't do anything about it anyway.'

'It's only promiscuous women who get it.'

'I wouldn't want to know if I had cancer anyhow.'

General practitioners also differ in their attitudes to the taking of cervical smears. Havelock *et al.* (JRCGP 1988) interviewed GPs in one area to investigate their attitudes. The large majority of the doctors interviewed were enthusiastic about screening and coped well with the demand for tests from those women requesting it. They made little effort, however, to persuade women to have a test, and many thought they were screening a majority of women over 35 but were in fact mainly screening those under 35.

Other objections raised by doctors include:

'It takes too much time.'

'Women aren't interested.'

'They don't turn up for appointments.'

'They ask for unnecessary smears.'

'It doesn't work anyway.'

Attitudes change. Many factors contribute to change. The way in which the service has been reorganized has effected change, if not in attitude certainly in practice, with more doctors taking more smears from more women since the computerization of the FHSA, a proper call/recall system, and the 1990 GP contract. There has also been good evidence in the past that the reason the majority of women never had a smear taken was that they were never asked to come forward and have one. There will always be women who do not want a smear, but they need to be given the relevant information and then be allowed to choose.

TAKING THE CERVICAL SMEAR

The objective of taking a smear is to identify women whose cytological pattern is suggestive of CIN. One of the key factors determining the effectiveness of a cervical screening programme is the quality of smear-taking. Poor smear-taking can miss 20 per cent or more of precancerous abnormalities in the cervix (BSCC 1989). The practicalities of exactly how to take a smear can be found in the second edition of *Cervical screening* (Austoker and McPherson 1992) and BSCC booklets. Whoever takes the smear should be adequately and appropriately trained whether a doctor or a nurse.

RESULTS

Explanation of the results

There is no point in taking cervical smears unless it is ensured that the results are transmitted to the women, who should be told how and when they are going to get their results at the time the smear is taken. Written information to this effect will avoid confusion, e.g. 'The result will be sent in four weeks; if you do not hear, please contact the practice.' The most commonly used system until now has been 'no news is good news'; or 'the test is normal unless you hear from us'. Unfortunately, this has resulted in poor follow-up of patients who have had abnormal smears. The ideal is to send out results to all women who have had a smear informing them whether it is negative or positive and when the next smear is due. Some practices ask women to leave a self-addressed envelope, some ask women to 'phone in', but all too often there is no check as to whether this has happened.

If women are told when the smear is taken that there may be a need to repeat it as it might be technically inadequate, or show a mild abnormality which does not indicate cancer, much anxiety can be avoided later. To put it into perspective: 5–10 per cent of all smears will be inadequate, 4–5 per cent will show borderline or mild dyskaryosis, and 1.5–2 per cent moderate or severe dyskaryosis.

Interpretation of smear results

Smear results can sometimes be difficult to interpret. The smear may be normal in that there is no nuclear abnormality, but other comments may be made. When a smear is reported with some abnormal cells the action required will depend on many factors, including the appearance of any previous smears. If you do not understand a smear result, contact your local cytopathologist for clarification.

It must be borne in mind that there is a whole spectrum of abnormality, from completely normal to definitely malignant, and cytological grading is an inexact science. The exact risk consequent on each grade is not clear either.

It also needs to be remembered, when recommending further action, that referral of *all* grades of abnormality would lead to considerable over-investigation and over-diagnosis. A careful balance thus has to be reached, taking into account both the benefits that are likely to ensue and the costs—to women and to the health service in terms of resource implications. Inevitably, opinions will differ on how such a balance is arrived at.

Tables 8.3 and 8.4 summarize the more commonly used terms in the reporting of cervical smears, with guidelines for action.

MANAGEMENT OF WOMEN WITH ABNORMAL CERVICAL SMEARS

The management of patients with abnormal smears is based on the limited available information about the behaviour of CIN. It is known that patients with severe dyskaryosis (suggesting CIN III) have a risk of progression to invasive cancer sufficiently high and immediate to merit early biopsy for histological confirmation followed by treatment. This action is also to exclude reliably the presence of an invasive carcinoma in such cases. The

Table 8.3 *Interpretation of smear results: result codes and action*

Result	Explanation	Action
Inadequate	Insufficient cellular material Inadequate fixation Smear consisting mainly of blood or inflammatory cell exudate Little or no material to suggest that the transformation zone has been sampled	Repeat smear
Negative	Normal. Includes simple inflammatory changes including a mild polymorph exudate.	Routine recall
Borderline changes, with or without HPV change	Cellular appearance that cannot be described as normal. Smears in which there is doubt as to whether the nuclear changes are inflammatory or dyskaryosis	Repeat smear at 6 months. Consider for colposcopy if changes persist.
Mild dyskaryosis with or without HPV change	Cellular appearances consistent with origin from CIN 1 (mild dysplasia)	Repeat smear at 6 months. Consider for colposcopy if changes persist.
Moderate dyskaryosis with or without HPV change	Cellular appearances consistent with origin from CIN 2 (moderate dysplasia)	Refer for colposcopy.
Severe dyskaryosis with or without HPV change	Cellular appearances consistent with origin from CIN 3 (severe dysplasia/carcinoma *in situ*)	Refer for colposcopy.
Severe dyskaryosis/? invasive carcinoma	Cellular appearances consistent with origin from CIN 3, but with additional features which suggest the possibility of invasive cancer	Refer for colposcopy.
Glandular neoplasia or suspicion of glandular neoplasia	Cellular appearances suggesting pre-cancer or cancer in the cervical canal or the endometrium	Refer for colposcopy.

Note: The use of the term 'atypical cells' is no longer recommended in the Result Codes and its use should be discontinued. The preferred term is 'Borderline changes' ('atypia' may still be used in the free-text comment, but the degree of atypia should be clarified in the Result Code).

Sources: BSCC, *Taking cervical smears*, 1989, p. 18;; A. McPherson, *Cervical screening: a practical guide* (first edition), (OUP 1985); I. Duncan (ed.), *Draft guidelines for clinical practice and programme management* (NHSCSP 1991).

Table 8.4 *Interpretation of specific negative cervical smear reports*

Result code	Explanation	Action
Specific infections	*Trichomonas*, *Candida*, and cell changes associated with *Herpes simplex* can be identified	*Trichomonas*—treat *Candida*—treat if symptoms *Herpes*—no treatment—discuss with patient
Actinomyces	Organisms associated with IUD	No consensus. Alternatives: 1. Do nothing unless other symptoms e.g. pain or discharge 2. Change coil and the actinomyces organisms will disappear
Endocervical cells	Cells from the glandular epithelium of the cervical canal. During its formation the transformation zone will include similar epithelium	No action needed
Metaplastic cells (metaplasia/squamous metaplasia)	Normal cells from the transformation zone	No action needed
Cytolysis	Normal process of cell disintegration	No action needed
Endometrial cells	Cells derived from the endometrial lining of the uterine cavity. Shed during menstruation and in some other circumstances	If IUD present—probably normal finding. If 1–12 day of 28 day cycle—normal finding. Otherwise discuss with laboratory or local gynaecologist.
Inflammatory changes	Cellular appearance present in some degree in many smears and not evidence of CIN	No consensus. Alternatives: 1. Do nothing 2. Take high vaginal swabs for culture and sensitivity and take chlamydial swabs. Then treat as necessary.
Atrophic smear	Common in postmenopausal smears, i.e. when oestrogen and progesterone levels are low. Similar changes are seen in postnatal smears	No action needed

behaviour of mild and moderate dyskaryosis is less certain, but there is no doubt that a number of these abnormalities will progress to invasive cancer if untreated. It is not possible at present to predict behaviour from morphological appearances, and there is disagreement as to whether all patients with mild dyskaryosis should be referred for further investigation (see p. 249).

Before the advent of colposcopy, cone biopsy or hysterectomy were the standard treatments for the most severe grades of CIN. These can be avoided in 80–90 per cent of patients by the use of colposcopically directed biopsies. CIN can be effectively destroyed by electro-diathemy, cryosurgery, laser evaporation, or cold coagulation. Alternatively, the transformation zone may be excised using a large cutting electro-surgical loop (laser loop excision). The benefit here is that it combines diagnosis and treatment in one visit which is advantageous to the patient. These procedures are usually associated with uterine pain. Local anaesthetic is of limited value and general anaesthesia is rarely required. These locally destructive methods have the advantage of preserving cervical function and have thus become acceptable in treating more minor degrees of CIN.

If the smear is reported as having malignant cells or carcinoma *in situ*, confirmation of the cytology report requires cervical biopsy. By arranging this quickly, the doctor can relieve the patient's anxiety about the extent of the disease as soon as possible. If the cervix looks malignant clinically, then it is best to prepare the woman for hearing this in hospital, possibly suggesting that she is accompanied there by her partner or a friend. If the cervix is clinically normal on examination by the naked eye, then the question of frank malignancy need not be raised and one should prepare the woman for colposcopy and/or biopsy.

Colposcopy

The colposcope is a low-powered microscope for viewing the cervix. During the investigation the patient lies on her back with her legs up in stirrups. A speculum is passed into the vagina to visualize the cervix before using the colposcope, which is mainly used for the investigation and management of cervical intraepithelial neoplasia (CIN).

Colposcopy takes about 15 minutes to carry out, and should not be painful, although it is uncomfortable. It allows the clinician to view the cervix very carefully in order to assess the extent and severity of any lesion properly and to provide appropriate treatment. A biopsy is usually taken and this can be acutely painful. Approximately 2–4 per cent of all smears will need referral of the woman for colposcopy, depending on what guide-lines for referral are used. Women having colposcopy may get very high levels of anxiety about both the procedure and the outcome, which can be decreased by adequate information and counselling before and during the procedure. In a study by Posner and Vessey (1988) many patients complained of the profuse vaginal discharge which lasted up to a month after the cryocautery as being particularly troublesome. Fifty-two per cent also had disturbed feelings about sexual relationships after colposcopy.

Follow-up after treatment

Follow-up is necessary to identify any residual disease, to identify new CIN or invasive disease, and, perhaps most important, to reassure the patient (and the doctor).

Duncan (1991) has recommended the following guide-lines:

1. Cytological follow-up is essential following treatment for CIN. Colposcopy is not essential, but may enhance detection of persistent disease at six months.
2. Following treatment, the first smear should be taken at six months and, if normal, repeated at 12 months.
3. More frequent surveillance need not be continued beyond five years of normal findings after conservative treatment for CIN III.
4. Women undergoing hysterectomy with a past or current history of CIN III need have no further smears if the cytology is normal six and 12 months after surgery.

THE NEGATIVE ASPECTS OF SCREENING

In evaluating any screening programme the negative aspects are sometimes forgotten and are rarely quantified. Campion *et al.* (1988) looked at women under investigation for CIN compared to women investigated as partners of men with sexually transmitted diseases, and found that CIN had a strong negative effect on sexual feelings and behaviour six months later, whereas the psychosexuality of those who had not had CIN treatment did not change.

There are many anecdotal stories and books now written of how women feel about having an abnormal smear, and the doctor should always be humble enough to listen to patients' opinions.

I felt dirty inside, as if I was rotten to the core. My imagination ran riot—I felt as if I was 'bad' in the most intimate and feminine part of my body. I was like an apple that looks crisp and juicy from the outside but inside is crawling with maggots. As you can imagine, this had a devastating effect on my sex life. Why wasn't I able to go to my doctors and tell them honestly how I felt?

CONTROVERSIES

Over the last few years there has been an attempt to get consensus in areas of screening policy. However, there are still many areas of uncertainty and further research and information is necessary to resolve these areas of controversy. Some of these issues are discussed below.

1. *Is screening cost-effective?*

The jury is still out. It has been argued by Skrabenek and others that the screening programme has failed in the UK, is not cost-effective, and should be stopped. This, of course, begs the question of who judges the cost-effectiveness, the women, the doctors or the politicians. It is true that the overall mortality from cervical cancer has not been significantly reduced in the UK compared to other countries, but until now the population coverage has been poor. A proper call and recall system has now been in place since March 1988 with coverage rates in 1990 showing:

England 74 per cent (79 per cent excluding Thames Region)
Wales 70 per cent
Northern Ireland 68 per cent

It is only by the late 1990s that the true cost-effectiveness data will start to be available (Farmery 1992).

2. *How often should smears be taken?*

The Department of Health has recommended that a smear should be taken 'at least every 5 years'. There is considerable local variation—some DHAs do five-yearly screening, some three-yearly, and some a mixture of both. This is further complicated by the fact that GP target payments relate to smears taken over a 5.5-year period. Because the natural history of the disease is not well understood, the optimum interval remains a subject of debate and an important research issue. Attempts have been made to show the effects on cervical cancer incidence of different screening policies.

As can be seen from Table 8.5, the advantage of one-year over three-year screening intervals is very small, whereas there is a significant difference between three and five yearly screening. This is the rationale for three-yearly screening.

3. *Should younger women be screened more frequently?*

For younger women, particularly those aged 25 to 34, there has been a significant increase in cervical cancer incidence and mortality rates over the past 10–15 years. Some DHAs screen women under 35 at three-yearly intervals, and women over 35 at five-year intervals. There is no evidence to support this decision one way or another. Further research on the natural history of the disease is necessary, for example to clarify whether the disease is more aggressive in younger women or not.

4. *Should high-risk women be screened more frequently?*

Although there are several risk factors associated with an increased risk of invasive cervical cancer (see p. 231), it is *not* possible to use these factors

Table 8.5 *Effects on cervical cancer incidence of different screening policies, starting at age 20*

Screening schedule	Reduction in rate (%)	No. of tests
Every 10 years, 25–64	61	4
Every 10 years, 35–64	55	3
Every 10 years, 45–64	43	2
Every 5 years, 20–64	84	9
Every 5 years, 30–64	81	7
Every 3 years, 20–64	91	15
Every year, 20–64	93	45

From IARC Working Group 1986; assuming incidence rates from Cali, Colombia. The first screening test is assumed to be 70 per cent sensitive.

reliably to predict which women will develop CIN. Moreover, there is no evidence that these risk factors affect the rate of progression of CIN. Thus it has been argued that there is little value in targeting these women for screening or selecting them for more frequent screening.

5. *Is screening teenagers worthwhile?*
The prevalence of invasive carcinoma of the cervix does not justify including women under the age of 20 in the routine screening programme, provided that there is good uptake in women aged 20 to 25. While CIN does exist in teenagers, invasive cancer is extremely rare. There is no rational basis for routinely screening teenagers, regardless of whether they are 'promiscuous' or not; a smear is not needed for at least two to three years after becoming sexually active. In particular cases an approach could be to take a smear where a teenage girl has had multiple sexual partners for over three years. This is *not* screening, but a matter of responding to individual cases on merit.

6. *Is screening 65-year-olds and over worthwhile?*
Although a substantial number of cases of cervical cancer occur in women aged 65 and over, an effective screening programme should detect pre-cancerous lesions in those under 65, and thus reduce the incidence of invasive disease in older women. Women aged 65 and over should be encouraged to have a smear if they have not previously been screened; but there is, of course, the added complication that the smear is more difficult to take for the smear-taker and the woman for physiological reasons.

7. *Which spatula?*

There are many different spatulae on the market. The Aylesbury spatula is most widely used and is a wooden spatula which has a tip larger than the old Ayres spatula and has been shown to be more likely to sample cervical cells as well as transformation zone squamous cells. The flatter reverse end may be used for a patulous cervix or a vault smear.

Recently, a study in GP practice showed that the newer plastic Cervex sampler gave a better pick-up of endocervical cells (78.2 per cent compared to 62.8 per cent) and fewer inadequate smears, although the percentage of abnormals was the same. Other studies have shown an increased number of blood-stained smears with the Cervex or other plastic samplers. The Cervex sampler costs about seven times as much as the Aylesbury type (20p compared to 3p). Furthermore, larger studies would be needed to evaluate properly the cost-benefit before any national change is recommended.

Another alternative is the cytobrush, which can also be used to sample the endocervix, and is mainly used in colposcopy clinics or when the cervix is distorted by surgery or local ablation. It may be used in addition to a spatula in some instances, for example when the woman has had two previous smears showing insufficient cells. Beware, as one is likely to get more bleeding; so get the spatula sample first. The cytobrush is *not* the method of choice in primary screening, because it does not always sample the transformation zone, and provides smears of sparse cellularity, which dry quickly and need very rapid fixation. It is also more expensive than the Aylesbury spatula.

8. *What is the best way to sterilize the equipment?*

It is important that the practice has adequate facilities for sterilizing the equipment used: soaking in Savlon and/or reusing a plastic speculum does *not* destroy the papilloma virus (Skegg and Paul 1986). Papilloma viruses are stable viruses and it is recommended that all instruments are autoclaved between patients. If this is not possible the instruments should be washed and put in boiling water for 10 minutes. The HIV virus will also be destroyed by these procedures.

9. *When in the menstrual cycle to take the smear?*

There are changes in the cervical epithelium during the menstrual cycle, although these do not reflect the hormonal changes as accurately as do the changes in the vaginal epithelium. Taking smears during menstruation is not a practice welcomed by most cytologists as erythrocytes, leucocytes, endometrial cells, and blood pigments obscure the field. However, in high-risk women any chance should be seized as they may not present again, and a note should be made about menstruation on the request form. Following menstruation and after ovulation, i.e. days 10–20 of the 28-day cycle, is probably the best time to take a smear as there are few polymorphs and the cells are mature. Histiocytes may be seen up to the 12th day of the cycle, which gives a dirty background to the smear. However, while in planning screening mid-cycle smears are ideal, rarely should a woman needing a smear (especially if high risk) be asked to return at another time.

10. *Is there a role for cervicography?*

Current studies of cervicography give a false-positive rate up to ten times higher than that for routine cervical smears, thereby leading to an unnecessarily high number of referrals for colposcopy. Cervicography may well pick up additional 'abnormalities', but the majority of these may be of no clinical significance. The cost of cervicography is higher than that for the cervical smear. So despite problems in the interpretation of cervical smears, cervicography cannot be seen at present as an alternative. There is currently no routine clinical role for cervicography in either primary cervical screening or in the assessment of patients with abnormal cytology.

11. *Do you need endocervical cells present on the smear for it to be adequate?*

A cervical smear if properly taken should contain cells from the whole of the transformation zone, which should therefore be adequately sampled (BSCC 1989). Squamous epithelial cells will normally be the most numerous cell type. The main evidence of an adequate smear is that it should contain a sufficient quantity of epithelial cells, taking into account a woman's age and her hormonal status.

An indication that the transformation zone has been properly sampled is the additional presence of endocervical columnar cells and recognizable metaplastic cells, but these can sometimes be difficult to identify as they become more mature. Owing to the variable nature of the transformation zone, *only one* of these cell types may be present on the smear. Endocervical cells may not always be seen in smears from postmenopausal women or those with atrophic smears. If the smear-taker is sure that the cervix was well sampled and the appropriate area was fully sampled, the absence of endocervical cells is not necessarily an indication to repeat the smear. But if the smear-taker feels there was a problem in sampling and there is no good evidence of transformation zone material in the smear, then an early repeat is necessary. Best to make a note at the time!

12. *How should HPV be managed?*

The role of HPV in cervical cancer causation is still uncertain. The apparent universal presence of the virus has been recognized, and adds to this uncertainty. Cell changes suggesting HPV infection are no longer in themselves considered an indication for more frequent screening. Therefore it is recommended that the management of women with HPV should be according to the CIN grade present, and not simply because of the presence of HPV (see Table 8.6). Smears showing viral change but no nuclear change should be considered normal and the woman recalled at normal frequency.

The presence of a particular strain of the virus, HPV16, may be an important prognostic marker for identifying women who are at risk of developing severe cervical disease. At some time in the future, viral typing may be a second discriminator in the process of deciding which lesions to treat. This is not the case at present. For treatment of the vulval warts see Chapter 10.

Table 8.6 *What women will need to know if the presence of HPV is reported*

- The wart virus in its subclinical state requires no specific treatment such as antibiotics. Referral to an STD/GUM clinic is not necessary.
- The changes are evidence of contact with the virus at some stage in the woman's life, and may not indicate an active infection.
- There are parallels with skin warts and many other viral conditions, where only very few contacts develop the clinical infection.
- The virus is usually transmitted sexually; but this is *not* the only way, as it has been isolated from other sites in the body and has also been found in children.
- The natural history of wart virus changes is to regress over a period of several years. One particular strain of the virus, HPV 16, may be an important prognostic marker for identifying patients who are at risk of developing severe cervical disease. Other factors such as smoking or lowered immunity may also come into play.
- In a steady relationship there is no need to change contraception; but if a woman is likely to have any sexual contact outside an established relationship, barrier methods might be used.
- Subclinical warts are not known to affect pregnancy, fertility, or the baby. Clinical warts should be treated prior to delivery.
- Visible cervical warts are thought to be more easily transmitted than subclinical HPV.

Note: Colposcopic treatment does not eradicate the presence of wart virus.

Source: Oxfordshire DHA 1991. *Cervical screening information factsheet.*

13. *What is the appropriate management of mild dyskaryosis?*

While the consensus view is that a single mildly dyskaryotic smear should be managed by a repeat smear at six months and only referred for colposcopy if the abnormality persists, there are those who believe that such smears should be referred immediately for colposcopy. This is because, while the majority of such smears will revert to normal or persist as mildly dyskaryotic, a small proportion may progress to severe dyskaryosis over a period of time. A balance obviously has to be achieved here between ensuring appropriate management and not subjecting too many women to unnecessary medical procedures. A study of over 200 patients by Jones *et al.* having cytological surveillance of mild dyskaryosis resulted in a 12 per cent risk of patients having a small CIN3 lesion after two years, but this risk was reduced to 4 per cent by the addition of a third repeat smear twelve months after the second. With such a policy only about a third of women would require colposcopy, and the risk of missing serious underlying precancerous changes would be low. Further research is clearly needed to assess the role of cytological surveillance in mild dyskaryosis and to determine its optimal management. The Aberdeen Birthright Project has been set up to evaluate the safety and effectiveness of a cytology-based approach to the management of both mild and moderate dyskaryosis.

14. *When should the cervix be treated?*

There is a whole spectrum of abnormality from completely normal to definitely malignant. Ideally, it is important to have some idea of the rate of progression of abnormalities. Currently, however, there is inadequate information available about the natural history of the lower grades of abnormality. A balance must thus be reached between potential overdiagnosis and overtreatment and the need to ensure that invasive cancer does not occur. A treatment policy cannot be defined with any degree of certainty. On balance the present belief is that CIN II and CIN III should be treated once diagnosed, while women with CIN I may be treated or keep under close surveillance.

CONCLUSION

In summary, what we perform in the way of cervical screening is the best we have at the moment, but we should not pretend that it is ideal. There are still many problems, not least the high false-positive and negative rates. In no way should the present screening programme lull us into a sense of 'doing OK'. What is needed is continuing research and evaluation into better, simpler, and cheaper methods for the early identification of cervical cancer; until then we must make the best of what we have.

REFERENCES AND FURTHER READING

Austoker, J. and McPherson, A. (1992). *Cervical screening*. Practical Guides for General Practice, No. 14. Oxford Medical Publications.

BSCC Booklet and Video (1989). *Taking cervical smears*. British Society for Clinical Colposcopy. (For further information contact Dr Keith Randall, Red Tree House, Pine Glade, Keston Park, Orpington, Kent BR6 8NT.)

Buckley, J. D., Harris, R. W. C., Doll, R., *et al.* (1981). Case control study of husbands of women with dysplasia or carcinoma of the cervix uteri. *Lancet,* **ii,** 1010–14.

Campion, M. J., Cuzick, J., McCance, D. J., *et al.* (1986). Progressive potential of mild cervical atypia: prospective cytological, colposcopic, and virological study. *Lancet,* **ii,** 237–40.

Campion, M. J., *et al.* (1988). Psychosexual trauma of an abnormal cervical smear. *British Journal of Obstetrics and Gynaecology,* **95,** 175–81.

Cancer Research Campaign Factsheets (1990). *Cervical cancer* (Factsheet 12). *Cervical cancer screening* (Factsheet 13).

Coney, S. (1988). *The unfortunate experiment*. Penguin, New Zealand.

Cumbrian Practice Research Group (1991). Sampling endocervical cells on cervical smears: a comparison of two instruments used in general practice. *British Journal of General Practice,* **41,** 192–3.

Cuzick, J. (1991). Organisation of cervical screening in England and Wales. In *Cancer screening* (ed. A. B. Miller, J. Chamberlain, N. E. Day, *et al.*). Cambridge University Press.

DHSS (Department of Health and Social Security) (1988). *Cervical cancer screening*. Health Circular HC(88)1.

DoH (Department of Health) (1988). *Cervical cytology and cervical cancer statistics 1976–1986, England and Wales*. Department of Health, London.

DoH (Department of Health) (1989). *Cervical cytology 1987/8*. Department of Health, London.

DoH (Department of Health) (1990). *Cervical cytology 1988/9*. Department of Health, London.

Duncan, I (ed.) (1991). *Guidelines for clinical practice and programme management*. NHS Cervical Screening Programme, Oxford.

Eardley, A., Elkind, A., and Thompson, R. (1990). HEA guidelines for a letter to invite women for a smear test: theory and practice. *Health Education Journal,* **49,** 51–6.

Elwood, J. M., Cotton, R. E., Johnson, J., *et al.* (1984). Are patients with abnormal cervical smears adequately managed? *British Medical Journal,* **289,** 891–4.

Farmery, Elaine (1992). Personal communication.

Harris, R. W. C., Brinton, L. A., Cowdell, R. H., *et al.* (1980). Characteristics of women with dysplasia or cancer *in situ* of the cervix uteri. *British Journal of Cancer,* **42,** 359–69.

Havelock, C. M., Edwards, R., Cuzick, J., *et al.* (1988). The organisation of cervical screening in general practice. *Journal of the Royal College of General Practitioners,* **38,** 207–11.

Jones, M. H., Jenkins, D., Cuzick, J., *et al.* (1992). Mild cervical dyskariosis: safety of cytological surveillance. *Lancet,* **339,** 1440–3.

Kinlen, L. and Spriggs, A. I. (1978). Women with positive smears but without surgical intervention. *Lancet,* **ii,** 463–5.

McAvoy, B. R. and Raza, R. (1991). Can health education increase uptake of cervical smear testing among Asian women? *British Medical Journal,* **302,** 833–6.

MacGregor, J. E., Moss, S. M., Parkin, D. M., *et al.* (1985). A case-control study of cervical screening in North-East Scotland. *British Medical Journal,* **290,** 1543–6.

NHSCSP (1991). Working Party Report.

Oxfordshire DHA (1991). Cervical Screening Information Factsheets. Cytology Department, John Radcliffe Hospital, Oxford.

Paul, C. (1988). The New Zealand Cervical Cancer Study: could it happen again? *British Medical Journal,* **297,** 533–53.

Posner, T. and Vessey, M. (1988). *Prevention of cervical cancer: the patient's view.* King Edward's Hospital Fund for London.

Robinson, J. (1982). Cancer of the cervix—occupational risks of husbands and wives and possible preventive strategies. In *Preclinical neoplasia of the cervix* (ed. J. Jordan, F. Sharp, and A. Singer), pp. 11–22. Royal College of Obstetricians and Gynaecologists, London.

Roberts, A. W., Lane, D. A., Buntine, D., *et al.* (1985). Invasive carcinoma of the cervix in young women. *Medical Journal of Australia,* **143,** 333–5.

Quilliam, S. (1989). *Positive smear.* Penguin Books, London.

Savage, W. and Schwartz, M. (1985). Letter. *Lancet,* **ii,** (8467), 1305.

Singer, A. and Szarewski, A. (1988). *Cervical smear test.* Macdonald, London.

Skegg, D. C. G. and Paul, C. (1986). Viruses, specular and cervical cancer. *Lancet,* **i,** 747.

Vessey, M. P., McPherson, K., Lawless, M., *et al.* (1983). Neoplasia of the cervix uteri and contraception: a possible adverse effect of the pill. *Lancet,* **ii,** 930–4.

Walker, E. M., Dodgson, J., and Duncan, I. D. (1986). Does mild atypia of cervical smear warrant further investigation? *Lancet,* **2,** 672–3.

WHO Collaborative Study (1985). Invasive cervical cancer and combined oral contraceptives. *British Medical Journal,* **290,** 961–5.

Wilkinson, C. (1992). Abnormal cervical smear test results: old dilemmas and new directions. *British Journal of General Practice,* **42,** 336–9.

Wilkinson, C., Jones, J. M., and McBridge, J. (1990). Anxiety caused by abnormal result of cervical smear test: a controlled trial. *British Medical Journal,* **300,** 440.

Wilson, A. and Leeming, A. (1987). Cervical cytology screening: a comparison of two call systems. *British Medical Journal,* **295,** 181–2.

Wolfendale, M., Howe-Guest, R., Usherwood, M., *et al.* (1987). Controlled trial of a new cervical spatula. *British Medical Journal,* **i,** 33–6.

Wright, N. H., Vessey, M. P., Kenward, K., *et al.* (1978). Neoplasia and dysplasia of the cervix uteri and contraception: a possible protective effect of the diaphragm. *British Journal of Cancer,* **38,** 273–9.

9. The 'ectomies

Ann McPherson

WHY DISCUSS 'ECTOMIES?

The idea that removing bits and pieces of the female reproductive system might have beneficial results arose from a variety of initial concepts, some of which are outlined below and most of which no doubt seemed valid at the time. Not surprisingly, many of these in retrospect had dubious scientific basis. The reasons for including a chapter on this subject are essentially that not only is a considerable amount of a general practitioner's time spent in dealing with the symptoms which will lead to these operations being performed, but nowadays even more time will be spent in dealing with their psychosocial consequences.

The operations discussed are hysterectomy, oophorectomy, and mastectomy, although it should be remembered that women are also twice as likely as men to have a cholecystectomy. Hysterectomy and oophorectomy will be dealt with in detail since they are not discussed in detail elsewhere in the book. Most of the discussion of women presenting with a breast lump is in Chapter 2 on breast cancer and benign breast disease, but there is included here a brief look at the psychological and social consequences of mastectomy and the role of the general practitioner in this sphere.

The general practitioner in deciding to refer a patient to a consultant will be aware that the very nature of a 'specialist' opinion means that the broader issues concerning the patient's needs may be focused on to the question of whether to have a specific organ in or out, on or off. Unless the GP indicates clearly what is wanted from the specialist referral, some women may end up with unnecessary surgery, as once referred the hospital machinery may take over. Even with referral, the GP's involvement has only just begun. Whether the decision is to operate or not to operate, the woman will always welcome the chance to have more extensive discussion than hospital consultations normally allow. Part of the reason for this chapter is to provide GPs with the facts which will allow both them and their patients to make better informed decisions themselves. A GP audit of referrals for menstrual disorders in patients aged 15–59 in the five years following referral showed that 81 per cent had been admitted to hospital, with 44 per cent having a hysterectomy and 48 per cent a D&C; 12 per cent received only drug therapy, and 5 per cent no active treatment at all (Coulter *et al.* 1991).

STATISTICS

The figures in this section try to give some sort of numerical perspective to the whole subject of 'ectomies. The number of women in a practice who will have had one of these operations will, of course, vary with the age and sex distribution of the patients. If one takes a so-called 'average' practice of 2000, then 64 women are likely to have had a hysterectomy and 16 a mastectomy (and 16 men a prostatectomy). By the age of 65, 20 per cent of women in the practice will have had a hysterectomy and 4.5 per cent a mastectomy. In 1984 in England and Wales (unfortunately there are no recent published figures available at present because of reorganization of data collection within the NHS), approximately 66 000 hysterectomies were performed, 37 500 mastectomies, 6000 oophorectomies (it is difficult to obtain exact numbers because of the method of coding operations in hospital statistics), and 34 500 prostatectomies. Each GP is likely to be involved in counselling only two women per year for hysterectomy, three women every two years for mastectomy, and one woman every two years for an oophorectomy (and one man every year for prostatectomy and rarely for orchidectomy). The reasons for doing any of the operations will, of course, be varied, particularly for hysterectomy.

If one looks in more detail at hysterectomy, most operations are done for benign disease. In 1984 in Scotland only 9.5 per cent of hysterectomies were for malignancies of the genital tract; 35 per cent were for disorders of menstruation, 20 per cent for fibroids, 9.3 per cent for prolapse, and 26.2 per cent were 'other' (Teo 1990). Whether differences in disease rates explain the variations across the world in hysterectomy rates (Fig. 9.1) is a matter for speculation (McPherson 1982), but it is of interest that the age-standardized hysterectomy rate is three times higher in the USA than in England and Wales. Hysterectomy rates vary widely across the regions, for example, from 180 per 100 000 population at risk per annum in Mersey to about 290 per 100 000 in North-East Thames. There is no social class gradient in hysterectomy rates in England and Wales (Coulter and McPherson 1986).

These differences undoubtedly have complex causes and may depend on factors that have little to do with disease. Women themselves may influence the rates depending on their perception about the need or otherwise for hysterectomy in their circumstances. But as stated earlier in the chapter, the general practitioner may play a central role in the decision-making about referral, and this will be a crucial factor in determining whether or not a woman has a hysterectomy.

HYSTERECTOMY/OOPHORECTOMY

Oophorectomy was first used in the mid-1800s for treatment of ovarian cysts and tumours—these had previously been treated by recurrent tapping.

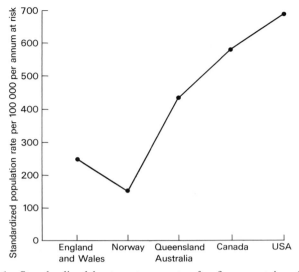

Fig. 9.1 Standardized hysterectomy rates for five countries. (From: McPherson 1982, with permission.)

As one would expect, the morbidity and mortality of the first operations were very high and within the profession there was considerable opposition to performing them. As the operation gradually became safer it was more widely performed. Although the first oophorectomies were performed for pathological disease of the ovaries, it soon became fashionable to do them for other problems. These included the treatment of epilepsy and insanity, and of nervous and psychological problems such as hysteria. It seems that people believed that a woman's personality was an orchestra conducted by her ovaries, and presumably any psychological problems with which a woman presented could be cured or controlled by performing oophorectomy. Clitoridectomy was an operation performed by nineteenth-century surgeons as a cure for another of women's evils—this time masturbation, which was thought to cause numerous physical disorders as well as dementia and overall moral decay. The fashion of clitoridectomy in this country lasted for a short time only and was never as popular as oophorectomy. Clitoridectomy is, however, still practised in some countries.

Female castration was largely superseded by other operations—including hysterectomy, as the womb then became seen as the seat of a woman's psychological problems. But many uteri were removed for pathology, much of it related to infection. The need and outcome were affected by safer surgery, antiseptics, anaesthesia, safer childbirth, fewer pregnancies, etc. Whereas in the nineteenth century, hysterectomy and oophorectomy were performed for psychological as well as pathological reasons, by the middle of the twentieth century hysterectomy, with or without oophorectomy, was often performed with little consideration for the psychological sequelae. It was a common practice to remove the ovaries at the same time as the uterus (a complete clean-out and a practice which has not been entirely abandoned) presumably because it was assumed that the ovaries had little function after the menopause and anyway they might become diseased in time.

Clinical perspective

The two 'ectomies hysterectomy and oophorectomy will be considered together for two reasons. First, it has been common in gynaecological practice for both the uterus and ovaries to be removed together, especially near or after the menopause. Second, it is important that the GP should feel able to discuss the pros and cons of oophorectomy when hysterectomy is being considered, particularly if it is being done for non-malignant reasons. Full discussion of exactly why hysterectomy with or without oophorectomy is required, how (by the vaginal or abdominal route) and by whom it is to be performed, and the after-effects of such surgery, should take place with the gynaecologist who recommends the operation; but many women leave the hospital clinic feeling that they failed to ask the crucial questions, or they cannot remember clearly afterwards what was discussed. These women are likely to seek further advice from their GP. In turn, the GP needs to know the views of the patient's gynaecologist on some of the more controversial issues concerning the operation, so the patient understands why she is receiving conflicting advice.

By and large the issues involved in performing hysterectomy and oophorectomy for malignant disease of the genital tract are clear-cut, although it is interesting that gynaecologists are debating whether one should remove at hysterectomy the ovaries of young women with carcinoma of the cervix, recognizing that this tumour is unlikely to be 'hormone-dependent' to the extent of others such as ovarian or endometrial carcinoma. Oophorectomy has recently become more selective with (1) the advent of ultrasound screening of women for ovarian cancer, and (2) meta-analysis of controlled trials showing that oophorectomy may be a useful adjuvant in the treatment of premenopausal breast cancer. Ovarian cancer has the poorest prognosis of all the gynaecological cancers, as 60 per cent of cases are picked up at an advanced stage and the five-year survival of stage III and IV is only 10 per cent. Five-year survival of greater than 95 per cent has been reported in those women diagnosed early with the cancer confined to the ovary. Trials are in progress using CA-125 tumour markers and ultrasound screening with special reference to women who have a family history of ovarian cancer. Unfortunately, to date the screening tests for ovarian cancer fall short on specificity or sensitivity thus causing many unnecessary abdominal operations because of false-positives. Routine screening is not recommended and large randomized studies are urgently needed to avoid screening being introduced into clinical practice without proper evaluation, making it difficult to examine its efficacy in an unbiased way.

Most hysterectomies are being done for non-malignant reasons, in particular disorders of menstruation, fibroids, and prolapse, and it is these women, especially if they are approaching the menopause, who are likely to be more concerned about their need for the operation and its long-term effects.

Gynaecologists and women themselves both vary enormously in their views. Thus some women will go to any lengths to avoid hysterectomy, even if their menstrual symptoms are severe, preferring to put up with them or control them with drug therapy for many years. Other women, even some in their twenties, almost beg the gynaecologist to remove their uterus, being unable to face endless years of menstrual problems once they have completed their family. These opposing views must be equally respected—being judgemental is not helpful, and each woman must be helped to think through the problem for herself. As in most areas of medicine, if the patient can share in the decision-making, she will be less likely to regret the outcome in the long term, especially when the treatment has implications for her sexuality.

Another option now available to some women is endometrial ablation (see p. 179). The long-term pros and cons of this procedure are not yet known, but in the short term some women will opt for it as it is less invasive and requires less time off work.

I will now try and deal with some of the main questions that women are likely to ask concerning hysterectomy. Some gynaecological departments have in recent years prepared leaflets for women about the operation and its after-effects; sadly, however, in the days of economic stringencies within the NHS it has become increasingly difficult to finance these, although studies have shown that they are much appreciated by women.

Anatomical

Some women may be unclear as to what will be removed at hysterectomy, being concerned in particular about whether or not their ovaries will be left and, if so, whether they will continue to function after removal of the uterus. Other areas of concern may relate to whether the cervix will be removed (almost certainly—subtotal hysterectomy is very rare now); and whether the vagina will be shortened by the surgical procedure (it should not be with a straightforward operation). For many patients a picture may be worth a thousand words, and a diagram of the pelvic organs can be useful on these occasions.

Oophorectomy

The vexed question of whether woman, especially those who are close to or beyond the menopause, should be castrated at the time of hysterectomy for non-malignant reasons has had many powerful advocates in the past. Some gynaecologists have set firm age limits, e.g. 45 years, beyond which they would always remove the ovaries at the time of hysterectomy. The two main arguments for advocating female castration near or after the menopause have been (1) that the ovaries have outlived their useful function, i.e. that their role relates only to reproduction; and (2), perhaps more important, that ovarian carcinoma is difficult to diagnose at an early stage and has, in the past, had a hopeless prognosis. Bilateral oophorectomy in middle-aged or older women has thus been regarded by some as a wise form of preventive surgery. It can also be argued that it does not increase the surgical risk associated with hysterectomy if the ovaries are also removed. Of course, the tempting anatomical proximity of the ovaries to the uterus is likely to be one factor militating against their conservation at abdominal hysterectomy. If women kept their ovaries in a pouch outside the pelvis, as men keep their testes in the scrotum, it is the author's hunch that there might be far less female castration!

The argument that the ovaries have no endocrine function after the menopause is no longer tenable, however. In recent years it has been clearly shown that the ovaries do not cease to be hormone-producing organs at the end of reproductive life. Thus removal of the ovaries even in postmenopausal women will deprive them of one source of both oestrogens and androgens (although of course there are others). Even when these no longer have any function in relation to reproduction, they might well have important implications for sexuality. Women should certainly not be told that they may as well have their ovaries removed at the time of hysterectomy in the belief that castration near or after the menopause will do them no harm. The truth is that we do not know the full long-term hormonal implications in older women of bilateral oophorectomy and it seems likely that the continued production of ovarian hormones serves some purpose. Hormone replacement therapy will replace oestrogens but will not address the other hormonal influences involved.

The most potent argument in favour of female castration is that one is removing a potential source of malignancy with the added problem that ovarian carcinoma is often not diagnosed until it has reached an advanced stage. On the other hand, ovarian carcinoma is a relatively rare disease—the mortality risk in a 40-year-old woman is of the order of 1.7 per 1000.

So what advice does the general practitioner give to the woman who wants to know whether or not to have her ovaries removed? As ever, there are no clear answers but at least some women will welcome a frank discussion on the pros and cons as set out in this chapter. The assumption cannot be made that women want and will give informed consent to having organs removed because of their potential to develop cancer. In particular, a woman who has not yet reached the menopause, or only recently so, may express the wish to conserve her ovaries more strongly than a woman several years past the menopause. The most embittered women in this respect are those who find out that they have been castrated at the time of hysterectomy only on coming round from the anaesthetic, and who rightly resent that prior discussion about oophorectomy was not entered into either by the gynaecologist or their GP. Obviously this resentment can easily be avoided if doctors invest a little more time in advance in discussing with women what their wishes are in this respect.

The general practitioner can reassure a woman opting for hysterectomy with conservation of the ovaries that her ovaries should continue to function normally up to when she would naturally have reached the menopause; although in clinical practice there is evidence that ovarian function can decline prematurely after hysterectomy alone, even in young women (see p. 201). The explanation may relate to a disturbance of the blood supply to the ovary, to the reasons for doing the hysterectomy in the first place, or it may have happened in any case. But the GP should be aware of the possibility of premature ovarian failure in a young woman who complains of 'menopausal symptoms' often with loss of libido as a dominant feature, even if her ovaries were not removed at hysterectomy. Measurement of her FSH levels (see Chapter 7 on the menopause) will aid the diagnosis, high levels indicating ovarian failure. Appropriate hormone therapy would be indicated in that event (see Chapter 7), and both oestrogens and testosterone may be replaced.

Psychological
The psychological effects of hysterectomy are still being debated and remain unclear. Some studies have suggested that a high proportion of women experience depression after a hysterectomy, others have challenged this conclusion. Probably no study is free of criticism over some aspects of its design (Meikle 1977), but there are so many variables to be considered that the perfect study may be too difficult to set up.

In a retrospective study in general practice, Richards (1973; 1974) found that 37 per cent of 200 women who had had a hysterectomy were treated for post-operative depression. Particularly vulnerable were women under 40, those with a history of depression, and those in whom there was no obvious pelvic pathology at hysterectomy. Prospective studies assessing the psychiatric state of women before and after hysterectomy in hospital practice have not confirmed these findings (Gath 1980; Coppen *et al.* 1981). In general their conclusions were of an improvement in the psychiatric state of many patients following hysterectomy when compared with the pre-operation assessment.

Because the debate about the psychological sequelae of hysterectomy continues, it is difficult to know what to tell patients, especially with so many conflicting data in the literature. Again, it is likely to be of importance that the woman comes to the decision herself that hysterectomy is what she wants, and does not feel 'browbeaten' by the medical profession. Doctors must also be aware of the implications of loss of the uterus for some women's sexuality (see below). Open discussion about how she feels about losing her womb may help to resolve such worries. One should, however, remain cautious about advocating hysterectomy in the young depressed woman with no obvious gynaecological pathology.

Sexual

Many women fear that a hysterectomy will ruin their sex lives by leading to loss of libido as well as physical discomfort during intercourse. On the whole, doctors can be reassuring if the operation is uncomplicated, if the ovaries are conserved, and if there is no shortening of the vagina. Prospective studies support the idea that sexual activity, assessed by the frequency of intercourse and of orgasm, does not decline after hysterectomy, whether or not oestrogen therapy is given (Coppen *et al.* 1981).

On the other hand, the general practitioner should be sympathetic to the woman with sexual problems after hysterectomy. Vault granulations can cause pain and even bleeding during intercourse in the early weeks, and because of this and other reasons it is usually advocated to abstain from intercourse for at least a month after operation. Granulations at the vaginal vault can be treated with silver nitrate on a stick. Later complaints of a dry vagina with failure to lubricate during sexual arousal, or loss of libido accompanied by menopausal symptoms, should alert the GP to the possibility of declining ovarian function. Clinical signs of atrophic vaginitis should be looked for and FSH levels measured if there are doubts. Local oestrogen cream or systemic hormone therapy may be required (see Chapter 7 on the menopause). In some women loss of the uterus and cervix may damp down sexual satisfaction during arousal and orgasm since, according to Masters and Johnson, both these organs may participate in normal sexual function. Of course, sexual problems following hysterectomy may not relate to the operation in any way and may have been present before it.

Women must be given the opportunity to discuss their worries about the effect of hysterectomy on their sexual feelings both before and after the operation. They may feel too embarrassed to raise the issues, yet would welcome discussion given the opportunity. It is therefore very important that the GP feels comfortable about opening up such a discussion with a woman, if that is what she wants, and is able to offer positive help and advice. This is discussed more fully in Chapter 14 on sexual problems.

Physical

Advice on when to return to full physical activity is often more readily offered by doctors than advice on other matters after hysterectomy, six to eight weeks being cited but many women need three months. This must vary enormously among individuals and it probably serves no purpose to set limits. The British Medical Association's booklet, *Women only*, suggests that in the early days of convalescence after hysterectomy some cooking, light dusting, or pushing the vacuum cleaner around are suitable activities for recuperating women, which might be interpreted by some as a particularly sexist view of women's daily activities! The fear that weight gain is an after-effect of hysterectomy is not upheld in recent studies.

MASTECTOMY

Mastectomy has been recognized as a therapeutic operation since the time of the ancient Greeks. Its more ancient phylogeny is probably because the pathology would be more visible and its removal more obviously feasible. Thus, since ancient times and through the ages it has been advocated with varying enthusiasm as a treatment—as well as having a vogue as a punitive measure. Renaissance times saw wide exclusion of breast tumours with ligatures to control bleeding, and in the 1890s Halsted advocated radical mastectomy.

Most breast lumps are found by the woman herself or by her husband or partner, and more rarely on routine examination by the doctor. The National Breast Screening Programme (see p. 22) means that many more 'lumps' will be identified via this procedure. But sooner or later these lumps will be brought to the GP. Unlike many other symptoms and signs, the patient is more aware of the implications of having a breast lump. Perhaps the most positive therapy to be offered at this stage is a realistic picture of the likely causes and a practical picture of future management based upon the information in Chapter 2 on breast cancer and benign breast disease. Referral may be needed and, if so, avoidance of delay is important to shorten the period of extreme anxiety that is bound to follow.

If the lump is found to be malignant some women will end up having a mastectomy, although lumpectomy is becoming more widely practised as a method of treatment. Mastectomy for breast cancer will be followed by a depressive illness in between 20 to 40 per cent of women. Most hospitals are involving specially trained nurse counsellors to help women who have to undergo a mastectomy, but as yet it is far from widespread. In one controlled study (Maguire *et al.* 1980) when a specialist nurse was employed to counsel women undergoing mastectomy in the hope of reducing morbidity, it was found that she failed to prevent immediate morbidity but, by its early recognition and referral for treatment, by 12–18 months after mastectomy there was much less psychiatric morbidity in the counselled group (12 per cent) than in the control group (39 per cent). The news that a woman has cancer and must lose a breast is a serious blow even when she is prepared for it. The woman has to deal with both the potentially life-threatening disease and the loss of a body part which may be important among other things to her femininity and sexuality. Whether a lumpectomy or mastectomy is medically recommended one also has to take into account the woman's own feelings. For instance, even if a lumpectomy were feasible some women might prefer a mastectomy, feeling that this would ensure more extensive removal of potentially abnormal tissue, while others would prefer the local less disfiguring operation. Whether the disease or the operation is the main worry varies in different women but Maguire (1978) showed that much of the distress experience (55 per cent) related to the fear of cancer. Women were questioned before and after the operation. Before the operation 18 per cent gave the loss of a breast as a main or subsidiary reason for anxiety, while after the operation this had increased to 35 per cent with special worries about the prosthesis and husbands' attitudes. The reactions experienced by women undergoing mastectomy for cancer are similar to those of bereavement, i.e. an initial phase of disbelief and often euphoria that it has been removed, followed by sadness and depression. Women often complained that they could not express their feelings to the medical staff, and follow-up studies at three to four months after operation showed that 26 per cent had experienced at least moderate depression during this time.

It does seem that patients can easily fall between two stools following the operation, with GPs feeling that they have little role to play and that everything is being taken care of by the hospital, and with the hospital not actually providing the support in the psychosocial areas where the patient needs it. Much is written about improving the communications between surgeons and patients, but when at least 25 per cent of women who undergo mastectomy complain of a lack of opportunity to discuss their worries, the GP has an important role to play in counselling before and after operation, to try and reduce psychiatric morbidity.

Recent reviews (Ramirez 1990) show that there is little difference in the sex or psychological problems experienced following a mastectomy, lumpectomy, or breast conservation. What does seem to be important is that the woman feels she has some part to play in the decision-making process, that she has some control and choices, and that the doctors involved are prepared to discuss the available options. As breast cancer can be considered a chronic disease, both the hospital and the GP could consider in each individual case how the follow-up could be best managed. Some patients may get reassurance from annual hospital visits, while for others it will be a source of anxiety which might be lessened by visiting their doctor instead. In order to do this it would be beneficial to indicate clearly what examinations and investigations need doing to minimize the chance of missing a recurrence. It does not seem that the hospital necessarily has more to offer. All too often routine hospital follow-up appears to be arranged without considering what the follow-up appointment is meant to achieve. On the other hand, general practice often fails to provide routine follow-up of patients, only seeing those that present with symptoms. If general practitioners are to take on more of the follow-up which is normally done at hospitals they need to organize themselves to ensure efficient and regular check-ups.

REFERENCES AND FURTHER READING

Bywaters, J. L. (1977). The incidence and management of female breast disease in a general practice. *Journal of the Royal College of General Practitioners,* **179,** 353–7.

Coppen, A., Bishop, M., Beard, R. J., *et al.* (1981). Hysterectomy, hormones and behaviour. *Lancet,* **i,** 126–8.

Coulter, A. and McPherson, K. (1986). The hysterectomy debate. *Quarterly Journal of Social Affairs,* **4,** 379–93.

Coulter, A., Bradlow, J., Agass, M., *et al.* (1991). Outcomes of referrals to gynaecology outpatient clinics for menstrual problems: an audit of general practice records. *British Journal of Obstetrics and Gynaecology,* **98,** 789–96.

Cuckle, H. and Wald, N. (1991). Screening for ovarian cancer. In *Cancer screening* (ed. A. B. Miller *et al.*). Cambridge University Press.

Fallowfield, L. J., Baum, M., and Maguire, G. P. (1986). Effects of breast conservation on psychological morbidity associated with diagnosis and treatment of early breast cancer. *British Medical Journal,* **293,** 1331–4.

Gath, D. H. (1980). Psychiatric aspects of hysterectomy. In *The social consequences of psychiatric illness* (ed. L. Robins). Brunner/Mazel, New York.

McPherson, K. (1982). Opting to operate. *Times Health Supplement,* 12 March, 12–13.

Maguire, P. (1978). The psychological and social sequelae of mastectomy. In *Modern perspectives in psychiatric aspects of surgery* (ed. J. G. Howells), Chapter 19. Macmillan Press, London.

Maguire, P., Tait, A., Brooke, M., *et al.* (1980). Effect of counselling on the psychiatric morbidity associated with mastectomy. *British Medical Journal,* **281,** 1454–6.

Meikle, S. (1977). The psychological effects of hysterectomy. *Canadian Psychological Review,* **18,** 128–41.

Ramirez, A. J. (1990). Psychological strategies. In *Detection and treatment of early breast cancer* (ed. I. Fentiman). Martin Duhitz, London.

Richards, D. H. (1973). Depression after hysterectomy. *Lancet,* **ii,** 430–2.

Richards, D. H. (1974). A post-hysterectomy syndrome. *Lancet,* **ii,** 983–5.

Teo, P. (1990). A change of trend or a change of heart? In *Women's health counts* (ed. Helen Roberts). Routledge, London.

10. Vaginal discharge

Penny Owen

INTRODUCTION

When a woman presents to her general practitioner with lower genital tract symptoms her doctor, as with all other problems seen in his or her clinical work, should attempt to understand both the patient and the disease; from that understanding comes the management of the problem (McWhinney 1989). Many of the illnesses seen in general practice cannot be fully understood unless they are viewed in their personal, family, and social context. General practitioners recognize that health and disease are strongly connected to personality, way of life, physical environment, and human relationships; and that understanding the meaning the illness has for the patient involves understanding the patient's expectations, feelings, and fears. This holistic approach to the consultation can be of particular value when dealing with the possibility of sexually transmitted disease, which can cause as many anxieties for the doctor as the patient.

Lower genital tract symptoms in women are common. The 1981–82 study of morbidity in general practice recorded 20.4 consultations for vaginitis per 1000 women (Third National Morbidity Survey 1986). The distribution of this symptom by age is shown in Table 10.1.

In a study from one suburban practice (O'Dowd *et al.* 1986) 80 per 1000 women aged 16 and over consulted with vaginal symptoms in one year.

CAUSES OF VAGINAL DISCHARGE

The symptoms of vaginal discharge may have a physiological or pathological basis; if pathological it may be due to an infective or non-infective cause.

Table 10.1 *Age distribution of the symptoms of vaginitis and pelvic inflammatory disease*

	Consultation rates per 1000 females at risk							
	All ages	0–4	5–14	15–24	25–44	45–64	65–74	75+
Vaginitis	20.4	8.4	6.9	31.5	35.0	13.3	10.8	9.5
PID	9.9	0.1	0.3	22.0	21.1	2.2	1.1	0.6

Source: Third National Morbidity Survey 1986.

Infective causes of vaginal discharge

Candida albicans
Bacterial vaginosis
Chlamydia trachomatis
Neisseria gonorrhoeae
Trichomonas vaginalis
Genital warts
Genital herpes
Group B streptococcus
Actinomyces.

In O'Dowd's study of women presenting to their GP with vaginal symptoms, and in whom a complete range of microbiological investigations were performed, only 20 per cent of the women were culture negative (O'Dowd *et al.* 1986). The results of this study are shown in Table 10.2.

Non-infective causes of vaginal discharge

Cervical erosion
Missed and incomplete abortions
Retained placenta
Cervical polyps
Genital tract malignancies (cervical, uterine, vaginal, vulval)

Table 10.2 *Organisms isolated from 154 patients with vaginitis*

	No. (%) of patients
Gardnerella vaginalis alone	30(20)
G. vaginalis + anaerobes	26(17)
G. vaginalis + known pathogens	
Yeasts	14(9)
Trichomonas	7(5)
Herpes	3(2)
Chlamydia	1(1)
Known pathogens	
Yeasts	30(19)
Trichomonas	2(1)
Anaerobes	7(5)
Escherichia coli	3(2)
Gonococcus	
Culture negative	31(120)
Total	154(100)

Atrophic vaginitis
Retained tampon
Irritants and allergic reactions.

ESTABLISHING AN INFECTIVE CAUSE FOR VAGINAL DISCHARGE

When a patient presents with the symptom of vaginal discharge the GP will face a number of management decisions. Firstly, does the patient's history indicate that an examination and microbiological investigations need to be performed? If so, what investigations are necessary and who should undertake them: the primary health care team or a genito-urinary medicine (GUM) department?

There are a number of symptoms which, if elicited from a patient presenting with vaginal discharge, should lead to microbiological investigation. These symptoms include the following:

(1) first presentation of vaginal discharge in a previously asymptomatic patient;

(2) blood-stained discharge;

(3) malodorous discharge;

(4) associated lower abdominal pain;

(5) intermenstrual bleeding or post-coital bleeding;

(6) IUD *in situ*;

(7) recent gynaecological surgery, e.g. termination of pregnancy, hysterectomy, or a delivery—whether vaginally or by Caesarian section;

(8) past history of a sexually transmitted disease;

(9) recent change of sexual partner(s);

(10) a partner with urethral symptoms, or who has recently attended a GUM clinic;

(11) presence of genital warts and/or genital herpes.

If the patient presents with a history of recurrent vaginal discharge which has previously been diagnosed by laboratory culture as either *Candida albicans* or bacterial vaginosis, and if none of the above more serious symptoms are present, then it would seem reasonable to treat the patient first and perform investigations only if the symptoms do not settle.

While the presence of vulval irritation or soreness, or the history of a recent course of antibiotics may make the diagnosis of *Candida albicans* more likely, if a definitive diagnosis is required then microbiological investigations will need to be performed.

Since practices can vary considerably in the socio-demographic characteristics of their patient populations, the range of investigations that a practice performs on patients presenting with vaginal discharge should be decided on by each practice, ideally after discussion with the local hospital laboratory consultant and GUM department. For example, a practice in which for many years no patient has been identified as having gonorrhoea may decide that cervical swabs for culture of the gonococcus are not warranted unless another sexually transmitted disease is found on investigating the patient. Also hospital laboratories vary in the type of swabs, transport medium, and non-culture tests they use. Communication with laboratory and GUM consultants who are aware of the nature and demands of primary care can assist the general practitioner in keeping up to date with new developments in the investigation of lower genital tract symptoms.

Practices and individual general practitioners will vary as to whether they carry out the investigations themselves or refer the patient to a GUM department. Patient preference may influence the referral decision. Ultimately, each consultation necessitates its own decision as to whether or not the patient requires investigation; the guidelines given in this section may be used to inform such decisions.

A comprehensive approach to investigating the symptom of vaginal discharge could involve taking the following swabs:

(1) one high vaginal swab (HVS) in Stuart's medium for culture of *Gardnerella vaginalis*, anaerobes, and *Candida albicans*;

(2) one HVS in trichomonas transport medium;

(3) one cervical swab in Stuart's medium for culture of *Neisseria gonorrhoeae*;

(4) one cervical swab plated on to a MicroTrak slide for identification of *Chlamydia trachomatis*;

(5) if vulval ulcers are present a swab from a lesion is placed in viral transport medium for isolation of *Herpes simplex* virus.

Infecting organisms

The following organisms are associated with lower genital tract symptoms in women:

Candida

Candida albicans is the commonest vaginal yeast pathogen. It is a dimorphic fungus which can grow in the form of budding yeast cells or hyphal filaments. Both forms are seen in infected tissues although hyphal forms are more successful at proliferating within vaginal epithelial cells. It has been suggested that recurrent infection with *C. albicans* is due to the organism living within the vaginal mucosa, protected from topical anti-fungal treatment, then emerging in the vaginal lumen some weeks or months later when the epithelial cells are shed. The intestinal tract is also a source of vaginal infection/re-infection, and most patients harbouring *C. albicans* in the genital tract are also harbouring the fungus in the gastro-intestinal tract. Typing the strains of *C. albicans* from male and female partners has revealed that both often harbour the same strain. However, evidence that the man is the source of vaginal infection rather than the recipient has still to be obtained.

Many people have within them an eco system of commensal yeasts which have a potential to become pathogenic. In most patients host defence mechanisms prevent the fungus from establishing an infection, but the balance between host and potential pathogen is a fine one. Although it has so far proved difficult to discover what host defects allow symptomatic vaginal infections with *C. albicans* to occur, candidosis has been associated with a number of predisposing factors:

1. Pregnancy. This is probably related to the increased proportion of large, glycogen-rich, vaginal epithelial cells.
2. Diabetes mellitus.
3. Broad spectrum antibiotics. The normal bacterial flora of the vagina is thought to form an important natural defence mechanism against *C. albicans*. Antibiotic treatment which causes the decrease or alteration of this flora could allow the proliferation of *C. albicans*.
4. Oral contraception. A possible association between the use of oral contraception and *C. albicans* has long been debated. It is likely that the combined pills containing lower amounts of oestrogen (i.e. 30 μg or less) do not cause the increased rates of candidal infection seen with the older 50 μg pills.

Incidence. O'Dowd *et al.* (1986) in their study from general practice isolated *C. albicans* in 28 per cent of women presenting with vaginal symptoms. In 1989 candidosis was diagnosed in 17 per cent of women attending GUM clinics in England and Wales (DoH 1991).

Symptoms and signs. The mechanisms by which *C. albicans* produces its classic symptom of pruritus, often with only minimal invasion of host cells, are not well understood. Other symptoms associated with candidal in-fection may include dysuria, dyspareunia, and vaginal discharge.

Signs that may be found on examination are predominantly those of vulval erythema, occasionally with fissuring of the skin. There may be a discharge present which is characteristically a curdy white material with adhering plaques on the vaginal walls. Chronic infection may lead to vulval lichenification. However, symptoms and signs do not correlate closely with laboratory findings and if a definitive diagnosis is required then a laboratory culture of a high vaginal swab should be performed (Berg *et al.* 1984; Reed *et al.* 1989).

Treatment.   The two main groups of drugs used in the treatment of candidosis are:

polyene antibiotics, e.g. nystatin and natamycin

imidazoles, e.g. clotrimazole, miconazole, econazole, and isoconazole.

For both groups, treatment is by vaginal pessaries or cream in courses of three to 14 days according to the preparation, although single-dose preparations are available.

Recurrence of symptoms is a major problem in the treatment of vaginal candidosis and various strategies have been suggested:

1. Concurrent treatment of the partner;
2. Intermittent prophylatic treatment, e.g. the use of antifungal pessaries once a week.
3. Systemic oral anti-fungals. Serious adverse side-effects, e.g. hepatitis, have been reported with the use of the oral antifungal ketoconazole. The hepatitis is not always reversible upon discontinuing therapy and fatalities have occurred. There is limited experience with the use of the newer systemic antifungals fluconazole and itraconazole. There is no good evidence that oral antifungal treatment with the specific intention of eliminating *C. albicans* from the gastrointestinal tract is useful.
4. Patient information leaflets may provide some women with helpful advice, for example the Health Education Authority publish a self-help guide to thrush (HEA n.d.). Advice given in this leaflet for women who suffer with recurrent thrush includes avoiding tights, nylon pants, and trousers—especially tight jeans; using pads rather than tampons; avoiding perfumed soaps, vaginal deodorants, and any other irritants such as disinfectants; always washing and wiping from 'front to back' to avoid contaminating the vulva with yeasts (or any other organisms) that may be present in the bowel; and avoiding antibiotics as far as possible. If an antibiotic has to be prescribed then the patient should ask for some medication against thrush at the same time.

Despite all the above precautions some patients with recurrent vaginal candidosis will continue to present difficult management problems.

Bacterial vaginosis

This condition is associated with the presence of *Gardnerella vaginalis* and mixed anaerobes. It was first described by Gardner and Dukes (1955), when it was thought to be due to a single pathogen known as *Haemophilus vaginalis*. This organism was later renamed *Gardnerella vaginalis*. It is now known that although *G. vaginalis* may be the only organism isolated by the laboratory there will often be an associated increase in anaerobic bacteria. *Gardnerella vaginalis* is a small Gram-variable facultative anaerobe.

Gardner and Dukes originally described the clinical features of this condition as a grey, homogeneous, and malodorous vaginal discharge with a higher than normal pH of 5–5.5 and minimal vaginal inflammation. The characteristic fishy odour of the discharge is probably due to the production of the amines putrescine and cadaverine. The cause of the change in the vaginal flora that is found in bacterial vaginosis is not known. Whether or not the condition should be viewed as a sexually transmitted disease is still not clear.

Incidence in general practice.   O'Dowd *et al.* (1986) reported the first study on bacterial vaginosis in general practice. In this study of 154 adult women who presented to their GP with vaginal symptoms, 30 (20 per cent) had *G. vaginalis* on its own; 26 (17 per cent) had *G. vaginalis* together with anaerobes; 25 (17 per cent) had *G. vaginalis* in combination with other known pathogens; and 7 (5 per cent) had anaerobes on their own. In 1989, women attending GUM clinics with a diagnosis of vaginosis or vaginitis comprised 11 per cent of the clinic's workload for women patients (DoH 1991).

Symptoms and signs.   The unpleasant-smelling vaginal discharge may sometimes be associated with an increase in the amount of discharge and a change in discharge colour. The characteristic smell has alternatively been described as either a fishy smell or a high cheese odour. The colour of the discharge has variously been reported as either grey or yellow. The unpleasant odour may often be noticed by the examiner, as may a watery frothy discharge. Vulval or vaginal erythema are not associated with bacterial vaginosis.

Investigations.   While symptoms and signs may point strongly to the condition of bacterial vaginosis, confirmation of the diagnosis will require laboratory culture of a high vaginal swab.

A couple of bedside tests are available which can be useful pointers to the condition. However, neither of these tests, the use of pH paper or the amine test, have been widely taken up in general practice. Vaginal pH can be measured using pH paper, with a value of 4.5 or less being normal. In bacterial vaginosis the pH will be 5 or above. However, pH paper can give a falsely high reading if blood or semen are present, the paper fades if left in sunlight, and colour changes are not always consistent along a strip of the paper. In the amine test a drop of 10 per cent potassium hydroxide is mixed with a drop of vaginal discharge on a glass slide. In bacterial vaginosis amines will be released by this procedure producing a very characteristic smell. A practical problem with the amine test is that safe storage of 10 per cent KOH in a GP's surgery may be difficult and render its regular use impractical.

O'Dowd *et al.* (1987) have reported that in a group of women with vaginal symptoms the clinical features of increased yellow discharge, high cheese odour, and pH greater than 5 were statistically strongly associated with the presence of *G. vaginalis* confirmed by microbiological culture. Another characteristic finding associated with bacterial vaginosis is the 'clue cell'. If a wet film of vaginal discharge is examined under the microscope then numerous bacteria will be seen adhering to vaginal epithelial cells. These cells are then called clue cells.

Treatment. The most commonly used regime for the treatment of bacterial vaginosis is metronidazole 400 mg t.d.s. for seven days. However, as with *Candida albicans* infections, a small number of patients do suffer with recurrent episodes of bacterial vaginosis. It seems reasonable in these patients to treat the partner with a concurrent course of metronidazole, although evidence is conflicting as to how successful this approach will be.

Chlamydia trachomatis

Chlamydia trachomatis is an important organism because of the long-term consequences of untreated infection, namely pelvic inflammatory disease, chronic pelvic pain, ectopic pregnancy, infertility, and perinatal transmission to infants. Several extensive reviews of chlamydial infections are available (Fraiz and Jones 1988; Stamm 1988; *Lancet* editorial 1986).

While classified as a bacterium, *C. trachomatis* is an obligate intracellular parasite. The endocervix is the anatomical site most frequently infected in women; ascending spread can then occur to the endometrium, fallopian tubes, and peritoneal cavity. The organism can also infect the urethra and rectum. Chlamydial infections in women may be asymptomatic, and patients can harbour the organism for a long time with few or no symptoms to suggest infection. When symptoms do occur they can often be fairly mild; typical complaints are vaginal discharge, dysuria, lower abdominal pain, and altered bleeding patterns. On examination mucopurulent cervitis may be present, although more commonly the cervix will appear normal. In chlamydial infection of the upper genital tract uterine and adnexal tenderness may be found together with cervical excitation. However, it is known that women with pelvic inflammatory disease associated with *C. trachomatis* have less severe symptoms and signs than when the pelvic inflammatory disease is due to *Neisseria gonorrhoeae* or anaerobic bacteria. Studies from the United States indicate that 30–50 per cent of women with laparoscope-confirmed pelvic inflammatory disease are infected with *Chlamydia*. After one episode of chlamydial cervicitis approximately 20 per cent of patients will develop pelvic inflammatory disease. Of the patients who have pelvic inflammatory disease 20 per cent will develop chronic pelvic pain, 15 per cent will be infertile (this number doubles for each subsequent attack of pelvic inflammatory disease), and 5 per cent will have an ectopic pregnancy. Chlamydial infection may spread from the fallopian tubes to the liver capsule giving rise to perihepatitis (Fitz-Hugh Curtis Syndrome) with its symptoms of right upper quadrant abdominal pain, nausea, vomiting, and pyrexia. Approximately 30 per cent of infants exposed to *C. trachomatis* during delivery will develop conjunctivitis, and 10 per cent will develop pneumonia.

Incidence of chlamydial infections.   In a study from an inner-London practice (Southgate *et al.* 1983), *C. trachomatis* was isolated by cell culture from 9 per cent of women with genito-urinary symptoms; and a study from a suburban practice using the MicroTrak test reported an incidence of 6 per cent (Owen *et al.* 1991). In the statistical returns from GUM clinics in England for 1989 (DoH 1991) 21 000 new cases of chlamydial infection (excluding pelvic inflammatory disease) were reported, representing 7 per cent of their total new cases workload for women. While changes in the GUM clinic reporting forms make direct comparisons between 1988 and 1989 difficult, the returns from 1989 indicate that the recent decline in chlamydial/non-specific genital infections did not continue. The clinics recorded nearly 5000 cases of pelvic inflammatory disease; 12 per cent were reported as chlamydial alone, 5 per cent as gonococcal alone, 2 per cent were mixed infections, and in 81 per cent of cases no organism was found.

Groups of patients who have traditionally been said to be more likely to have chlamydial infections are younger women, patients with a recent change of sexual partner, those taking the combined contraceptive pill, and non-Caucasians. However, it is possible that these sub-groups may only reflect the selected populations in which the majority of studies have so far been carried out.

Diagnostic methods.   The isolation of *C. trachomatis* requires cell culture methods which are costly, technically difficult, and take up to four to seven days. Specimens have to be refrigerated and transported at 4 °C to the laboratory the same day. Routine use of cell culture has therefore not been feasible for the majority of general practitioners. However, recent advances have been made in the development of two methods of non-culture antigen detection tests for *C. trachomatis*. One method is by direct immunofluorescence staining of smears using monoclonal antibodies (e.g. the MicroTrak test); and the other method uses the detection of chlamydial antigen eluted from swabs and measured by enzyme-linked immunoassay (ELISA) methods (e.g. the Chlamydiazyme test). When the MicroTrak test is compared with cell culture (Stamm 1988) a median sensitivity of 77 per cent and specificity of 97 per cent have been reported in intermediate prevalence populations of women. Taylor Robinson has reported the Micro-Trak test to be as sensitive and specific as cell culture, but the ELISA test to have a lower sensitivity of approximately 70 per cent and specificity of approximately 90 per cent (Taylor Robinson *et al.* 1987). Therefore, when the MicroTrak or Chlamydiazyme test are used some patients will be incorrectly identified as positive and a smaller number incorrectly identified as negative. A description of the problems of false positives and false negatives, and how the prevalence of disease affects the usefulness of a test, can be found in a clinical epidemiology textbook by Sackett *et al.* (1985). A review of these problems with specific reference to chlamydial infections is also available (Southgate 1990). Collaboration with the local laboratory will be useful in deciding which of the diagnostic methods is suitable for each practice. However, the resolution of this diagnostic problem awaits the introduction of second-generation non-culture methods of diagnosis with higher sensitivity and specificity. The use of serology is of little value in the diagnosis of uncomplicated chlamydial genital infections. General guide-lines as to which patients may require investigating for chlamydial disease are given on pages 266–7.

Treatment.   Treatment involves the co-operation of both the patient and her current and/or recent sexual partner(s). Chlamydial cervicitis can be treated with doxycycline 100 mg b.d. for seven days or erythromycin 250–500 mg q.d.s. for seven days. Longer courses of antibiotics may be required in pelvic inflammatory disease (a standard regime for the treatment of pelvic inflammatory disease is provided in the section on gonococcal disease). Following treatment a test of cure investigation should be carried out, although the limitations of non-culture methods of diagnosis discussed previously still apply. In a study from general practice (Owen *et al.* 1991) 9 per cent of women with chlamydial cervicitis had a positive MicroTrak test after treatment, and therefore required re-treatment. Hospital studies have reported re-isolation rates following treatment of chlamydial cervicitis of between 27 and 0 per cent.

Contact tracing requires the patient to inform her current and/or recent partner(s) that they have been in contact with a chlamydial infection and should therefore seek medical advice. The address of the nearest GUM clinic can be provided or the partner(s) can see their own general practitioner. Because of the possibility of latent infection with *Chlamydia* it cannot be said with certainty when the infection was transmitted to the patient. This may need to be discussed. The wider role of the health adviser in GUM departments in discussing health education and lifestyle, and decreasing the risk of acquiring further sexually transmitted infections is now well established.

Although the sequelae of untreated chlamydial infections in women are known to be serious, the low incidence of the disease in primary care together with diagnostic tests that are not yet highly accurate leaves the role of the general practitioner in managing chlamydial disease in a considerable state of flux. It has been suggested (Owen *et al.* 1991) that chlamydial cervicitis can be managed in general practice, although this is still hotly disputed by GUM departments (White and Radcliffe 1991).

Gonorrhoea

Gonorrhoea is an uncommon diagnosis to make in general practice, with incidence rates of 2 per cent (Southgate *et al.* 1983) and 0 per cent (O'Dowd *et al.* 1986) in women presenting with lower genital tract symptoms. Statistical returns from GUM clinics in 1989 (DoH 1991) indicated that approximately 8,400 cases were diagnosed in women, representing 3 per cent of the total new female cases seen in GUM clinics. Also in 1989, for the first time in many years, there was a rise in the number of cases of gonorrhoea with a 3 per cent increase in women and a 4 per cent increase in men. There was an associated increase in the number of cases of gonoccocal pelvic inflammatory disease seen in GUM clinics, from 88 in the first two quarters of 1989 to 143 in the last two quarters of that year.

Neisseria gonorrhoeae is a Gram-negative diplococcus which infects mucosal surfaces, most commonly the cervix, but also the endometrium and fallopian tubes, the urethra, and rectum. Approximately 10 per cent of women with gonorrhoea will develop pelvic inflammatory disease, which in turn can lead to chronic pelvic pain, ectopic pregnancy, and infertility. Disseminated gonococcal infection can lead to septic arthritis. Perinatal transmission has long been associated with gonococcal conjunctivitis in the newborn.

Approximately 70 per cent of women with gonococcal infections will be asymptomatic. When they do occur symptoms include vaginal discharge, dysuria and frequency, lower abdominal pain, and abnormal bleeding patterns. The affected cervix may appear normal on examination, or there may be a mucopurulent cervicitis. Diagnosis of gonorrhoea in general practice will be by culture. While direct plating and immediate incubation achieves the best isolation rates, this will be impractical for most surgeries. Instead a cervical swab can be placed in Stuart's medium and transported to the laboratory the same day. If *Neisseria gonorrhoeae* is isolated then other sexually transmitted diseases, particularly *Chlamydia*, need to be looked for if this has not already been done.

Uncomplicated gonorrhoea is treated with a single dose of oral ampicillin 2 g and oral probenecid 1 g. In patients allergic to penicillin, ciprofloxacin in a single dose of 250 g can be used. Acute pelvic inflammatory disease, unless the patient requires hospital admission, can be treated with a loading dose of oral ampicillin 2 g and oral probenecid 1 g, followed by doxycycline

100 mg b.d. and metronidazole 400 g t.d.s. for ten days. A test of cure investigation should be carried out after treatment; and contact tracing must be discussed with the patient so that she is aware that she should inform her current and/or recent sexual partner(s) that they have been in contact with gonorrhoea and need to seek medical attention. Advice about the prevention of contracting gonorrhoea and other sexually transmitted diseases should also be discussed with the patient.

Trichomoniasis

Trichomonas vaginalis is a flagellate protozoon, and infection with the organism is generally regarded as being sexually transmitted. An incidence rate of 6 per cent has been described for the isolation of *T. vaginalis* in patients presenting to their general practitioner with lower genital tract symptoms (O'Dowd *et al*. 1986). In 1989, GUM clinics in England reported approximately 7500 new cases of trichomoniasis in women (DoH 1991), representing 3 per cent of the total new female cases seen. GUM clinic reports of trichomoniasis have been decreasing since the early 1980s.

The clinical features of trichomoniasis are very variable; although vaginal discharge is the commonest symptom, not all patients will complain of a discharge. Classically the discharge is said to be frothy and yellow, but again the type of discharge varies. Vulvitis and vaginitis may be present, and sometimes this inflammation produces marked symptoms. Dysuria may also occur. Up to two-thirds of the male partners of infected women may harbour the parasite, although the organism's presence is short-lived and rarely causes symptoms in men.

Diagnosis. *T. vaginalis* can be diagnosed either by microscopy or culture. Trichomonas transport medium is available, although Stuart's medium can also be used.

Treatment. *T. vaginalis* is treated with metronidazole 200 mg t.d.s. for seven days, or alternatively a single oral dose of 2 g can be used. Metronidazole should not be given during the first trimester of pregnancy, and patients should be warned to avoid alcohol. Nimorazole, a nitromidazole similar to metronidzole, can be used as an alternative treatment, in a regime of three oral doses of 500 mg at 12-hourly intervals, or a single 2-g dose. If *T. vaginalis* recurs then the current sexual partner(s) should be treated.

Syphilis

The trend in the incidence of infectious syphilis in women reported from GUM clinics since 1977 has been downwards, from 468 cases in 1977 to 160 in 1987 and 117 in 1988. However, in 1989 the number of cases of infectious syphilis in women remained stable (DoH 1991) at 122.

Syphilis is an infectious disease caused by the bacterium *Treponema pallidum*. The principal method of spread is sexual transmission, although it can be acquired congenitally. Syphilis can be divided into an early infectious stage and a late non-infectious stage. The primary lesion that develops at the site of inoculation of *T. pallidum* is characteristically a painless ulcer. If such a lesion is noted the patient should be referred to a GUM clinic. There is as yet no evidence to suggest that women presenting to their general practitioner with lower genital tract symptoms require routine serological testing for syphilis.

Genital warts

Genital warts are usually sexually acquired and are caused by infection with the human papilloma virus (HPV). The commonest sites for genital warts are the introitus and vulva; they may also affect the vagina and cervix. HPV infection of the cervix often produces lesions which are not visible to naked eye inspection, rather requiring colposcopy for detection. Such cervical lesions can produce a vaginal discharge. Other areas that may be infected are the perineum, anus, and rectum.

The incubation period is long, varying from two weeks to eight months, with a mean of three months. Up to 60 per cent of sexual partners can acquire warts. A rare complication of genital warts in pregnancy is the development of laryngeal papillomas in the infant.

Up-to-date information on how often patients with genital warts are seen in general practice is not available. Genital warts account for about 10 per cent of the workload of GUM clinics, partly owing to the need for re-attendance for treatment. There has been a steady increase during the 1980s in the number of women seen in GUM clinics with genital warts, which in 1989 reached a total of just over 32 000 (DoH 1991).

Treatment. Genital warts are diagnosed solely from their clinical appearance. They are difficult and time-consuming to treat, and some will regress spontaneously. Treatment is usually started with podophyllin paint, provided the woman is not pregnant when its use is contraindicated because of a possible mutagenic action. Having protected the skin adjacent to the warts, for example with vaseline, 25 per cent podophyllin should be applied to the warts and then washed off after six hours. Re-application of podophyllin can be undertaken every three to seven days, but if it is ineffective after three to four weeks then alternative forms of treatment should be considered. Trichloracetic acid is an even more caustic substance which has been used for local application to warts. Other methods for removal of genital warts include electrocautery, cryotherapy, and excision.

Women with genital warts should be investigated to exclude concurrent sexually acquired conditions. The recognition of penile warts in the partners of infected women often requires magnified observation after acetic acid preparation.

Another viral infection molluscum contagiosum, which causes characteristic umbilicated lesions, may also be sexually transmitted.

The role of HPV as a possible aetiological agent for cervical cancer has been the cause of much debate (Singer and Jenkins 1991), see p. 233.

Genital herpes

Genital herpes is caused by the *Herpes simplex* virus (HSV). HSV can be divided into two types, HSV-1 and HSV-2. Both cause genital infection but HSV-1 is predominantly associated with facial lesions. Genital herpes is usually sexually transmitted. A first episode of genital herpes (i.e. primary herpes) in a patient usually presents with multiple painful genital ulcers after an incubation period of under seven days. In most primary attacks both the vulva and cervix are affected; lesions may also be seen perianally and on the thighs. Cervical lesions can cause vaginal discharge. The lesions begin as erythematous areas which then blister, ulcerate, and finally crust over, the whole process lasting about two to three weeks. Patients may be systemically unwell with a temperature and malaise. Dysuria may occur, and inguinal lymphadenopathy is often present. Viral shedding usually begins a few days before any lesions are noted and continues for up to a fortnight.

Recurrent infections are less severe and are not due to re-infection. The mean time interval between initial and recurrent infection is about 120 days, with a range of 25–360 days. Patients often notice prodromal symptoms of local tingling and paraesthesiae for 24–48 hours before the onset of lesions. The recurrent infection is usually both milder and shorter than the initial attack. Both initial and recurrent attacks of herpes may be asymptomatic in women and men.

Diagnosis. Accurate information on the number of patients with genital herpes who are seen in general practice is not available. Diagnosis of genital herpes is by culture. A swab should be taken from any suspicious lesions and sent to the laboratory in viral transport medium. If HSV is isolated the patient should be investigated to exclude the presence of any other sexually transmitted disease. Current and/or recent sexual partners should be advised to seek medical advice. Patients need to be warned that they are infectious when lesions are present. They should therefore abstain from sexual intercourse once lesions are noted or sooner if prodromal symptoms are present. The sheath is not effective in preventing transmission of the virus.

Treatment. Symptomatic treatment involves the use of analgesics; saline baths may be helpful, and if lesions become secondarily infected then antibiotics should be used. Severe, uncontrolled pain or urinary retention may lead to hospital admission. Acyclovir can be used for the treatment of initial and recurrent genital herpes (BNF 1991), and treatment should be started as early as possible in an attack. Oral acyclovir is used in a dosage of 200 mg, five times daily for five days for each attack. Although acyclovir given in five-day courses speeds the rate of healing, shortens the duration and lessens the severity of symptoms, and decreases the duration of viral shedding, it does not seem to decrease the likelihood of subsequent recurrences when used to treat patients either during a primary attack or a recurrence.

For the prevention of severe and frequent recurrent herpes acyclovir can be given either as 200 mg q.d.s. or 400 mg b.d., reducing to 200 mg two or three times daily, with a break in treatment every 6–12 months. Neonatal herpes can occur if the mother has active herpes at the time of delivery. The risk to the neonate is greater from primary than from recurrent episodes in the mother. If viral shedding is found at 39–40 weeks a Caesarean section should be considered.

Streptococcus

Group B streptococci are a serious cause of bacteraemia and other invasive infections in the newborn within the first few days of life. Heavy vaginal colonization seems to make transmission more likely, and prematurity and a prolonged labour after rupture of the membranes are important risk factors. If this organism is isolated from a high vaginal swab during the puerperium, both mother and baby should be treated with penicillin.

Actinomyces

Actinomyces are Gram-positive filamentous fungi which may colonize the genital tract in the presence of a plastic IUD. Current opinion is that if patients are asymptomatic then no action need be taken on identification of this organism. However, rarely it can be associated with pelvic inflammatory disease and in a symptomatic patient the coil should be removed and antibiotic usage considered. The organism is sensitive to penicillin and tetracycline.

MANAGEMENT OF PATIENTS WITH A SEXUALLY TRANSMITTED DISEASE

For a patient with a sexually transmitted disease the diagnosis and treatment are often the simplest part of management. The patient's anxieties about having acquired the infection, the difficulties contact tracing may cause, and educating the patient on how to prevent further infections may all present the doctor with more complicated and often fraught management problems. The general practitioner will need to feel at ease when discussing sexual lifestyle and anxieties with the patient, so that there can be an open discussion on the implications for the patient of having a sexually transmitted disease. General practitioners have available the option of referring to GUM clinics patients whom they suspect or in whom they have diagnosed a sexually transmitted disease. Some patients will be concerned that they may have acquired HIV infection as well, and may require counselling about testing.

When providing patients with information about the prevention of further sexually transmitted diseases the risks of multiple partners, or a partner with multiple partners, and the use of barrier contraception to help reduce the risk, can all be discussed. A useful patient booklet called *Guide to a healthy sex life* is produced by the Health Education Authority. It contains information on symptoms and treatment of sexually transmitted diseases, how to get help, telling partners, and how to avoid catching an infection.

STRATEGIES FOR THE PREVENTION OF SEXUALLY TRANSMITTED DISEASES

In the report *The nation's health: a strategy for the 1990s* (Jacobson *et al.* 1991) the current state of Britain's health is outlined and strategies put forward for how it can be changed for the better. The report recommends that instead of considering the prevention of one disease in isolation from others, attempts need to be made to unify policies on the prevention of sexually transmitted diseases and cervical cancer with those concerning the prevention of the spread of AIDS.

As well as a politically co-ordinated strategy, the report recommends that a fundamental part of school education should be the provision of information on personal relationships, contraception, and the prevention of sexually transmitted disease. Health authorities and FHSAs should have quantified objectives for the promotion of safe and effective forms of contraception and for the reduction of sexually transmitted disease, and they should liaise with local authorities and other community agencies in planning information and advisory services. Effective mass media campaigns should avoid arousing a combination of fear and helplessness, and focus instead on giving unambiguous, direct information on sexual practices that confer a high or low risk of sexually transmitted disease. The two behaviour changes which are most likely to have an impact on sexually transmitted disease are a reduction in the number of sexual partners and the use of barrier methods of contraception.

TRENDS IN SEXUALLY TRANSMITTED DISEASE

Trends in sexually transmitted disease are often difficult to interpret because of the reliance on selective information from attendance at genito-urinary medicine clinics. Numerous factors, such as changing social perceptions and improved professional recognition and diagnosis, can artificially boost the numbers coming forward to such clinics. Analysis of the information by the Communicable Disease Surveillance Centre (CDSC 1985) shows that the large increase in the numbers of reported new cases for herpes and non-specific genital infections are exaggerated by other factors, and that the only real increases in incidence that have taken place are for genital warts and AIDS. Monitoring of representative samples of the whole community is needed in order to be able to predict more accurately the future impact of sexually transmitted disease.

Non-infective causes of vaginal discharge

Cervical erosion

An erosion is the term applied when the stratified epithelium normally lining the vaginal portion of the cervix is replaced by columnar epithelium from the cervical canal. An erosion is commonly seen in women taking the combined oral contraceptive pill. An erosion may cause a mucoid discharge, and on examination a red granular area is seen around the external os replacing the usual pink appearance of the stratified epithelium. If the patient requests treatment the erosion can be cauterized.

Cervical polyps

Cervical polyps may be asymptomatic or they can cause a discharge which becomes bloodstained if they are ulcerated. They are treated by surgical removal (see p. 195).

Cervical carcinoma

The earliest symptoms of carcinoma of the cervix are irregular bleeding and a vaginal discharge often of a watery, offensive nature. On examination of the cervix there may be an ulcerated lesion, pronounced bleeding on light touch, a hard module may be palpable, and friability may be noted with small fragments of the growth breaking away on touch. Endocervical carcinoma may be more difficult to diagnose because speculum examination may not reveal any abnormality, and the diagnosis may only be made when a D and C is performed.

Endometrial carcinoma

The commonest symptoms of endometrial carcinoma are irregular bleeding and a vaginal discharge, usually brown, watery, and offensive. A bimanual examination of the pelvis may not reveal any abnormality; the only reliable method of making the diagnosis is by curettage.

Vaginal carcinoma

Primary squamous cell carcinoma of the vagina is rare. Malignant disease is usually secondaries from a primary growth elsewhere, e.g. the cervix or endometrium. A patient with carcinoma of the vagina usually presents with irregular bleeding and an offensive discharge. The growth often takes the form of an ulcer with a hard base and raised edges. The surface is friable and bleeds easily; the lesion may be fixed.

Vulva carcinoma

In carcinoma of the vulva the symptoms are those of a vulval swelling or soreness, bleeding, and a purulent discharge. An ulcerated lesion with raised, everted, irregular margins will be noted.

Atrophic vaginitis

Atrophic vaginitis is caused by the vulva and vagina losing their resistance to infection as part of the ageing process. The patient presents with a discharge, sometimes bloodstained, and vulval soreness. On examination the vulva and vagina appear inflamed, often with small, multiple, reddened areas. When malignant disease has been excluded as a cause of the discharge the vaginitis can be treated with oestrogen, either orally or topically.

Retained tampon

A forgotten tampon will soon cause a very offensive discharge, which quickly settles on removal of the tampon. Antibiotics should be given if there are symptoms or signs of a pelvic infection.

Retained products—postnatal or post-abortion

This can cause a vaginal discharge, particularly if complicated by an infection. Both uterine curettage and antibiotics will need to be considered in the management of each patient.

MANAGEMENT OF PATIENTS WITH NO PHYSICAL CAUSE FOR THEIR SYMPTOMS

Occasionally, a patient presenting with the symptom of vaginal discharge will have no abnormalities detected either on examination or microbiological investigation. Such patients can be reassured there is no serious cause for the discharge, and an explanation should be provided that some women have a heavier discharge than others without this meaning that anything is wrong. GPs may occasionally find themselves dealing with patients with somatic fixation, in which a variety of mutually reinforcing factors can continually prevent the creation of conditions necessary for recovery (Grol 1981). The doctor can try to limit his or her own contribution to this process by the appropriate use of investigations, by paying sufficient attention to psychological signs, and by attempting to maintain a satisfactory doctor–patient relationship.

In other patients the symptom of vaginal discharge may be the method of presentation of a psychological or psychosexual problem. Such patients may require time and a supportive atmosphere in which to discuss their difficulties.

REFERENCES AND FURTHER READING

Berg, A. O., Heidrich, F. E., Fihn, S. D., *et al.* (1984). Establishing the cause of genitourinary symptoms in women in a family practice. *Journal of the American Medical Association,* **251,** 620–5.

British National Formulary (BNF) (1991). British Medical Association.

Communicable Disease Surveillance Centre (CDSC) (1985). Sexually transmitted disease surveillance in Britain. *British Medical Journal,* **291,** 528–30.

DoH (Department of Health) (1991). *On the state of the public health.* HMSO, London.

Fraiz, J. and Jones, R. B. (1988). Chlamydial infections. *Annual Review of Medicine,* **39,** 357–70.

Gardner, H. L. and Dukes, C. D. (1955). *Haemophilus vaginalis* vaginitis. A newly defined specific infection previously classified as 'non-specific vaginitis'. *American Journal of Obstetrics and Gynecology,* **69,** 962–76.

Grol, R. (1981). *To heal or to harm.* Royal College of General Practitioners, London.

Health Education Authority (n.d.). *A self-help guide to thrush.* HEA, London.

Health Education Authority (n.d.). *Guide to a healthy sex life.* HEA, London.

Jacobson, B., Smith, A., and Whitehead, M. (1991). *The nation's health: a strategy for the 1990s.* King Edward's Hospital Fund for London.

Lancet editorial (1986). Chlamydia in women: a case for more action? *Lancet,* **i,** 892–4.

McWhinney, I. R. (1989). *A textbook of family medicine.* Oxford University Press, New York.

O'Dowd, T. C., West, R. R., Ribeiro, C. D., *et al.* (1986). Contribution of *Gardnerella vaginalis* to vaginitis in a general practice study. *British Medical Journal,* **292,** 1640–2.

O'Dowd, T. C. and West, R. R. (1987). Clinical prediction of *Gardnerella vaginalis* in general practice. *Journal of the Royal College of General Practitioners,* **37,** 59–61.

Owen, P. A., Hughes, M. G., and Munro, J. A. (1991). A study of the management of chlamydial cervicitis in general practice. *British Journal of General Practice,* **41,** 279–81.

Reed, B. D., Werner, H., and Zazove, P. (1989). Differentiation of *Gardnerella vaginalis, Candida albicans,* and *Trichomonas vaginalis* infections of the vagina. *Journal of Family Practice,* **28,** 673–80.

Sackett, D. L., Haynes, R. B., and Tugwell, P. (1985). *Clinical epidemiology: a basic science for clinical medicine.* Little Brown, Boston/Toronto.

Singer, A. and Jenkins, D. (1991). Viruses and cervical cancer. *British Medical Journal*, **302**, 251–2.

Southgate, L. (1990). The diagnosis and management of chlamydial cervicitis: a test of cure. *Journal of Family Practice*, **31**, 33–5.

Southgate, L. J., Treharne, J. D., and Forsey, T. (1983). *Chlamydia trachomatis* and *Neisseria gonorrhoeae* infections in women attending inner city general practices. *British Medical Journal*, **287**, 879–81.

Stamm, W. E. (1988). Diagnosis of *Chlamydia trachomatis* genitourinary infections. *Annals of Internal Medicine*, **108**, 710–17.

Taylor-Robinson, D., Thomas, B. J., and Osborn, M. F. (1987). Evaluation of enzyme immunoassay (Chlamydiazyme) for detecting *Chlamydia trachomatis* in genital tract specimens. *Journal of Clinical Pathology*, **40**, 194–9.

Third National Morbidity Survey (1986). *Morbidity statistics from general practice 1981–82*. RCGP/OPCS/DHSS. HMSO, London.

White, D. and Radcliffe, K. (1991). Management of chlamydial cervicitis in general practice. *British Journal of General Practice*, **41**, 434–5.

11. Cystitis

Tom O'Dowd

HISTORICAL ASPECTS

There has always been a lot of cystitis about. *The Hearst collection of old Egyptian papyri* (1550 BC) was a doctors' formulary which gave no less than fifteen possible recipes for urinary problems. One such prescription of juniper berries, cumin, and coriander was 'to cure the sending forth heat from the bladder' which is probably the earliest known reference to dysuria. Hippocrates (500 BC) made many references to urinary disorders and urged close inspection of the urine for sediment, particles, and pus. In *Epidemics* Book 1 he tells of 'many cases of perineal abscess accompanied by strangury and a painful, bilious, watery discharge containing particles and pus. There was no disease of the kidneys in these cases.' Thus Hippocrates separated the upper from the lower renal tract nearly one hundred and fifty years before Aristotle (384–322 BC) described the (predictably) male urogenital system with such perceptive and accurate detail!

The sixteenth-century Tudor physicians recognized frequency and dysuria but directed most of their attention to the collection of urine; indeed the urine flask became the pictorial symbol of the physician much as the stethoscope is today. This ritual naked eye inspection of urine—urinoscopy—did nothing to advance the understanding of disease. In 1653 the famous herbalist Nicholas Culpeper advised red coral, marshmallow in goat's milk, and burnt mice in milk for urinary tract symptoms. This concoction had less therapeutic rationale than that of the Egyptian papyrus 3000 years before. However Culpeper did recognize lower urinary tract symptoms of 'strangury' and also 'inflammation in the bladder'.

MODERN CONCEPTS

In 1863 Pasteur observed that urine was a good culture medium and in 1881 Roberts (1881) made the association between bacteriuria and urinary symptoms of frequency and dysuria especially in the female. In 1894 Escherich was to describe similar organisms in children's urines and these organisms become eponymously known as *Escherichia coli*.

The observations of Pasteur, Roberts, and Escherich gave an important impetus to scientific research into urinary tract infections (UTI). In a classic series of *in vitro* experiments Stohl and Janney (1917) successfully demonstrated that the growth of *E. coli* is inhibited between pH 4.6 and pH 5. Using this knowledge a ketogenic diet was tried for the treatment of UTI and it was demonstrated that the active agent was oxybutyric acid. This led Rosenheim (1935) to search for an organic acid that would be a bacteriostatic agent excreted unchanged by the kidneys. Using *in vivo* and *in vitro* experiments he developed the effective use of mandelic acid for urine infections. Thus for the first time in the history of UTI, research led to rational therapy. The advent of sulphonamides in 1935 meant, however, that therapeutics had outstripped knowledge about the aetiology and natural history of UTI.

A faulty numerator

Because Richard Bright (of Bright's disease) in 1827 had advanced the knowledge of kidney pathology so much, it is perhaps small wonder that pathologists a century later felt sufficiently competent to study chronic pyelonephritis. Weiss and Parker (1939) established criteria for the diagnosis of pyelonephritis based on 100 necropsies. They pointed out that only 20 per cent of their series had an accurate diagnosis made during life. Their criteria were uncritically accepted for many years and led to a rather sepulchral view of UTIs. In an audit of necropsies in a hospital in Connecticut between 1957 and 1964 Freedman (1967) noticed a progressive decline in the frequency of the diagnosis of chronic pyelonephritis from 2.4 per cent to 0.5 per cent. This decline was mainly due to a growing realization that such a diagnosis should be made only if there were changes in both the renal parenchyma and the pelvicalyceal system.

Screening

Because Weiss and Parker's criteria were uncritically accepted for about forty years it was only natural that investigators should search for what they thought was a large reservoir of undiagnosed urinary infection. They were hampered by the lack of agreed criteria for diagnosis and plagued by the need to separate contaminants from true bacteriuria. In 1956 Edward Kass developed a reproducible quantitative method of separating contaminants from true bacteriuria; a count of 10^5 bacteria or more per millilitre of urine was designated arbitrarily as the dividing line between true bacilluria and contamination in asymptomatic females. Kass's criterion was exactly what was needed for screening purposes (Kass 1956). Researcher's now had high hopes of eradicating pyelonephritis and unravelling the natural history of urinary infection by using a non-invasive urine test.

Screening revealed that there was a higher prevalence of UTI in neonatal males than in females which parallels their greater incidence of congenital urinary tract abnormalities. Covert or symptomless infections are the commonest infection of the urinary tract. Studies among adults demonstrated that about 5 per cent of females between 16 and 65 years had significant bacteriuria. In an imaginative study of nuns and black and white working women, Kunin (1968) demonstrated a significantly higher incidence of bacteriuria in working women and postulated the protectiveness of celibacy in UTIs. Kass himself demonstrated a link between asymptomatic bacteriuria (ASB) of pregnancy and acute pyelonephritis (1960) while Little (1966) in a randomized controlled trial of 5000 pregnant women demonstrated that treatment of ASB prevented pyelonephritis.

False promises

Now that screening had established the frequency of ASB, and fortified by the success of treating ASB in pregnancy, researchers argued for the need to detect and treat ASB in the general female population. Cochrane, an epidemiologist, argued that there were two basic requirements for a screening test, namely the detection of disease before irreversible damage had occurred and that the disease so detected could be effectively treated (Cochrane 1972). Fry, in a six-year follow-up of acute UTI in general practice, did not observe any of the serious sequelae feared by contemporary observers (Fry *et al.* 1962). Little, a radiologist, in a small follow-up study of acute pyelonephritis, using intravenous pyelography, three months to two years after the initial episode, observed that the kidneys had become smaller but noted an absence of scarring or calyceal damage (Little *et al.* 1965). Asscher put Cochrane's criteria to the test in a randomized controlled double-blind trial of 107 non-pregnant adult females with ASB (Asscher *et al.* 1969). Follow-up at one year showed that treatment failed to prevent recurrence and he concluded that screening the adult female for ASB was unlikely to be of value as a preventative measure since it failed to detect UTI at an early and reversible stage of its natural history; treatment was ineffective for larger scale use.

TERMINOLOGY

It would be reasonable to expect urinary symptoms to be derived from the genito-urinary tract. This is not the case, although the term 'cystitis' seems to be common ground between doctors and patients. Patients and doctors will speak of a 'kidney infection' when they mean a lower urinary tract infection without any renal signs or symptoms being present. Some patients will speak about having a 'cold in the kidneys', again meaning they have contracted lower urinary tract symptoms. Part of the difficulty in arriving at precise terminology is that diagnosis is based on history and occasional examination of the urine. Patients complaining of urinary symptoms rarely have a physical examination mainly because it is not usually warranted. The term 'urethral syndrome' is applicable to half the female patients consulting their GP with lower urinary tract symptoms, but without any evidence of infection (see below).

WHO CONSULTS?

In a community prevalence study in a South Wales mining valley, Waters (1969) found that one in five adult women had experienced dysuria in the previous year; one in ten suffered dysuria for two weeks or longer. Interestingly less than half the women had consulted their doctor about the problem; the study does not say how long those who did consult suffered before seeking medical attention. A general practice-based study in London has demonstrated that 52 per cent of women get cystitis at some stage in their lives (Walker *et al.* 1983). However, the study also demonstrated that 27 per cent of all women had experienced three or more episodes of dysuria in their lives. Sadly some 6 per cent had experienced three or more episodes during the previous 12 months. Again this study demonstrated that despite a 20 per cent prevalence rate for recent dysuria only 6 per cent had visited the doctor because of dysuria.

SEX AND COFFEE

Cystitis is 12.8 times commoner in the general female population than in nuns, who are assumed to be celibate (Kunin *et al.* 1968). Prevalence studies confirm that about one woman in five will have had a recent episode of dysuria (Kunin 1978). Lower urinary tract symptoms seem to parallel the onset of sexual activity, and post-intercourse bacteriuria is common in women prone to post-coital UTIs (Kass 1956).

A clear association has now been shown between diaphragm use and UTI (Fihn *et al.* 1985). Vaginal colonization with *E. coli* was significantly greater in diaphragm users in an American study. Uro-dynamic studies demonstrated that the diaphragm was causing a severe distortion of urinary flow and elevation of the bladder neck angle. By changing diaphragm size or method of contraception virtually all patients were infection free on follow-up.

Patients with symptoms of frequency and urgency often complain that their symptoms are exacerbated by tea or coffee. Caffeine-containing compounds do have a diuretic effect and there is also evidence that caffeine has an effect on the detrusor muscle in the bladder which causes excitation which is exhibited as frequency of micturition (Creighton and Stanton

1990). Advising women to reduce their caffeine intake, which incidentally also includes cola drinks, may cause a reduction in frequency.

URETHRAL SYNDROME

While trying to establish the place of sulphonamides in the treatment of UTI, a group of New Zealand general practitioners made a classic observation (Aarnoudse *et al.* 1980; Gallagher *et al.* 1965). They prospectively studied all adults presenting with lower urinary tract symptoms to their GPs. Using Kass's criterion (10^5 organisms per millilitre) they found that only half their patients had conventional UTI while the other half had $<10^5$ typical organisms per millilitre of urine or sterile urines. They called this the 'urethral syndrome' postulating that the urethra was involved in this new condition which predominantly affects females.

In the past decade research into the urethral syndrome has been based in specialist, genito-urinary, or campus clinics and in laboratories with minimal clinical information. This shift in research from the bedside and community to the laboratory, while following a general trend in medicine, is very noticeable in studies on the urethral syndrome. These studies have employed micro-biological skills and techniques not normally available in the community. Microaerophilic and fastidious organisms have been implicated and dismissed as causative organisms. There is broad agreement that *Chlamydia* is associated with the urethral syndrome in genito-urinary and campus clinics. The causation of the urethral syndrome in general practice is more difficult to fathom. Detailed microbiological investigations of general practice patients with the urethral syndrome failed to find any *Chlamydia* (O'Dowd *et al.* 1985*a*). Indeed the *Chlamydia* positive studies are really describing chlamy-dial cervicitis, urethritis, or vaginitis and not the urethral syndrome.

It has been shown that the urethral syndrome is a short self-limiting illness and that dysuria is much less in the urethral syndrome than in conventional UTI (O'Dowd *et al.* 1984*a*). Women with the urethral syndrome have a higher consultation rate than women with UTI. They tend to suffer from anxiety, have relationship problems (O'Dowd *et al.* 1984*b*) and generally feel less healthy than UTI or control patients (O'Dowd *et al.* 1986). The syndrome has much more in common with the irritable bowel syndrome than it has with UTI. Indeed both conditions commonly coexist in the same patient and can be a great drain on time and investigations. It has been suggested that it should be thought of as the irritable urethral syndrome in order to recognize the psychosomatic aspect of the condition (O'Dowd 1985*b*). Too often patients with urethral syndrome receive serial courses of antibiotics and the occasional MSU. It is unusual to see the urethral syndrome made as a positive diagnosis in patients' GP files, which means that it is a diagnosis of omission which does not have a management plan or indeed a clear approach in the GP's mind. Sufferers can remain an angry and mismanaged group as they are usually told by the receptionist over the telephone that 'your water test was perfectly all right, nothing to worry about.'

The unkindest thing that can be done to a women with the urethral syndrome is to refer her to an invasive specialist. In the past such women have been subjected to treatments like urethrotomy, urethral dilatation, and steroid injections into the urethra. The urethral syndrome has been labelled as lower urinary tract symptoms in an anxious woman who is prone to other psychosomatic difficulties, but recent studies have shown that this is not so. It is rather a suitable and appropriate condition to be managed in general practice.

FEMALE URINE

Vulnerability to infection

Whereas tears, saliva, and bronchial secretions contain lysozyme and immunoglobulins, human urine lacks both these mechanisms against bacterial invasion. There is a range of pH for normal urine which is between 4.6 and 7.25. The optimal growth for the commonest urinary pathogen *E. coli* is obtained between a pH 6.0 and 7.0. At pH values less than 5.5 or greater than 7.5 bacterial growth is inhibited. This factor is exploited in many home remedies which try to make the urine very acid or very alkaline.

The osmolality of human urine also has a range depending on the state of hydration. The usual physiological range is between 300 and 1200 mosmol/ litre. However, if the urine is very dilute—below 200 mosmol—growth is reduced irrespective of pH. This is the basis for the advice to increase fluids during episodes of cystitis. It is interesting that the urine of females is significantly more often at a suitable pH and osmolality for the growth of *E. coli* than urine obtained from males. These factors taken in combination with a short anatomical urethra go a long way towards explaining the greater susceptibility of the female to cystitis. Indeed urine obtained from pregnant women is almost invariably at a suitable pH for the growth of urinary pathogens at all stages of pregnancy. There is a theoretical possibility that a patient on antibiotics who consumes gallons of fluids could dilute the antibiotic to the point of ineffectiveness. However, since the concentration of most antibiotics in urine is far in excess of the minimum inhibitory concentration needed to kill off bacteria this is an unlikely occurrence and the benefits of high fluid intake outweigh the fears of diluted antibiotics.

Ascending infection

The organisms causing UTI are mostly derived from the patient's own faecal flora. This bald fact is of great importance in giving advice to women with recurrent infections. In hospital practice, of course, infections are often acquired from outside sources like instrumentation, catheterization, surgical procedures, and cytoscopy.

The presence of faecal organisms is encouraged by incontinence and in some women *E. coli* has the ability to adhere to peri-urethral epithelial cells through special receptor sites. Sexual intercourse plays an important part in the ascent of organisms from the perineum to the bladder (Fihn *et al.* 1985). It is likely that clumsy sexual techniques in furtive surroundings may play an important part in a first UTI. This factor was well recognized in advance of epidemiological studies by the (now) quaint bitter-sweet term 'honeymoon cystitis'. In adult women most of the organisms stay in the bladder and do not ascend any further to the ureters or kidneys unless there are pre-existing problems like vesicoureteric reflux.

ANTIBIOTIC TREATMENT

Indications for using drug therapy

It seems obvious to the traditional medical mind that all urine infection should be treated with antibiotics. However, it is well known that a proportion of UTIs, particularly in adult females, will clear up on their own regardless of treatment. In a placebo-controlled study of antibiotics, Mabeck (1972) found that of 63 women on placebo 43 attained sterile urine without active treatment. He also noted that in 21 out of 23 patients with four weeks' bacteriuria the symptoms disappeared before the infection was eliminated. Indeed in covert infections spontaneous remissions and new infections occur at the rate of 1 per cent per annum (Asscher 1980). It is also true that treatment does not prevent relapse and there are groups of patients who are particularly prone to relapse.

Patients who are prone to recurrent UTIs are in need of special management plans of which drug treatment is an important part. Such patients can be given permission and instructions to start their own courses of antibiotics from supplies that they keep in a safe place at home. Such a plan can minimize further structural damage and decrease morbidity. Similarly, such patients can send the occasional MSU to the laboratory to check that their urine hasn't become resistant to their favourite antibiotic.

Hallmarks of a good antibiotic for UTIs

A good antibiotic preparation for urinary tract infections should ideally be excreted unaltered in the urine. It should have a long half-life, should be effective in either single dose or short (three-day) courses (Bailey and Ross 1983), and have a low incidence of side-effects. Such antibiotics need to overcome local resistance patterns and the prescriber needs to know the prevalence of resistance to different antibiotics. Resistance is a major problem with different patterns emerging for hospital and general practice. Cost is a debatable factor because there is no more expensive antibiotic than the one that doesn't work.

Antibiotics in use for UTIs

Trimethoprim

Trimethoprim fulfils many of the hallmarks of a good antibiotic by indeed reaching the parts not reached by others. It is excreted in the urine and has a long half-life. Over 80 per cent of urinary pathogens in general practice are susceptible to trimethoprim although this figure used to be over 90 per cent in the 1970s. In adult females it is ideal as a short dose treatment of either one or three days. There is probably little advantage in using co-trimoxazole which is a combination of trimethoprim and sulphonamide. Co-trimoxazole can occasionally cause allergic reactions and neither co-trimoxazole or trimethoprim are advisable in pregnancy.

The ampicillins

The ampicillins, including amoxycillin, have fallen out of favour because resistance is now at about 40 per cent of urinary pathogens in general practice. The percentage is higher still in hospitals. However, the addition of clavulinic acid to amoxycillin has made it more powerful.

Clavulinic acid is an inhibitor of the bacterial beta-lactamase. Amoxycillin can give rise to gastrointestinal side-effects and must be used with caution in patients who declare that they are allergic to penicillin.

Nitrofurantoin

Nitrofurantoin can be very effective in long-term treatment of recurrent urinary tract infections or in post-coital UTIs. However, it is ineffective against *Proteus mirabilis* which is a common pathogen in both hospital and general practice.

The B-lactams

Cefuroxime axetil and cefixime are third generation cephalosporins which are active against a wide range of bacteria. At present they demonstrate excellent effectiveness against the common organisms in general practice but cefixime is inactive against pseudomonas, staphylococci, and the enterococci. Cefuroxime can be given twice daily and cefixime can be given once a day.

The new Quinolone antibiotics

Ciprofloxacin, ofloxacin, enoxacin, and norfloxacin are examples of this group of drugs. These are very effective against the organisms involved in urinary tract infections. However, at present they are excluded in children and pregnancy and can interact with theophyllines and caffeine. Central nervous system side-effects have been occasionally reported.

How long should treatment last?

Patients have always been admonished by doctors to 'finish the course of antibiotics'. Now that we have a greater appreciation of compliance we know that patients take antibiotics for as long as they are feeling unwell and then stop them. It used to be quite common for women to be given 10 days' treatment for urinary tract infection but in recent times this has come down to a three-day course of treatment or even a one-off single dose of antibiotic (Bailey 1983). There is ample evidence to show that 10 days' treatment is no better than eight days' treatment with respect to eradication of organisms, relief of symptoms, and prevention of reinfection. The eradication of organisms is often much easier to achieve than the relief of symptoms. When prescribing a short dose of antibiotics it is worth telling patients that their symptoms may persist after the antibiotic course has been completed.

Single doses of 2 g of sulfadoxine, 3 g of amoxycillan, and 2.88 g of co-trimoxazole have all been tried against conventional treatment and found to be successful. The striking feature of such a regimen is the size of the dose. More recently 1 g of amoxycillan has been found to be effective, and four tablets of trimethoprim (400 mg), or four tablets of co-trimaxazole are as effective as the seven days' treatment. The advantages of short or single dose therapy are fewer side-effects and better compliance. There is also a considerable saving to be made which may make the PACT data on our prescribing just a little less depressing.

SPECIAL PROBLEMS

Chronic UTI

There is a minority of women in every practice whose records are full of MSU reports and haphazard notes recording a variety of antibiotics. The file will also contain a referral letter and a consultation opinion about an essentially normal genito-urinary tract. It is worthwhile having a management strategy for such patients. Nowadays we trust patients to measure their own blood glucose, adjust their anti-coagulation treatment, and check their IUDs. Women with chronic UTI can become much more self-reliant if allowed to initiate their own antibiotic treatment at the onset of symptoms. An occasional MSU may be needed to check the organism present and the development of any antibiotic resistance. The doctor need only be visited for repeat MSU bottles, laboratory forms, and antibiotics for the bathroom shelf. If the pattern of infection and symptoms shows any changes, or resistance emerges, then re-evaluation of the treatment is needed. Otherwise such patients can manage quite well on their own.

Post-coital and adolescent UTI

A UTI in a young girl is often an indication of the commencement of sexual activity and a shrewd clinician will always make tactful enquiry about contraception in such cases. If further attacks occur sensitive advice may be offered about hygiene, sexual technique, and prevention. Emptying the bladder after intercourse helps to flush out any organisms that have ascended the short female urethra during intercourse. Indeed, French women consider their British counterparts as bereft in not having a bidet in the bedroom for the purpose of douching. If sexual intercourse continues to be a trigger for UTI it is worth giving such women an antibiotic such as trimethoprim or nalidixic acid to take after intercourse.

SELF-HELP AND GENTLE REMEDIES

Books and leaflets on self-help and cystitis seemed to abound in the early 1980s after Angela Kilmartin published her self-help book on cystitis and founded the U and I Club. Angela Kilmartin's acting career was ruined by cystitis and she sought the help of many doctors. Her book is quite critical of the medical profession and she advocates self-help where possible (Kilmartin 1973). The U and I Club has since been disbanded but it helped to popularize self-help remedies for many women fed up with recurrent cystitis. Leaflets on cystitis come and go and always include the caveat to 'call your doctor if in doubt', which is hardly the way to empower the individual patient. One of the best HEA leaflets available is *Understanding cystitis*.

Most self-help remedies are a combination of increased fluids to dilute the bacteria, alkalinization of the urine to inhibit bacterial growth, and common sense. Bicarbonate of soda used to be widely available in the kitchen but has virtually disappeared in many homes with the decline in baking at home. It is a good cheap way of alkalinization of the urine but many women will have to rely on Mist. Pot. Cit. which is effective but unpleasant to taste. The role of coffee has been discussed and avoiding alcohol is often found to be helpful, as is the avoidance of acidic fruits and juices. The use of antiseptics like mandelamine is a useful ploy as it also helps to inhibit bacterial growth. Women with cystitis can feel very unwell and lethargic. Nowadays doctors are less willing to prescribe rest than before but taking painkillers and retiring to bed with a hot water bottle across the lower abdomen is found to be soothing and recuperative by some women.

Before advising a patient with reported UTI to stop using a diaphragm as her method of contraception it may be worth reviewing the fitting technique and also bearing in mind that allergies to the rubber and contraceptive gel can occur. It is worth changing the contraceptive cream or gel initially and if UTI persists then changing the brand of diaphragm. However, it is likely that only a patient woman or a strong devotee of the diaphragm will tolerate such a level of experimentation.

SUMMARY

Female urine has always been known to be susceptible to infection and it has surprised modern doctors that there is a huge reservoir of infection in the community which they do not see in their clinics. Screening for UTI has had its day, being motivated by a desire to eradicate kidney damage. However, there is no association between cystitis and kidney damage in non-pregnant adult females. Another surprising factor is that half the women consulting with symptoms of cystitis do not have demonstrable infection. This, the urethral syndrome, has had very bizarre and invasive treatments to no avail. The modern GP would do well to protect such women by recognizing the syndrome. Antibiotic treatment of UTI has gradually shortened over the years and a single dose of antibiotic is now advocated with substantial research backing. Self-help and gentle remedies can empower those women whose lives are made miserable by lower urinary tract symptoms.

REFERENCES AND FURTHER READING

Aarnoudse, J. G., Meyer-Scuers, G. J., and Dankert, J. (1980). Do anaerobes cause urinary tract infections? *Lancet,* **i,** 368–9.

Asscher, A. W. (1980). *The challenge of urinary tract infections,* pp. 59–60. Academic Press, London.

Asscher, A. W., Sussman, M., Water, W. E., *et al.* (1969). Asymptomatic significant bacteriuria in the non-pregnant woman. Response to treatment on follow-up. *British Medical Journal,* **1,** 804–6.

Bailey, Ross R. (1983). *Single dose therapy of urinary tract infection.* AIDS Health Science Press, Sydney.

Cochrane, A. L. (1972). *Effectiveness and efficiency: random reflections on health services.* Nuffield Provincial Hospitals Trust, London.

Creighton, S. M. and Stanton, S. L. (1990). Caffeine: does it affect your bladder? *British Journal of Urology,* **66,** 613–14.

Fihn, S. D., Latham, R. H., Roberts, P., *et al.* (1985). Association between diaphragm use and urinary infection. *Journal of the Association of Medical Advisers,* **254, (2),** 240–5.

Freedman, L. R. (1967). Chronic pyelonephritis at autopsy. *Annual International Medicine,* **66,** 697–710.

Fry, J., Dillane, J. B., Joiner, C. L., *et al.* (1962). Acute urinary infections, their course and outcome in general practice with special reference to chronic pyelonephritis. *Lancet,* **1**, 1318–21.

Gallagher, D. J. A., Montgomerie, J. Z., and North, J. D. K. (1965). Acute infections of the urinary tract and the urethral syndrome in general practice. *British Medical Journal,* **1**, 622–6.

Health Education Authority (n.d.). *Understanding cystitis.* HEA, London.

Kass, E. H. (1956). Asymptomatic infections of the urinary tract. *Transatlantic Association of American Physicians,* **69**, 56–63.

Kass, E. H. (1960). Bacteriuria and pyelonephritis of pregnancy. *Archives of International Medicine,* **105**, 194–8.

Kilmartin, A. (1973). *Understanding cystitis.* Pan Books, London.

Kunin, C. M. (1978). Sexual intercourse and urinary infections. *New England Journal of Medicine,* **298**, 336.

Kunin, C. M. and McCormack, R. C. (1968). An epidemiological study of bacteriuria and blood pressure among nuns and working women. *New England Journal of Medicine,* **278**, 635–42.

Little, P. J. (1966). The incidence of urinary infection in 5000 pregnant women. *Lancet,* **2**, 925–8.

Little, P. J., McPherson, D. R., and de Wardner, H. E. (1965). The appearance of the intravenous pyelogram during and after acute pyelonephritis. *Lancet,* **1**, 1186–8.

Mabeck, C. E. (1972). Treatment of uncomplicated urinary tract infection in non-pregnant women. *Postgraduate Medical Journal,* **48**, 69–75.

O'Dowd, T. C., Ribeiro, C. D., Munro, J. A., *et al.* (1984*a*). The urethral syndrome—a self-limiting illness. *British Medical Journal,* **288**, 1349–52.

O'Dowd, T. C., Smail, J. E., and West, R. R. (1984*b*). Clinical judgement in the management of frequency and dysuria in general practice. *British Medical Journal,* **288**, 1347–9.

O'Dowd, T. C., Munro, J. A., and Parton, D. (1985*a*). *Chlamydia trachomatis* infection in women: a case for more action? *Lancet,* **i**, 1215–16.

O'Dowd, T. C. (1985*b*). The irritable urethral syndrome: discussion. *Journal of the Royal College of General Practitioners,* **35**, 140–1.

O'Dowd, T. C., Pill, R., Smail, J. E., *et al.* (1986). The irritable urethral syndrome: a two-year follow-up study in general practice. *British Medical Journal,* **292**, 30–2.

Roberts, W. (1881). On the occurrence of microorganisms in fresh urine. *British Medical Journal,* **2**, 623–5.

Rosenheim, M. L. (1935). Mandelic acid in the treatment of urinary infections. *Lancet,* **i**, 1032–7.

Stohl, A. T. and Janney, J. H. (1917). The growth of *Bacillus coli* in urine at varying hydrogen ion concentrations. *Journal of Urology,* **i**, 211–29.

Walker, M., Heady, J. A., and Shaper, A. G. (1983). The prevalence of dysuria in women in London. *Journal of the Royal College of General Practitioners,* **33**, 411–15.

Waters, W. E. (1969). Prevalence of symptoms of urinary tract infection in women. *British Journal of Preventative and Social Medicine,* **23**, 263–6.

Weiss, S. and Parker, F. (1939). Pyelonephritis: its relation to vascular lesions and to arterial hypertension. *Medicine,* (Baltimore), **18**, 221–5.

12. Endometriosis

Stephen Kennedy

INTRODUCTION

Endometriosis is an enigma as virtually nothing is known about its aetiology or pathophysiology. Therefore, the management of the disease can be intensely frustrating as its behaviour refuses to conform to any textbook norms. The frustration is most keenly felt by patients who come to realize there is no magical cure for their debilitating symptoms.

Numerous unsubstantiated myths have arisen about endometriosis: for example, delayed childbearing is a risk factor or pregnancy is a cure. The aims of this chapter are to dispel some of these myths and to give guidelines on the diagnosis and management of the disease.

As the diagnosis is usually made at laparoscopy, the incidence of endometriosis in general practice will depend upon how readily symptomatic women are referred for a gynaecological opinion. As a general rule, pelvic pain and dyspareunia are abnormal and warrant referral to a gynaecologist, as does dysmenorrhoea that fails to respond to conventional therapy. Endometriosis must always be considered whenever repeated episodes of pelvic pain fail to respond to antibiotic treatment.

After a laparoscopic diagnosis has been made, surgery is usually recommended or medical treatment commenced in hospital. The subsequent management of endometriosis should be in general practice unless the woman is also infertile, or unless her symptoms fail to improve or recur. Successful management requires an understanding of the efficacy and side-effects of the drugs currently being used.

DEFINITION AND AETIOLOGY

Endometriosis is defined histologically as the presence of endometrial glands and stroma outside the uterine cavity. The definition excludes adenomyosis which is considered to be a separate pathological entity. The most commonly affected pelvic sites are the ovaries, peritoneum, and utero-sacral ligaments. Intestinal involvement occurs in approximately 12 per cent of women with endometriosis and most commonly affects the sigmoid colon and/or rectum. Endometriosis involving extra-pelvic sites such as the lungs and central nervous system is exceedingly rare.

Ectopic endometrium was first described in 1860 and since then there have been many theories to explain its occurrence. These include:

(1) stimulation of embryonal cell rests;

(2) coelomic metaplasia of cells lining the pelvic peritoneum;

(3) blood or lymph borne spread;

(4) mechanical implantation;

(5) retrograde menstruation.

One theory may appeal more than others as an explanation for rare manifestations of the disease: for example, the theory of vascular spread to explain a lesion on the thumb, or mechanical implantation to explain endometriosis in an abdominal wall scar following mid-trimester hysterotomy. However, no single theory adequately explains the majority of cases. The most attractive is coelomic metaplasia as metaplastic change is so common throughout the genital tract, but there is little scientific support for this theory.

Currently, the most favoured theory is retrograde menstruation. Sampson (1940) first suggested that endometriosis develops as a result of the implantation of endometrial tissue that is regurgitated through the fallopian tubes during menstruation. Modern advocates of Sampson's theory have had to explain why the disease is not more common given that retrograde menstruation occurs in so many women (Liu and Hitchcock 1986) and as commonly in women with endometriosis as in those with a normal pelvis (Bartosik *et al.* 1986).

An answer may be that endometriosis only develops if the amount of retrograde flow exceeds the immune system's capacity to eliminate the menstrual debris. Causes include excessive regurgitation due to heavy periods or outflow obstruction. The clinical evidence certainly suggests that short menstrual cycles and heavy, prolonged menstrual loss are risk factors for endometriosis and that the disease is common in women with patent fallopian tubes and outflow obstruction, i.e. congenital atresia of the cervix. Another cause is a deficient immune system: women who develop endometriosis may have a specific cell-mediated immunodeficiency, probably genetically transmitted, that prevents the lysis of menstrual debris and endometrial cells in the peritoneal cavity (Steele *et al.* 1984).

Prevalence

All estimates of the prevalence of endometriosis are purely speculative as the diagnosis can only be made at laparoscopy or laparotomy. Most women who undergo surgery have pain and/or infertility and therefore represent a highly selected population. The range of prevalence figures is wide: for example, in 860 laparoscopies performed in eight studies to investigate pelvic pain the range was 4.5–32.0 per cent. One explanation for this apparent discrepancy may be that some surgeons are unfamiliar with the disease and its numerous atypical manifestations (see 'Histological criteria' below).

There is certainly no evidence that endometriosis has a predilection for middle-aged, upper-class, ambitious, white women as suggested in many gynaecology textbooks. This stereotype probably only demonstrates that such women have greater access to medical care and a laparoscopic diagnosis.

Many authors have claimed that endometriosis is hereditary but their claims have relied upon poorly controlled data and the studies have often not included laparoscopic assessment. The true prevalence can only be determined if all the women in a study have surgery to exclude the diagnosis; the presence or absence of symptoms is insufficient evidence. Bias in the selection of study populations is common: if a mother is found to have endometriosis it is possible that she will advise her daughter to seek gynaecological advice for any number of symptoms that may or may not be related to the disease.

DIAGNOSIS

Clinical criteria

Numerous symptoms are attributed to endometriosis. The most common is pelvic pain which usually starts one to two days before, and lasts throughout, a period. Many women also complain of concomitant rectal pressure, pain on defecation, and low backache which radiates to the anterior thigh. Deep dyspareunia is common due to involvement of the rectovaginal septum.

Despite the association, there is little conclusive evidence that endometriosis causes pain. In a study of 1000 consecutive diagnostic laparoscopies, the incidence of endometriosis was only 8.2 per cent (11/135) in women with pelvic pain or dyspareunia and 7.4 per cent (2/27) in those with dysmenorrhoea or mid-cycle pain (Duignan *et al.* 1972). The severity of symptoms rarely correlates with the extent of endometriosis; in fact, women with severe diseases are often asymptomatic.

Abnormal vaginal bleeding may occur, often in the form of premenstrual spotting and staining. Approximately 20 per cent of women with intestinal involvement will also have rectal bleeding. Endometriosis in the urinary tract is rare but may cause haematuria, loin pain, and hydronephrosis. Women occasionally present with an acute abdomen due to intra-abdominal haemorrhage from a ruptured endometrioma.

Physical findings

The physical findings are extremely variable and depend upon the extent of the disease. The most common sign is cul-de-sac tenderness often associated with tender nodules in the rectovaginal septum and on the utero-sacral ligaments. The uterus may be fixed, tender, and retroverted. Adnexal masses due to ovarian endometriomas may be palpable. Speculum examination may reveal a bluish nodule on the cervix or the posterior vaginal wall. Alternatively, the examination may be entirely normal.

Differential diagnosis

So variable is the presentation of endometriosis that it must be considered in the differential diagnosis of nearly all pelvic pathology. Thus, similar symptoms may be associated with primary dysmenorrhoea, pelvic inflammatory disease, ovarian tumours, uterine fibroids, and gastrointestinal disorders, e.g. irritable bowel disease. Pelvic inflammatory disease is the condition most frequently confused with endometriosis. Many women attain a diagnosis only after numerous antibiotic courses have failed to relieve their symptoms. Odendaal (1990) has written a comprehensive guide to the management of acute pelvic inflammatory disease which lists the minimum criteria required for a firm diagnosis.

Diagnostic methods

A blood test for endometriosis would be useful and would allow screening of at-risk populations such as infertile women, but a test with sufficient sensitivity and specificity awaits development. The test that has received the most attention is an immunoradiometric assay for serum CA-125 levels. CA-125 is a membrane antigen expressed on a variety of gynaecological malignancies and on endometriotic tissue. Serum CA-125 levels are elevated in women with ovarian carcinoma and levels can be mildly elevated in women with endometriosis, especially those with extensive disease (Barbieri *et al.* 1986). Despite initial optimism, diagnostic sensitivities of only 14–53 per cent have been reported for endometriosis.

In vivo antigen expression in ovarian carcinoma can be demonstrated by immunoscintigraphy using radiolabelled monoclonal antibody fragments directed against CA-125. Our group in Oxford has recently reported similar findings for pelvic and pulmonary endometriosis (Kennedy *et al.* 1990*a*, 1991).

Histological criteria

Endometrial glands and stroma are required for a definite histological diagnosis. Sometimes tissue that resembles endometriosis macroscopically is excised, but the diagnosis cannot be confirmed histologically; for such cases, the term 'presumptive endometriosis' has been coined. The use of scanning electron microscopy has helped the histological diagnosis of endometriosis. Three different types of endometriotic lesion are now recognized: (1) intraperitoneal polyps in continuity with deep lesions, (2) intraperitoneal foci with surface epithelium, glands, and stroma, and (3) small retroperitoneal foci with few glands and scanty stroma (Vasquez *et al.* 1984).

Laparoscopy

In the past, the diagnosis of endometriosis based upon histological criteria required women to undergo laparotomy. With the advent of laparoscopy, visual assessment of the pelvis has become the gold standard for diagnosis and it is currently the best method available. Typical ovarian 'chocolate' cysts and 'powder-burn' peritoneal lesions are easily diagnosed and it is arguable whether these lesions should routinely be biopsied (*Lancet* 1986). Subtle appearances of endometriosis are now recognized such as non-pigmented lesions (Jansen and Russell 1986). Most authors favour biopsy of these suspicious foci although in many British hospitals facilities for laparoscopic biopsy are not available.

Despite its diagnostic usefulness, laparoscopy has a number of inherent faults and it is associated with significant morbidity. The diagnostic accuracy of laparoscopy relies upon the operator's purely visual and very subjective assessment of the pelvis (Dmowski 1987). Consequently, subtle changes can be overlooked or misinterpreted. In addition, microscopic disease in visually normal peritoneum can theoretically be missed at laparoscopy (Murphy *et al.* 1986). If microscopic disease does exist, then normal laparoscopic findings do not exclude the diagnosis and the prevalence of endometriosis may be higher than previously estimated even by the most meticulous laparoscopists.

An answer to this confusing issue may be that laparoscopy is simply too primitive a tool for diagnosing endometriosis and evaluating its severity. The recent innovation of 'photoradiation diagnosis' (Vancaillie *et al.* 1989) illustrates how laparoscopy may be improved in the future. The method relies on the ability of certain drugs ('photo-enhancers') to concentrate in endometriotic tissue and emit a characteristic laser-induced fluorescence, which can be seen at laparoscopy.

Dmowski (1987) emhasized the relative crudity of laparoscopy as a diagnostic tool by comparing endometriosis with systemic lupus erythematosus (SLE):

... counting the number and cumulative size of peritoneal implants to stage the disease may be analogous to evaluating skin lesions to assess the severity of SLE.

The analogy is valuable as Dmowski and others now consider endometriosis to be a systemic autoimmune disease like SLE.

Weed and Arquembourg (1980) first suggested that endometriosis may be an autoimmune disease, based upon finding complement component C3 only in the endometrium of women with endometriosis. They speculated that menstrual proteins released from endometriotic tissue may be recognized as foreign, triggering an immune response. A clinical association between SLE and endometriosis has been reported in one study (Grimes *et al.* 1985).

Further evidence for such an immune response is the presence of a wide variety of auto-antibodies in the serum of women with endometriosis, suggesting polyclonal B-cell activation. Serum levels of auto-antibodies against histones, nucleotides, and phospholipids, including cardiolipin, were significantly higher in women with endometriosis than in a control population (Gleicher *et al.* 1987). Organ-specific auto-antibodies, mainly against endometrium, have also been described and their detection has been advocated as a diagnostic test and as a means of monitoring the effects of treatment (Chihal *et al.* 1986).

INFERTILITY AND ENDOMETRIOSIS

Endometriosis is associated with infertility: 30–70 per cent of women investigated for infertility are found to have endometriosis in varying degrees of severity. This may be a chance finding as there is little evidence of a causal link between endometriosis and infertility; though this does not apply to severe disease which destroys normal pelvic anatomy. Densely adherent fallopian tubes cannot pick up an egg, nor can an egg easily be released from an ovary containing large chocolate cysts.

Research into mild endometriosis as a cause of infertility has concentrated on three main areas: ovarian function, gamete transport, and altered immunity.

Ovarian function

The following disturbances in ovarian function may occur in endometriosis:

(1) anovulation
(2) the luteinized unruptured follicle syndrome
(3) luteal phase deficiency.

Abnormal follicular growth patterns in endometriosis have been described and some women with the disease are anovulatory; however, anovulation is a common finding in infertile women. Despite suggestions to the contrary, there is little evidence that ovulation induction is unsuccessful in women with untreated endometriosis.

Luteinized unruptured follicle syndrome (LUFS) may occur more commonly in women with endometriosis: the follicle responds to the LH surge but fails to rupture, despite ovarian steroidogenesis and a mid-cycle body temperature rise suggestive of ovulation. Diagnosis can be made at laparoscopy only by noting an absent stigma or by serial ultrasound measurements of follicular diameter. As some studies have reported a strong association between LUFS and endometriosis, it has even been suggested that LUFS is a cause of the disease.

Corpus luteum deficiency is another possible cause of infertility. This may result in decreased progesterone production in the luteal phase, shortened menstrual cycles, and reduced implantation rates. However, most studies overwhelmingly refute the hypothesis that luteal phase progesterone production is abnormal in women with endometriosis. All the evidence suggests that women with endometriosis have normal FSH, LH, oestrogen, and progesterone profiles.

Gamete transport

The passage of gametes through the upper genital tract is aided by muscular contractions of the fallopian tubes. The strength of these contractions is mediated by many factors including prostaglandins which are synthesized by endometriotic tissue. Theoretically therefore, altered tubal transport of ova or sperm could cause the embryo to arrive in the uterus at a suboptimal time for implantation.

Endometriosis causes an inflammatory reaction: there are therefore increased numbers of activated macrophages in peritoneal fluid which results in sperm phagocytosis. *In vitro* studies consequently demonstrate that sperm motility and survival are reduced in peritoneal fluid taken from women with endometriosis.

Immunology

The significance of auto-antibodies in endometriosis is unclear. They may be a primary phenomenon involved in the aetiology of the disease; alternatively, their production may be secondary to the presence of ectopic endometrium. It has been suggested that auto-antibodies may cause infertility and early pregnancy loss in women with endometriosis by interfering with implantation (Gleicher *et al.* 1989). Although there may be an association between some auto-antibodies, infertility, and miscarriage as in the cardiolipin syndrome, there is no evidence of a causal effect, nor even any evidence that miscarriage is more common in women with endometriosis (Pittaway *et al.* 1988). Given the present level of knowledge, the most rational approach to the problem is to consider auto-antibody abnormalities in endometriosis an epiphenomenon until the evidence proves otherwise.

Does mild endometriosis cause infertility?

There is no easy answer to this question. The evidence is often unhelpful as it is difficult to distinguish between cause and effect; for example, all the disturbances outlined above can occur in women with severe disease and in infertile women who do not have endometriosis. These disturbances could just as easily be major causes of infertility in their own right, rather than ways in which endometriosis adversely affects fertility. Finding endometriosis during the investigation of women with infertility may just be a coincidence; the disease is after all quite commonly found at laparoscopic sterilization in women who never had problems conceiving. Perhaps the strongest evidence against endometriosis as a cause of infertility emerges from the few double-blind placebo-controlled studies that have failed to show increased pregnancy rates in treatment groups. In fact, non-treatment groups achieve comparable fertility rates in most treatment studies (Evers 1989). Therefore, expectant management, i.e. merely waiting for conception to occur naturally, with the reassurance that it will with time, is increasingly being recommended to infertile couples in whom the only problem is mild endometriosis.

TREATMENT

Principles of treatment

Treatment for endometriosis varies greatly. It depends upon the severity of the disease, the woman's symptoms, and fertility problems. It will also be influenced by an individual gynaecologist's experience and the facilities available in his hospital.

Radical surgery is the best advice for a symptomatic woman over the age of 40 who wants a permanent cure, i.e. total abdominal hysterectomy, bilateral salpingo-oophorectomy, and resection of all residual disease. (Note that if endometriotic ovaries are conserved at hysterectomy, there is a 50 per cent likelihood of further surgery being needed.) Most cases, however, involve much more complex management decisions. For example, how should young symptomatic women with severe disease be treated or infertile women who fail to conceive despite conservative surgery and months of medical treatment?

The decisions need to be taken after lengthy discussion, especially if radical surgery is being considered for a young woman. Years after a surgical cure, some women forget their past pain and deeply regret the decision to be castrated.

Surgery for infertility

The best hope of treating severe disease is to remove as much endometriotic tissue and as many adhesions as possible so as to restore normal pelvic anatomy. This can be achieved at laparotomy with conventional surgery or laparoscopically with the use of a laser or specially designed instruments. The advantages of laparoscopic surgery are a much shorter hospital stay and a speedier recovery. Drugs may be prescribed before and/or after surgery. Theoretically, pre-operative medical treatment reduces the volume of endometriotic tissue and makes surgery easier. Unfortunately, endometriotic cysts rarely shrink and adhesions hardly ever disappear on medical treatment alone.

Mild endometriosis in women with infertility can be treated with drugs and/or surgery. Surgery is usually restricted to cauterizing endometriotic foci at laparoscopy. Although this has been common practice for many years, its value has never been established. Cautery may be performed at the initial laparoscopy and be the only treatment given. A range of drugs may then be offered, with the recommendation that they be taken for six to nine months. Obviously, this has the disadvantage of delaying attempts to conceive until after treatment.

All the drugs available for the treatment of endometriosis seem equally effective at relieving pain and improving fertility. Therefore what matters most is choosing the drug that is likely to have the fewest side-effects in that patient, i.e. avoiding danazol if the woman is already hirsute.

Medical treatment

Traditionally, hormonal treatments for endometriosis have attempted to mimic pregnancy or the menopause, based upon the clinical impression that the disease regresses during these physiological states. There is scanty evidence of a therapeutic effect for pregnancy: however, the hypo-oestrogenic state induced by lactation may, like the menopause, be beneficial. The modern aim of hormonal treatment is still to induce ovarian suppression in the hope that this will lead to atrophy of endometriotic implants.

The therapeutic options include:

(1) non-steroidal anti-inflammatory drugs such as mefenamic acid (Ponstan) or naproxen (Naprosyn);

(2) a combined oral contraceptive pill (usually one with a high progestogen content, such as Eugynon 30);

(3) a high-dose progestogen such as dydrogesterone (Duphaston) or medroxyprogesterone (Provera).

If fertility is not an issue and if PID has been excluded clinically, then there is an argument for a therapeutic trial of any of these drugs *without a definite laparoscopic diagnosis*. The COC pill, for example, will provide excellent symptomatic relief for many women.

The most commonly used drugs, danazol and gonadotrophin-releasing hormone agonists, are associated with numerous side-effects and therefore ideally should not be used until laparoscopy has been performed.

Danazol

Danazol (a derivative of 17α ethinyl testosterone) has several possible modes of action. These include direct effects on ovarian steroidogenesis, and raising free testosterone levels via testosterone displacement from sex hormone binding globulin (SHBG) and SHBG suppression. A specific antigonadotrophin effect is unlikely, although danazol does suppress the mid-cycle rise. Atrophy of endometriotic implants after danazol treatment has been demonstrated by both laparoscopy and histology.

Danazol's side-effects are largely androgenic; the most common are listed in Table 12.1. Women must be warned that the voice changes may be irreversible. Barrier forms of contraception are advisable as there are case reports of female pseudohermaphroditism on treatment.

Standard medical treatment is 200 mg t.d.s. for six months, but 800 mg daily may be required in some women; a dose as low as 100 mg daily may be effective in others. The GP may wish to titrate the dose by balancing symptom relief against side-effects. Amenorrhoea is not a prerequisite for effective treatment. Long-term therapy is theoretically inadvisable as danazol reduces high-density lipoprotein levels, but many women remain on treatment for years without any apparent clinical ill-effect. Gestrinone is a recently introduced alternative to danazol; it has a similar side-effect profile but the advantage of a twice-weekly dosage.

Pain relief after danazol is reported in more than 90 per cent of women and in the largest studies, 28–47 per cent of women conceived after danazol alone. The only randomized trial comparing danazol with expectant management failed to show any significant difference in pregnancy rates between the two treatments in minimal endometriosis (Seibel *et al.* 1982).

Table 12.1 *Possible side-effects of danazol*

Weight gain	Muscle cramps
↓ breast size	Hot flushes
Mood changes	Oily skin
Depression	Oedema
Acne	Hirsutism
↓ libido	Nausea
Headaches	Deep voice

The clinician wishing to use medical therapy in an infertile woman with endometriosis may be influenced by the suggestion that danazol will affect one of the possible causes of infertility, namely auto-antibody levels. Lower anti-endometrial antibody levels have been reported in women treated with danazol compared with untreated women (Chihal *et al.* 1986).

In a prospective study, El-Roeiy *et al.* (1988) demonstrated reduced levels of some non-specific auto-antibodies after treatment with danazol. Although these authors speculated on the influence of auto-antibodies on infertility and miscarriage rate, suggesting, for example, that the chances of maintaining a successful pregnancy would be greater after treatment with danazol, those clinical end-points in their study involved very small numbers of women.

These authors have presumed a specific immunosuppressive effect for danazol; however, other evidence suggests that gonadotrophin-releasing hormone agonists can also lower auto-antibody levels (Kennedy *et al.* 1990*b*).

Gonadotrophin-releasing hormone (GnRH) agonists

GnRH agonists induce hypo-oestrogenism by reversible suppression of gonadotrophin secretion—a form of medical oophorectomy. At present, they are taken by nasal spray (Nafarelin) or subcutaneous injection (Zoladex). The first action of these drugs is agonistic; therefore some women will notice an exacerbation of their symptoms caused by an initial rise in gonadotrophin levels that results in high oestradiol levels.

The side-effects of GnRH agonists are those of the menopause and the most common are listed in Table 12.2.

Therapy should not last longer than six months because studies have demonstrated a significant, but reversible, reduction in trabecular bone density on treatment. Adding an androgenic progestogen, such as norethisterone, may protect against bone loss and will reduce the intensity of the menopausal side-effects.

GnRH agonists seem as effective as danazol in relieving symptoms and in causing distress regression. In most double-blind studies, GnRH agonists are associated with more hot flushes and headaches, and danazol with greater weight gain. Clinicians must, therefore, estimate which set of side-

Table 12.2   *Possible side-effects of GnRHa*

Vaginal dryness	Hot flushes
↓ libido	Breast tenderness
Headaches	Insomnia
Depression	Irritability
Joint stiffness	Skin changes

effects will be better tolerated. My clinical impression is that GnRH agonists are well tolerated in women who have previously stopped taking danazol because of androgenic side-effects.

Alternative treatments

These are summarized very well in *Understanding endometriosis* by Caroline Hawkridge. Evening primrose oil (EPO), a rich source of gamma-linolenic acid, blocks leukotrine production and is said to be effective treatment for abdominal pain in endometriosis sufferers. In addition, it reduces some side-effects of danazol such as muscle spasms. Other treatments recommended by the Endometriosis Society include selenium, magnesium, calcium, vitamin E, and zinc.

Assisted conception

Assisted conception techniques such as *in vitro* fertilization (IVF) and gamete intrafallopian transfer (GIFT) are increasingly being offered as treatment for infertility associated with endometriosis. However, the efficacy of such treatment is difficult to assess as individual centres around the world report their figures in different ways. No study has ever compared assisted conception to conventional treatment or expectant management.

Some centres have reported that ovarian stimulation with human menopausal gonadotrophins (hMG) is impaired in women with endometriosis, especially in those with extensive disease and adhesions. As the number and quality of oocytes obtained has a direct bearing upon the success of treatment, such centres have understandably reported lower clinical pregnancy rates for women with endometriosis.

Lastly, Wardle *et al.* (1986) have reported lower fertilization rates in women with untreated endometriosis than in women who have been treated or who have tubal damage. However, this may become less problematic now that most IVF units use a regime of pituitary downregulation with a GnRH agonist (which of course is a treatment for endometriosis) before ovarian stimulation with hMG.

If a couple have other causes for their infertility, such as a low sperm count or cervical hostility then assisted conception may very well be indicated. Whether a woman with mild endometriosis as the only apparent cause of her infertility should be offered assisted conception is highly controversial.

Hormone replacement therapy

Whether or not a woman is offered HRT after a total abdominal hysterectomy and bilateral salpino-oophorectomy depends upon the severity of the disease and the personal preferences of the surgeon.

The fear is that exogenous oestrogens will stimulate residual disease and cause symptoms to recur; in the worst cases, ureteric or bowel obstruction occur. For this reason, HRT may be denied women or they may be advised to endure 6–12 months of hypo-oestrogenism before commencing HRT. Fortunately, reactivation is rare: for the majority of women there is no evidence that HRT is harmful irrespective of the route of administration employed. Some gynaecologists strongly favour the use of implants as testosterone can be added, which improves libido and may suppress residual disease. However, a disadvantage of oestradiol implants is that they cannot easily be removed if the disease is reactivated.

As a general rule, endometriosis is *not* a contraindication to HRT. In fact, as there is some evidence that women with endometriosis are at increased risk of osteoporosis, they should be actively encouraged to take HRT.

SUMMARY

Life for endometriosis sufferers can be unbearable as they struggle to endure the misery of intractable pain or prolonged infertility. Many women are embittered by the treatment they receive from the medical profession, without realizing the difficulties inherent in making an accurate diagnosis and in treating the condition. Therefore patient education is a vital part of the management of a chronic problem such as endometriosis. Advising women to join the Endometriosis Society may also be helpful. This self-help group often provides considerable relief as it gives fellow sufferers an opportunity to share their experiences and voice their grievances.

USEFUL ADDRESSES

Endometriosis Society, 65 Holmdene Avenue, Herne Hill, London SE24 9LD.

Hysterectomy Support Group, 11 Henryson Road, London SE4 1HL.

National Association for the Childless, 318 Summer Lane, Birmingham B19 3RL.

Women's Health Information Centre, 52–54 Featherstone Street, London EC1.

REFERENCES AND FURTHER READING

Barbieri, R. L., Niloff, J. M., Bast, R. C., *et al.* (1986). Elevated serum concentrations of CA-125 in patients with advanced endometriosis. *Fertility and Sterility,* **45,** 630–4.

Bartosik, D., Jacobs, S. L., and Kelly, L. J. (1986). Endometrial tissue in peritoneal fluid. *Fertility and Sterility,* **46,** 796–800.

Chihal, H. J., Mathur, S., Holtz, G. L., *et al.* (1986). An endometrial antibody assay in the clinical diagnosis and management of endometriosis. *Fertility and Sterility,* **46,** 408–11.

Dmowski, W. P. (1987). Visual asessment of peritoneal implants for staging endometriosis: do number and cumulative size of lesions reflect the severity of a systemic disease? *Fertility and Sterility,* **47,** 382–4.

Duignan, N. M., Jordan, J. A., Coughlan, B. M., *et al.* (1972). One thousand consecutive cases of diagnostic laparoscopy. *Journal of Obstetrics and Gynaecology of the British Commonwealth,* **79,** 1016–24.

El-Roeiy, A., Dmowski, W. P., Gleicher, N., *et al.* (1988). Danazol but not gonadotropin-releasing hormone agonists suppresses autoantibodies in endometriosis. *Fertility and Sterility,* **50,** 864–71.

Evers, J. L. H. (1989). The pregnancy rate of the no-treatment group in randomized clinical trials of endometriosis therapy. *Fertility and Sterility,* **52,** 906–7.

Gleicher, N., El-Roeiy, A., Confino, E., *et al.* (1987). Is endometriosis an autoimmune disease? *Obstetrics and Gynecology,* **70,** 115–22.

Gleicher, N., El-Roeiy, A., Confino, E., *et al.* (1989). Reproductive failure because of autoantibodies: unexplained infertility and pregnancy wastage. *American Journal of Obstetrics and Gynecology,* **160,** 1376–85.

Grimes, D. A., LeBolt, S. A., Grimes, K. R., *et al.* (1985). Systemic lupus erythematosus and reproductive function: a case control study. *American Journal of Obstetrics and Gynecology,* **153,** 179–86.

Hawkridge, C. (1989). *Understanding endometriosis.* Macdonald Optima, London.

Jansen, R. P. S. and Russell, P. (1986). Nonpigmented endometriosis: clinical, laparoscopic, and pathologic definition. *American Journal of Obstetrics and Gynecology,* **155,** 1154–9.

Kennedy, S. H., Mojiminiyi, O. A., Soper, N. D. W., *et al.* (1990*a*). Immunoscintigraphy of endometriosis. *British Journal of Obstetrics and Gynaecology,* **97,** 667–70.

Kennedy, S. H., Starkey, P. M., Sargent, I. L., *et al.* (1990*b*). Antiendometrial antibodies in endometriosis measured by an enzyme-linked immunoabsorbent assay in women with endometriosis before and after treatment with danazol and nafarelin acetate. *Obstetrics and Gynecology,* **75,** 914–18.

Kennedy, S. H., Mojiminiyi, O. A., Soper, N. D. W., *et al.* (1991). Imaging of pulmonary endometriosis by immunoscintigraphy. *British Journal of Obstetrics and Gynaecology,* **98,** 600–1.

Lancet Editorial (1986). LHRH analogues in endometriosis. *Lancet,* **ii,** 1016–18.

Liu, D. T. Y. and Hitchock, A. (1986). Endometriosis: its association with retrograde menstruation, dysmenorrhoea and tubal pathology. *British Journal of Obstetrics and Gynaecology,* **93,** 859–62.

Murphy, A. A., Green, W. R., Bobbie, D., *et al.* (1986). Unsuspected endometriosis documented by scanning electron microscopy in visually normal peritoneum. *Fertility and Sterility,* **46,** 522–4.

Odendaal, H. J. (1990). The management of acute pelvic inflammatory disease. In *Recent advances in obstetrics and gynaecology,* Vol. 16 (ed. J. Bonnar), pp. 165–83. Churchill Livingstone, Edinburgh.

Pittaway, D. E., Ellington, C. P., and Klimek, M. (1988). Preclinical abortions and endometriosis. *Fertility and Sterility,* **49,** 221–3.

Sampson, J. A. (1940). The development of the implantation theory for the origin of peritoneal endometriosis. *American Journal of Obstetrics and Gynecology*, **40**, 549–57.

Seibel, M. M., Berger, M. J., Weinstein, F. G., *et al.* (1982). The effectiveness of danazol on subsequent fertility in minimal endometriosis. *Fertility and Sterility*, **38**, 534–7.

Steele, R. W., Dmowski, W. P., and Marmer, D. J. (1984). Immunologic aspects of human endometriosis. *American Journal of Reproduction and Immunology*, **6**, 33–6.

Vancaillie, T. G., Hill, R. H., Riehl, R. M., *et al.* (1989). Laser-induced fluorescence of ectopic endometrium in rabbits. *Obstetrics and Gynecology*, **74**, 225–30.

Vasquez, G., Cornillie, F., and Brosens, I. O. (1984). Peritoneal endometriosis: scanning electron microscopy and histology of minimal pelvic endometriotic lesions. *Fertility and Sterility*, **42**, 696–703.

Wardle, P. G., Foster, P. A., Mitchell, J. D., *et al.* (1986). Endometriosis and IVF: effect of prior therapy. *Lancet*, **i**, 276.

Weed, J. C. and Arquembourg, P. C. (1980). Endometriosis: can it produce an autoimmune response resulting in infertility? *Clinical Obstetrics and Gynecology*, **23**, 885–93.

Further reading for patients

Ballweg, M. and Deutsch, S. (1988). *Overcoming endometriosis*. Arlington, London.

Breitkopf, L. J. and Bakoulis, M. G. (1988). *Coping with endometriosis*. Grapevine.

13. Urinary incontinence

Jacqueline Jolleys

DEFINITION

The International Continence Society defined incontinence as: 'The condition in which the involuntary loss of urine is a social or hygienic problem and is objectively demonstrable.'

PREVALENCE

Urinary incontinence in women is a common symptom. The reported prevalence varies according to the population studied, and the definition used, but is usually given as 10 per cent or more (McGrother *et al.* 1987*a*; Thomas *et al.* 1980). The exact prevalence of women suffering from incontinence is not known due to reticence and embarrassment which ensures that for a significant proportion of sufferers the condition remains unrecognized by doctors. Thomas *et al.* (1980) in a study of over 22 000 people on the practice lists of 12 general practitioners in London showed that in patients aged 15 to 64 years the prevalence was 8.5 per cent in women. This rose to 11.6 per cent in women aged 65 and over. The health care and social services agencies were aware of approximately one-quarter of these sufferers. Similarly, in a Mori Poll published in February 1991, 14 per cent of women aged 30–70 years admitted to suffering from incontinence ($n =$ 2980); however, only one-third sought medical advice at the onset of the complaint, although a further third later consulted a doctor.

Several studies have shown the incidence of urinary incontinence to be very high in selected populations. Brocklehurst *et al.* (1972) in a community-based study of women aged 45–64 years found a prevalence of 57 per cent ($n = 454$); a study of women in Edinburgh aged 62–90 found a prevalence of 42 per cent ($n = 272$); Nemir and Middleton (1984) looked at nulliparous American students and found a prevalence of 52 per cent ($n =$ 1327); Wolin (1969) studied nulliparous women and found a prevalence of 51 per cent incontinence; whereas Crist *et al.* (1972) reported an incidence of 30 per cent in their study of nulliparous women aged 21–63 years. These apparent variations may partly be due to differing definitions and methods of eliciting the presence of incontinence. Another study looked at working women aged 35–60 years and found a prevalence of incontinence of 26 per cent ($n = 600$). Incontinence is usually thought of as a condition associated with the process of ageing as the prevalence increases with age, however, urinary incontinence is common not only in the elderly, but also in the middle-aged and young female. Thomas *et al.* (1980) in their community prevalence study showed the incidence of urinary incontinence (inappropriate loss of urine twice or more per month) to be high in all age groups. The study showed that once over the age of 25 years women have a 30 per cent chance of suffering incontinence. In a prevalence study of women aged 25 years and over registered with my practice 43 per cent were regularly incontinent (Jolleys 1988).

FACTORS ASSOCIATED WITH THE ONSET OF INCONTINENCE

Incontinence is often an age-related complaint with the majority of patients suffering from urge incontinence. Many young women develop stress incontinence through pregnancy and childbirth. Despite the high prevalence, research has not determined the aetiology of the symptom and further studies are being conducted. There have been community studies using postal questionnaires which have made some attempt to establish the associated factors (Jolleys 1988; Yarnell *et al.* 1982), but these have merely proposed links between the onset of incontinence and obesity, the type of delivery, vaginal suturing, parity, previous gynaecological surgery, etc.

The multifactorial aetiology of the different types of incontinence has still to be established, and the varying degree to which women are susceptible to the development of incontinence explained.

ANATOMY AND PHYSIOLOGY OF THE FEMALE UROGENITAL TRACT

The challenge of treating incontinence cannot be met without prior consideration of continence. An understanding of the anatomical structure and the physiological control of the bladder and urethra is essential if the complexities of continence are to be appreciated (see Fig. 13.1). With new technology and methods of investigation knowledge of bladder and urethral function has increased. Gosling's (1979) work with the electron microscope has been notable here. The formation of the International Continence Society 20 years ago confirmed the extent of interest in the study of continence, and the increasing membership bears witness to the growth of activity and commitment in this field.

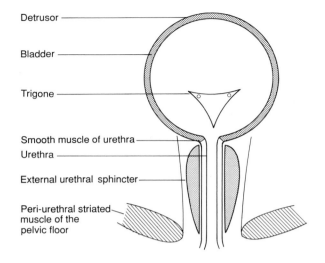

Detrusor

Bladder

Trigone

Smooth muscle of urethra

Urethra

External urethral sphincter

Peri-urethral striated
muscle of the
pelvic floor

Fig. 13.1 A coronal section of the female lower urinary tract.

The bladder

The lower urinary tract basically comprises the bladder, the urethra, and the surrounding sphincter mechanism. The function of the bladder is to store urine and expel it when socially appropriate. The bladder is a muscular sac, the wall of which is composed of a meshwork of interlacing bundles of smooth muscle fibres, not clearly defined into layers, forming the detrusor muscle. This muscle has the physical property of compliance, which means that during the storage phase of micturition, the muscle accommodates an increasing volume of urine with the pressure remaining fairly constant. Compliance indicates the relationship between change in volume and pressure during filling. During normal filling, until almost the limit of distension of the bladder is reached, the compliance remains at infinity. On voiding, the interwoven muscle bundles contract causing a reduction in all dimensions of the bladder enabling complete emptying to occur. The detrusor muscle is innervated by parasympathetic fibres arising from the 2nd, 3rd, and 4th sacral segments of the spinal cord via the pelvic nerve. The trigone of the bladder forms a firm muscular base for this structure and has orifices for the ureters and urethra. On contraction during micturition the trigone forms an open funnel leading into the urethra, but at rest it is flat. The flat base plate formed is essential for the maintenance of continence. It is composed of two distinct muscular layers, and it is to the deep trigonal muscle that the detrusor of the bladder is anchored. Some refer to this layer as the detrusor muscle of the trigone (Gosling 1979). The superficial trigonal muscle extends to the proximal urethra from the longitudinal layer of the ureteric muscle in continuity with it. The angle between the bladder base and the urethra is known as the posterior urethro-vesical angle. Disturbance of this angle at rest coupled with downward movement of the bladder base on straining could result in incontinence because of resulting urethral sphincter dysfunction.

The urethra

The watertight closure of the urethra is mainly due to compression of the folded urethral mucosa. The mucosa is entirely transitional cell epithelium in males, but in females the lower one-third of the urethra is lined with stratified squamous cell epithelium which is under the hormonal influence of oestrogen. Thus it may be affected by hormonal changes around the menopause, and atrophic changes occurring postmenopausally may result in incontinence.

The proximal bladder neck sphincter, sometimes known as the internal sphincter, is formed from loops of detrusor muscle and elastic tissue which fold around the internal meatus and the urethral smooth muscle. The external sphincter is composed of striated muscle and its contraction between voids prevents the passage of urine through the urethra. In women there is no equivalent to the male internal sphincter around the proximal urethra, which is composed of circular smooth muscle richly supplied by sympathetic nerves. This additional sphincter in men is involved in the mechanism of ejaculation and prevents retrograde flow of seminal fluid into the bladder. This means that the urethral closure pressure in women is lower than that in men. Instead, the smooth muscle runs in a longitudinal or oblique direction. The intrinsic muscle of the urethra is striated slow-twitch musculature which surrounds the urethra exerting an influence on its whole length, although it is most prominent in the middle third. Slow-twitch muscle is capable of sustained contraction for prolonged periods and is innervated by the parasympathetic autonomic nervous system.

The balance between sphincter and detrusor mechanisms is maintained by a co-ordinated reflex involving both autonomic and somatic nerves. The urethral sphincter mechanism has both parasympathetic and adrenergic innervation. The striated muscle of the pelvic floor which lies outside the urethra is supplied by the pudendal nerve (S2, S3, and S4). This is fast-twitch muscle capable of rapid but short-lived contraction. Reflex contraction of this muscle, which occurs on sudden coughing and straining in response to stimulation of the muscle spindles of the pelvic floor which are sensitive to changes in tension reflecting alterations in intra-abdominal pressure, can stop micturition.

The neurological control

Co-ordinated reflex activity of the autonomic and somatic nerves maintains the balance between the detrusor and sphincter mechanisms (see Fig. 13.2). Peripherally these are mediated by efferent and afferent pathways between the micturition centre in the 2nd, 3rd, and 4th sacral segments of the spinal cord and the lower urinary tract, and centrally by inhibitory and facilitatory influence of the higher centres of the nervous system. The parasympathetic fibres supply the detrusor muscle stimulating contraction, the smooth muscle of the urethra, and the intramural striated muscle of the external urethral sphincter. Thus the cholinergic endings of the para-sympathetic nerves in the urethral sphincter maintain urethral closure. If these become damaged, as in diabetic neuropathy or during pelvic surgery, urethral closing mechanisms may be affected. Alpha-adrenergic receptors of the sympathetic nerves from the thoraco-lumbar region (T11–L1) are found in the smooth muscle of the proximal urethra, with beta receptors in the fundus of the bladder. Alpha receptors contract muscle fibres in response to noradrenaline release, whereas beta receptors respond by

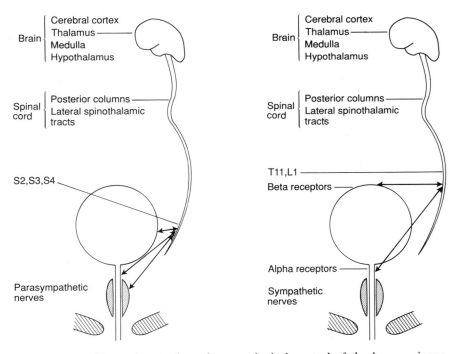

Fig. 13.2 An illustration to show the neurological control of the lower urinary tract.

relaxing smooth muscle. Thus sympathetic nervous activity promotes urine storage. Pudendal nerves from the 2nd, 3rd, and 4th sacral segments of the spinal cord supply the striated musculature of the pelvic floor. Proprioceptive and exteroceptive sensory impulses from the lower urinary tract and pelvic floor are carried in both pudendal and parasympathetic nerve pathways. These maintain cerebral cortex awareness and are an essential component of the feedback mechanism of the spinal cord. Increasing intra-abdominal pressure causes afferent stimulation from the muscle spindles in the pelvic floor and the abdominal cavity resulting in reflex contraction of the pelvic floor. Bladder filling causes afferent discharge which stimulates pelvic floor contraction. This contraction supports the bladder and also potentiates inhibition of detrusor contraction.

Mechanism of micturition

The normal micturition cycle comprises the storage of urine until it can be voided at a convenient time in a suitable place. There is individual variation within the limits of normality as some people need to void more frequently than others and the bladder capacity is variable. Continence is maintained, in dynamic terms, when the pressure in the bladder is lower than the urethral resistance, and urine is voided when this is reversed. Damage to the structures of the lower urinary tract, the urethral mucosa, or the bladder neck, dyssynergism causing increased pressure to be exerted by the detrusor muscle, or from within the abdominal cavity, deficient proximal and distal urethral sphincter mechanisms, can all result in incontinence. Incontinence can also result from disturbances to the neurological control of micturition. Afferent information is relayed back from the lower urinary tract to the central nervous system, at all levels between the spinal cord and the cerebral cortex but especially to the medulla and thalamus, by sensory nerves in the posterior columns and the lateral spinothalamic tracts. Bladder sensation of fullness and voiding is perceived bilaterally in the spinal thalamic tracts, so that damage to both tracts must occur before normal bladder awareness is lost. Any disturbance of the central nervous system may cause disorders of micturition. The hypothalamus controls autonomic nervous function and the higher centres suppress detrusor contractions. The main influence of the brain is to inhibit micturition but it also allows co-ordination of the voiding mechanisms in the pons and voluntary inhibition of the reflex in the cerebral cortex.

Normally the higher centres of the brain inhibit reflex voiding until it is socially appropriate and control the voiding reflex to initiate micturition. As the bladder fills the sensory stretch receptors in the bladder wall are stimulated, the first sensation occurring at approximately 150–200 ml. This sensation of filling is transmitted to the spinal cord via afferent nerves which in turn synapse with motor nerves which stimulate the reflex contraction of the detrusor muscle initiating micturition. Reflex information is transmitted in the normal patient to and from the cerebral cortex and pons via pathways in the spinal cord allowing inhibition of the reflex between voids. This also co-ordinates the reflex preventing dyssynergia. As the higher centres reduce or cease inhibition of the reflex, micturition is initiated. This occurs normally during voluntary voiding but may possibly be a cause of incontinence. The initiation of micturition involves a co-ordinated relaxation of the pelvic floor, relaxation of the urethral sphincter, and then contraction of the detrusor muscle. In women voiding in the absence of the detrusor muscle, contraction is possible with merely the relaxation of the pelvic floor and urethra.

Mechanism of continence

Continence is maintained when the urethral pressure is higher than the pressure within the bladder. There are several aspects of bladder and urethral function which are essential for maintaining continence. The bladder is a highly compliant organ and can fill with only a small rise in internal pressure. The urethral sphincter contracts to impart a positive pressure sufficient to ensure urethral closure. The urethral sphincter should not relax inappropriately or incontinence may occur.

Voluntary inhibition of the voiding reflex is continued between voids. During coughing, sneezing, and physical exertion which all result in a rise in the intra-abdominal pressure, sensory information is also transmitted to the proximal urethra and peri-urethral skeletal musculature of the pelvic floor to initiate further contraction in order to prevent a pressure differential occurring and possible leakage of urine.

CLASSIFICATION OF INCONTINENCE

A classification of types of incontinence based on presentation is useful in that it helps the clinician identify the possible cause of incontinence and from there decide a management plan. In order of frequency of occurrence, the causes of incontinence in females are:

(1) stress incontinence

(2) urge incontinence

(3) overflow

(4) enuresis

(5) passive or reflex incontinence

(6) other—e.g. constipation, urinary tract infection, anxiety, oestrogen deficiency.

Stress incontinence

Stress incontinence is the term used to describe the symptom of involuntary loss of urine on exertion in the absence of bladder contraction—associated with laughing, coughing, sneezing, or physical exertion. The cause is the overstretching or laxity of the supporting structures of the urethra or bladder neck and the weakness of the pelvic floor muscles.

It can be observed as loss of urine from the urethra when the patient raises the intra-abdominal pressure by straining or coughing. If this does not occur when the patient is lying on the couch, it may be demonstrated with the patient standing. Genuine stress incontinence, as defined by the International Continence Society, is the involuntary loss of urine which occurs when the intravesical pressure exceeds the maximum urethral pressure in the absence of detrusor contraction. Without conducting urodynamic studies, it is impossible to determine who has stress incontinence with detrusor muscle contraction occurring on coughing, and who suffers from genuine stress incontinence. Genuine stress incontinence is associated with urethral sphincter defect. It may occur during intercourse on penetration. Giggle incontinence is a form of stress incontinence which occurs when laughing.

Urge incontinence

Urge incontinence is the condition characterized by involuntary loss of urine accompanied by a strong desire to void. It can be subdivided into two types.

Sensory urge incontinence is the involuntary loss of urine associated with urgency, and a strong desire to void urine immediately due to hypersensitivity of the bladder and urethral sensory receptors which may prevent the bladder filling normally. The cause may be infection (cystitis), irritation of the lining of the bladder or its outlet, e.g. calculus, diuretics, or emotions, e.g. anxiety or excitement.

Motor urge incontinence (unstable bladder) is when urgency, bladder contraction, and leakage occur simultaneously owing to unstable detrusor muscle contractions. This is the common cause of urge incontinence. It is characterized by urgency, frequency, nocturia, and incontinence. The cause may be cerebrovascular atherosclerosis, a cerebrovascular accident, diseases affecting the nervous system, e.g. multiple sclerosis or Parkinson's disease, or injury to the higher nervous centres. Diuretics will often precipitate this form of incontinence. Detrusor instability can also occur at orgasm causing incontinence during intercourse.

Although an unstable bladder cannot be demonstrated clinically, it can be through cystometry. An unstable bladder will be shown by cystometry to contract spontaneously, or on provocation during filling (International Continence Society definition). In a stable bladder the volume of urine filling the bladder increases without causing a significant rise in pressure and no voluntary contraction of the bladder wall is seen on the cystometry tracing. The incontinent patient may experience the unstable bladder contractions as urgency—an excessive desire to micturate—or may be unaware until leakage occurs. A bladder may become unstable after bladder neck surgery, and urgency is sometimes reported post-hysterectomy (Jequier 1976).

Overflow incontinence

This is due to the over-distension of the bladder resulting in involuntary loss of urine and dribbling resulting in constant dampness. It occurs when the intravesical pressure exceeds the maximum urethral pressure. Long-standing obstruction to the outlet of the bladder results in bladder distension and loss of compliance. Effective detrusor muscle contractions can no longer occur and continuous leakage of urine results. This retention with overflow can occur when uterine fibroids or uterine prolapse obstruct urine outflow.

The raised intravesical pressure can lead to impaired renal function if not corrected as the pressure may result in obstruction of the upper urinary tract. The neurogenic bladder can also present like this owing to detrusor failure following trauma to or lesions of the cauda equina. Faecal impaction is a common cause of overflow incontinence in the elderly, often immobile patient. Diabetic neuropathy and tabes dorsalis also cause overflow incontinence, as can multiple sclerosis and Parkinson's disease.

Enuresis

Although 'enuresis' means incontinence it is generally understood to apply to nocturnal enuresis, or bed-wetting. Bed-wetting is very common in children, though all but 1 per cent have gained total bladder control by puberty. Usually urodynamic assessment will show these patients to have bladder instability.

Continuous (passive or reflex) incontinence

Continuous incontinence can occur through a variety of conditions. If the patient is conscious of the loss (rare) it may be due to sphincter damage or degenerative changes. More usually the patient is unaware and emptying of the bladder occurs with no conscious awareness. Neuropathic bladder usually results from damage to the central nervous system due to illness, an accident, spinal injuries, spina bifida or cerebrovascular atherosclerosis, or stroke. Functional passive incontinence can also occur in the absence of neurological or urodynamic disorder due to psychiatric and emotional disorders, chronic immobility, physical disability, or drug-induced (sedatives and tranquillizers) drowsiness and confusion states.

THE EFFECTS OF INCONTINENCE ON PATIENTS AND THEIR LIFESTYLE

Incontinence causes embarrassment and anxiety. Patients fear 'accidents' and worry about smelling of urine. As a result people who suffer from incontinence lose their confidence, socialize less, reduce their fluid intake, and cease participating in sports. Some may make dramatic changes to their lifestyle, planning their entire lives around fears of having an accident in public and even confining themselves to their own home. For some the expense of pads and additional washing causes hardship.

The 1991 BACC Mori Poll found that 14 per cent of incontinence sufferers said their lifestyle had been greatly affected, 24 per cent said a fair amount, 38 per cent said not very much and 24 per cent said not at all. Although only 3 per cent had had to cease employment through incontinence, 15 per cent stated that they went out less as a result, and it had made 4 per cent housebound. Incontinence can affect personal relationships. Indeed 2 per cent reported seeing less of their friends and 1 per cent less of the family owing to incontinence. 5 per cent said that they had given up sporting activities such as aerobics or running, and 4 per cent social activities such as dancing. One in ten reported restricting lifting activities. One-third drank less when going out, and one in three made a conscious effort to locate public toilets in advance.

Only 46 per cent of people with incontinence said that they were very confident about going to the supermarket, with 12 per cent not very or not at all confident. For going on a long car journey, the proportion of sufferers who were very confident fell to 33 per cent with 28 per cent not confident to do so. One in three were able to go to the cinema or the theatre and use public transport, one in four were unable to do so. Less than half felt very confident about visiting friends or going out to dinner, and only one in three felt very confident about going to work.

Those with incontinence reported carrying spare underwear (10 per cent), wearing pads (16 per cent), wearing incontinence underwear (3 per cent), using sanitary towels or nappies (8 per cent), self-medicating (3 per cent), learning pelvic floor exercises (11 per cent), and reading information on the problem (6 per cent). Similarly, 6 per cent of women registered with my practice permanently wore protection against urine leakage, and 15 per cent when participating in sporting activities (Jolleys 1988). The frequent use of self-care measures by incontinent women has been reported in other studies (Brink *et al.* 1987; Herzog *et al.* 1989; Jeter and Wagner 1990; McGrother *et al.* 1987*a*). These studies also confirmed that many of the products used were not designed as continence aids, and may therefore not be as effective as pants and pads designed for the purpose. However, the former are more easily purchased and are less indicative of a continence problem.

The results of the Mori Poll show that only 10 per cent of patients with incontinence tell their spouses, and less than 10 per cent tell a close friend or relative. Encouragingly, two-thirds of sufferers had consulted their general practitioners although nearly one-third only after they had had the problem for some time.

Incontinence frequently affects sexual relationships. Women who are embarrassed and ashamed often feel dirty and lose their sexuality. Not uncommonly, women who have stress incontinence fear intercourse since they may experience leakage of urine with orgasm.

For the elderly, incontinence may jeopardize the chance to live in the place of their choice be it sheltered housing, an old people's home, with the family, or in their own home.

THE ROLE OF THE PRIMARY CARE TEAM

There is a place for the management of urinary incontinence in the setting of general practice. Doctors, health visitors (if concerned with care of the elderly), community nurses, physiotherapists, practice nurses, midwives, and social workers may all be involved in various capacities. These will include detection, giving simple or more detailed advice, providing supplies and aids, and so on, and will be complementary to the service of gynaecologists, urologists, and continence clinics. The prevalence of urinary incontinence is such that continence services in England are already fully stretched, even though the majority of women with incontinence problems probably do not present to the family doctor.

Even in the enlightened nineties, when people talk readily and openly about sex, they are embarrassed to talk about bodily functions. It is up to the GP to adopt a respectful and empathic approach to encourage patients to discuss these sorts of personal problems, and to use routine screening (Well Woman Clinics) and special clinic opportunities (pre-conception counselling, antenatal and postnatal appointments) to help identify sufferers.

Incontinence is rarely presented as a dominant symptom and it may be introduced by a query relating to a physical symptom, e.g. 'something is coming down in front'. Presenting symptoms may be frequency, urgency and associated urge incontinence, leakage/stress incontinence associated with posture change or physical exertion, and incontinence during intercourse.

Having elicited a continence problem, the GP can take a history and medically assess the patient. In the majority of cases the doctor will be able to diagnose the continence condition and offer a management plan in the form of treatment and advice. If s/he is unable to provide the necessary treatment at the practice, or is unable to reach a diagnosis, s/he can then refer the patient to the appropriate health care professional—urologist, gynaecologist, continence adviser, or a nurse with an interest in incontinence.

The GP can use the doctor–patient relationship developed through continuing care to give support and understanding, encourage self-help, and restore the patient's self-esteem and self-confidence. The patient can be given literature which reinforces the doctor's explanation of the common causes of incontinence, its prevalence and its treatability, and provides lifestyle advice.

THE DIAGNOSIS OF URINARY INCONTINENCE IN THE PRIMARY CARE SETTING

Urinary incontinence can usually be diagnosed from history and examination, provided that the general practitioner understands the mechanism of continence. GPs who wish to promote continence in the community can manage and treat many of their patients in the setting of general practice, referring only those who require specialist treatments and urodynamic assessment. The initial history and examination will ensure appropriate referral and optimal use of resources.

History

The majority of diagnoses can be reached from the history alone and confirmed by examination. The history must elicit:

The exact nature of the incontinence, the onset, and related or precipitating factors. It will not be necessary to ask all the questions below in every case. The patient may describe classical stress incontinence which can be confirmed by appropriate questions and an examination. However, often mixed incontinence is present so it is advisable to ask the questions relating to urge incontinence as well.

Questions relating to control of micturition
1. Do you normally get a feeling of wanting to pass urine? (Absence of feeling may indicate neuropathy.)
2. Will the first feeling go away before you eventually pass water? (The first feeling usually comes and goes. Persistent feeling before and/or after voiding suggests bladder pathology, e.g. cystitis.)

3. Does the feeling disappear after passing water? (The feeling should disappear or there is a suggestion of bladder pathology.)

4. Is there any pain associated with urine leakage? (Pain is indicative of urinary tract infection, atrophic vaginitis/urethritis, and occasionally of obstruction.)

5. When you are ready to pass water does it come straight away? (Hesitancy indicates dysfunction or neurological problems of MS.)

6. Do you feel you empty your bladder completely? (Negative response may indicate obstruction or residual urine volume.)

Questions relating to the severity of the incontinence

1. How bad is your leakage? How much do you lose? How often?

2. Do you have to change your under/outer clothes or wear pads? If so, how many?

Questions to confirm stress incontinence

Replies in the affirmative indicate stress incontinence.

1. Do you leak urine when you cough, sneeze, or laugh without having the feeling of wanting to pass urine?

2. Do you leak urine when you play sport, run, or jump without having the feeling of wanting to pass urine?

3. Do you leak if you make a sudden movement?

4. When you leak do you lose small amounts of urine?

Questions to confirm urge incontinence/detrusor instability

Replies in the affirmative indicate urge incontinence/detrusor instability.

1. Do you go to the toilet more than six times a day?

2. Do you have to hurry to reach the toilet in time?

3. Do you leak before you can get there?

4. Do you wet the bed in your sleep or do you leak before you can get to the toilet?

5. Do you have to get up to pass water three or more times at night?

Questions to confirm passive incontinence

Replies in the affirmative indicate passive incontinence.

1. Have you ever passed water without knowing it?

2. Do you have accidents when you are in bed at night?

3. Do you have frequent accidents?

Questions to confirm overflow incontinence
Replies in the affirmative indicate overflow incontinence.

1. Do you have to strain to pass water?
2. Do you dribble after you have passed water?
3. After you have passed water do you ever feel as if your bladder is still full?

The history must also elicit:

Fluid intake history—volume and type. Alcohol and coffee can have diuretic effects. In some cases the balance between continence and incontinence can be altered simply by cutting down on liquid intake.

Drug history. A drug history is important since diuretics, antidepressants, hypnotics, tranquillizers, anti-parkinsonian drugs, and anti-oestrogens can all affect continence.

Medical history.

Examination

Included in the physical examination should be the height and weight of the patient, abdominal and where appropriate rectal or vaginal examination, a urinalysis for sugar, protein, and nitrites, and a neurological examination of the patient if indicated. Further examination of the urine is indicated if urinary tract infection is suspected.

A palpable loaded colon indicating constipation, or a palpable enlarged bladder after micturition, found on abdominal examination indicate retention. If there is a palpable bladder after micturition the patient needs urgent referral to a urologist. It is useful to pass a catheter post-micturition to establish the residual volume of urine.

On vaginal examination there may be atrophy vaginitis which can result in urge incontinence. Stress incontinence may be demonstrated on cough voiding. The ability to contract the levator ani muscle can be confirmed by asking the patient to squeeze your finger. The presence of a large prolapse, cystocoele, rectocoele, or fibroids, which can be associated with either urge or stress incontinence, would suggest the need for referral to a gynaecologist.

Having completed the history and examination, any urinary tract infection or constipation should be treated. The GP should then be able to place the patient in one of the following diagnostic/management categories:

stress incontinence
urge incontinence
atrophic vaginitis
stress/urge incontinence.

Exclusion criteria for primary care management

The following conditions are unsuitable for primary care management and require specialist opinion:

1. Vesico-vaginal fistula—refer to a urologist or gynaecologist.
2. Palpable bladder or large residual volume of urine after micturition— refer to a urologist.
3. Disease of the central nervous system—refer to a urologist or continence clinic.
4. Certain gynaecological conditions, e.g. procidentia, rectocoele, cystocoele, and fibroids of a size requiring surgical intervention—refer to a gynaecologist.
5. Failure to reach a diagnosis—refer to a continence clinic or urologist.

Who to refer for urodynamic investigation

Many female patients present not only with stress incontinence but also with urge incontinence or frequency and nocturia. These patients ideally require urodynamic assessment to establish the diagnosis. This is not necessary for patients with stress incontinence alone as they are usually found to have genuine stress incontinence due to pelvic floor weakness. However, when stress symptoms are accompanied by urgency or voiding difficulties, urodynamic tests will assist with the selection of appropriate treatment. Apparent stress incontinence may be found on urodynamic investigation to be due to bladder instability.

Indications for urodynamic assessement
Groups of patients with the following problems may be helped by urodynamic assessment:

(1) stress incontinence complicated by coexistence of other symptoms;
(2) incontinence following previous unsuccessful surgery;
(3) voiding problems—difficulty with emptying the bladder and retention;
(4) unstable bladder which fails to respond to treatment in general practice;
(5) neurological problems, spinal injuries.

Jarvis (1980) looked at the correlation between the diagnosis given to the patients based on clinical symptoms and a final diagnosis based on cystometry in 100 incontinent women. Following urodynamics the diagnosis made on clinical grounds alone was confirmed in only 68 per cent of cases. 25 per cent of women who were eventually diagnosed as having genuine stress incontinence presented with urgency. The conclusion drawn was that accurate diagnosis based on clinical symptoms alone is difficult since patients with either detrusor instability or stress incontinence often present with symptoms indicative of both disorders. Despite taking a careful history and examination, further investigation is almost always necessary; the bladder tends to be an unreliable witness in that symptoms often do not mirror the underlying cause. Jarvis concluded that generally the correlation between clinical diagnosis and urodynamic diagnosis is poor. This may be correct, but from my experience of treating women with incontinence in general practice without access to urodynamic tests, treatment regimes chosen on the basis of a diagnosis reached through history and examination alone were successful in promoting continence in the majority of cases which had previously been selected as suitable for management in the community.

Since many patients requiring urodynamic assessment have to go on a waiting list in order to be seen, in some cases it may be appropriate and beneficial to commence management of the condition prior to the diagnosis being confirmed since pelvic floor exercises, frequency/volume charts, and habit retraining cannot have deleterious effects.

MANAGEMENT

Figure 13.3 gives a broad management algorithm.

Published literature reveals one study which assesses the efficacy of treatment of urinary incontinence in general practice (Jolleys 1989), though there are many other hospital studies assessing similar treatment regimes. Physiotherapy as management of stress incontinence is well documented and the literature is encouraging in giving suggestions for a simple and practical approach for the diagnosis and management of urinary incontinence in general practice (Giesy 1986; Mohr *et al.* 1983).

Mangement of stress incontinence

Conservative management

A programme of pelvic floor exercises is an effective treatment for stress incontinence irrespective of the age of the patient and the duration of incontinence. Since the treatment of incontinence is quite time-consuming and requires various skills, it is appropriate that management of the incontinent patient is conducted by the primary health care team. After the doctor has diagnosed the patient and counselled her, depending on availability and interest, a joint approach to management may be adopted by the doctor, practice nurse, physiotherapist, dietician, and community nurse. Initially an explanation of stress incontinence is required so that the patient fully understands the condition and is highly motivated to be compliant with instructions. The overweight patient is put on a *reducing*

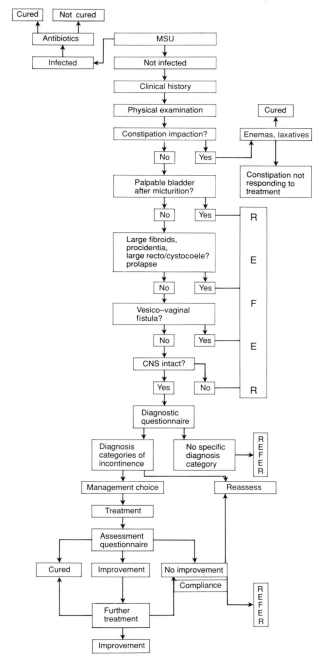

Fig. 13.3 Female patients with urinary incontinence who wish to be treated.

diet. Having checked the patient's current understanding of them, the patient is instructed on how to do *pelvic floor exercises*, i.e. isolated contraction of the levator ani muscle for four seconds four times every hour while breathing normally. This means that there should be no simultaneous contraction of the abdominal or gluteal muscles. Confirmation of active contraction of the levator ani can be obtained on vaginal examination if necessary. It is essential to explain that initially the exercise may be difficult to do for four seconds owing to the weakness of the muscle, but that with practice and in time it will become easier. Offering patients written instructions (see Table 13.1) improves compliance since many patients forget the content of the consultation after leaving the surgery.

Table 13.1   *Pelvic floor exercises*

The muscles that form the floor of your pelvis have been very stretched during your life by pregnancy, delivery, and lifting. If they are allowed to remain weak, leaking of urine, vaginal prolapse, or slackness may result.

Practise the exercises sitting with the thighs apart as follows: close your back and front passages, now draw them up inside you and HOLD. Count to 4 then let go slowly.

Repeat 4 times.

Do 4 pelvic floor exercises every hour.

A time to do these exercises might be after passing water.

AFTER THREE MONTHS test your pelvic floor muscles like this:

Ensure your bladder is nearly full (about 3 hours from last empty)

Stand feet apart and bounce up and down on the spot and cough deeply twice
Dry pants indicate recovery.
If leakage of urine occurs continue exercises for 3 more months.

Retest.

It is advisable to do some pelvic floor exercises for the rest of your life.

As well as the exercise programme it is essential to give advice on lifting correctly, and avoidance of heavy lifting since this increases intra-abdominal pressure and stretches the muscles of the pelvic floor. For this reason, it is advisable to instruct the patient to avoid the activities which precipitate incontinence until total control of urine flow has been regained.

Patients can be reviewed at intervals for a subjective assessment of their continence status and a weight check. This serves to encourage compliance and perseverance with the exercise programme. Although it often requires three months or less of exercising to regain continence, pelvic floor exercises should be practised at regular intervals throughout the patient's lifetime for the continued maintenance of continence.

Vaginal cones are increasing in popularity as a method for retraining the pelvic floor muscles and for continued exercising of the pelvic floor. This method has the advantage that the patient can appreciate progress made and measure it objectively. The GP should encourage patients to present for diagosis prior to embarking on treatment with cones in order to assess the appropriateness of the therapy.

Surgical treatment

Should conservative management not significantly improve the symptom of incontinence or fail to cure it, it may be that:

(1) the diagnosis is incorrect;

(2) the patient is not compliant with the management programme;

(3) severe damage to the pelvic floor muscles exists.

The patient will thus require referral to a gynaecologist for urodynamic tests and for a surgical opinion. There is no one procedure which is suitable for treating all women with stress incontinence. The principal indication for surgery is urethral sphincter incompetence. The surgical aims are to elevate the bladder neck and raise bladder resistance, simultaneously correcting anterior vaginal wall prolapse. The choice of procedure is affected by the following considerations:

(1) the surgeon's expertise in the procedures;

(2) the surgical history of the patient;

(3) the fitness of the patient;

(4) the need to treat other pathology;

(5) the success rates for the different operations;

(6) the incidence of post-operative bladder instability;

(7) the mobility of the bladder neck at operation.

If childbearing is not complete, although it is appropriate to refer the patient and have a urodynamic assessment to confirm the diagnosis, the woman should be warned that surgery is likely to be deferred until her family is complete, as a subsequent vaginal delivery is likely to produce a recurrence of the incontinence.

The main procedures for the treatment of stress incontinence are suprapubic urethrovesical suspension operations (Burch colposuspension whereby the vaginal fornices are used to support the bladder base, sling procedure, and the Marshall–Marchetti–Krantz operation) or an endoscopic bladder neck suspension such as the Stamey procedure. In the Stamey procedure sutures are passed under endoscopic guidance on both sides of the bladder neck and tied anteriorly to the rectus sheath. This is an effective and successful operation in the majority of female patients. Gynaecologists are more likely to prefer the first procedures, urologists more frequently offer the Stamey. The vaginal approach anterior repair is often used but is less successful than the other procedures, and in many centres has been replaced by the suprapubic approach procedures.

Marshall–Marchetti–Krantz, Burch, and sling operations are carried out via an abdominal incision (a sling procedure requires a vaginal incision too) and are major procedures—more major than an anterior repair. The operation is usually followed by a brief period of catheter drainage and the patient may expect to remain in hospital for a week to ten days. Reported cure rates vary, depending on the centre, from 35–75 per cent. If there is vaginal wall prolapse as well as incontinence a variation on the Burch procedure—when additional sutures inserted alongside the bladder base between the paravaginal fascia and ileo-pectineal ligaments provide additional support for the anterior vaginal wall—is particularly effective. Stanton and Cardoza (1979) reported an 86 per cent overall cure rate at two-year post-operation follow-up.

Patients need to be informed that post-operatively a gradual return to normal activity within three months is recommended, but that heavy lifting is to be permanently eschewed. Intercourse should not be resumed until healing is complete, two months after surgery.

Management of urge incontinence

Conservative treatment

Initially a frequency/volume chart (urinary output diary) should be completed for a period of three days to a week (see Chart 13.1). This helps to identify the frequency and pattern of voiding, as well as providing information relating to the volume of urine in the bladder prior to micturition (assuming complete voiding). Subsequently bladder retraining and psychological support is the treatment of choice. In bladder retraining the patient is encouraged to void increasingly larger volumes of urine, gradually increasing the intervals between micturition, so relearning inhibition of abnormal detrusor muscle contractions. A rigid toileting regime should not be imposed on patients who are commencing habit retraining as too frequent emptying of the bladder (more than two-hourly) without adjustments to suit individual need may mitigate against restoration of continence by reducing the effective capacity of the bladder. The starting interval between voiding is taken from the frequency/volume chart. If a patient is able to go two hours between voids then this would be a suitable interval; however, if the chart shows that the bladder is usually emptied at hourly intervals or less, then hourly micturition would be appropriate.

On introduction of the toileting schedule, the patient is instructed to go to the toilet to pass urine every half hour or hour initially, depending on the severity of the condition. She must go to the toilet whether or not she

Chart 13.1   A record of the frequency/volume of urine passed. (Used with permission of Leicester General Hospital Continence Clinic.)

Go to the toilet when you want to go.
Measure the amount passed each time.

Date:													
Time	Vol.	Time	Vol.	Time	Vol.	Time	Vol.	Time	Vol.	Time	Vol.	Time	Vol.

needs to, even if she is already wet (see Chart 13.2). The patient is instructed not to go to the toilet in advance of this time even if she fears an incontinence episode. She is instructed to keep to this toiletting schedule until two whole days have elapsed without incontinence. The micturition interval is then increased by half an hour and the process repeated until an

Chart 13.2   Daily record of micturation. (Used with permission of Leicester General Hospital Continence Clinic.)

Go to the toilet every ....hours,
whether you want to or not, and whether you
are wet or dry.

Date: Day:	Wet or dry	Was urine passed	Wet or dry	Was urine passed	Wet or dry	Was urine passed	Wet or dry	Was urine passed	Wet or dry	Was urine passed	Wet or dry	Was urine passed	Wet or dry	Was urine passed
12 midnight														
1 am														
2 am														
3 am														
4 am														
5 am														
6 am														
7 am														
8 am														
9 am														
10 am														
11 am														
12 noon														
1 pm														
2 pm														
3 pm														
4 pm														
5 pm														
6 pm														
7 pm														
8 pm														
9 pm														
10 pm														
11 pm														

interval of four hours is achieved. Patients are seen at regular intervals to assess progress.

Habit retraining instructions for patients
1. Start by going to the toilet to pass urine every . . . hours.

2. *You must go* to pass urine whether you want to or not.
   You must go to pass urine even if you are already wet.
   You must not cheat and go before the time is up.

3. Keep to this toiletting time until you have gone two whole days without being wet. Don't worry about the night-time at this stage.

4. When you can manage two consecutive dry days, extend your time between visits to the toilet by half an hour. You will probably find that you initially become wet again on occasion but *do not go back* to the previous short time. Persist with this new time strictly as before.

5. When you have had two dry days at this new time, extend the time again by half an hour, and so on until you reach four hours between visits to the toilet.

6. When you can wait four hours between visits to pass urine, stop watching the clock and regard yourself as normal.

7. Do keep a check on yourself and do not allow yourself to go back to your old way of going so frequently.

By this time you should be able to go without a pad quite confidently.

The patient should be referred to a gynaecologist or urologist if home or family circumstances render this treatment impossible to prevent further loss of morale.

The unstable bladder is most successfully treated by a combination of retraining and drug therapy. (See Table 13.2.) Drug therapy aims to inhibit involuntary detrusor contractions in the bladder. Since the bladder has complex innervation, no one single drug may be entirely effective. Available drug therapy lacks specificity and the unwanted anticholinergic side-effects limit their use. As with other drug therapy there may be initially a placebo response with apparent success, which rapidly falls off after several weeks as the placebo effect wanes.

Bladder retraining combined with anticholinergic pharmacological treatment aims to increase the time between voids by suppression of the reflex motor output to the bladder thus stabilizing the detrusor muscle. Drug treatment may be particularly helpful during the first two weeks of therapy when the patient's confidence is low and the clinical benefits of the training programme have not yet become apparent. At this time the placebo effect is also maximal.

If the patient is unable to increase the time interval, adjuvent drug therapy may be commenced, e.g. antidepressant imipramine 25 mg nocte or b.d., or anticholinergic/smooth muscle relaxants oxybutynin 5 mg b.d.–t.d.s. or propantheline 15 mg max. 8 daily. Once continence has been regained many patients are able to sustain the improvement without the continued requirement of medication. All overweight patients will benefit from weight reduction.

Table 13.2   *Pharmacological preparations used in the treatment of incontinence*

Generic name	Dosage
Anticholinergics Propantheline bromide	15 mg tablets Adults: up to 8 tablets
Anticholinergic antispasmodic Oxybutynin hydrochloride	2.5 mg, 5 mg tablets Adults: 5 mg two or three times daily Elderly: 5 mg twice daily
Tricyclic antidepressants Amitryptyline hydrochloride	10.25 mg, 50 mg tablets, 10 mg/ml syrup Adults: not recommended
Imipramine	10 mg, 25 mg tablets Adults: 25 mg three times a day; increase to 50 mg three times a day if necessary. Elderly: 10 mg nocte to 10–25 mg three times a day
Vasopressin analogues Desmopressin	10 μg spray metered dose Adults: 1–2 sprays each nostril before retiring. After three months, reassess need for continued treatment by a week free of treatment NB. Contraindicated in patients with raised blood pressure

Surgical treatment

Detrusor instability should be treated surgically only after failure of conservative management. Referral to a specialist urological centre is advised since the only reliable procedure is augmentation ileocystoplasty, when a section of the ileum is used to enlarge the bladder capacity.

Management of stress and urge incontinence

The treatment here is a combination of pelvic floor exercises, bladder retraining, psychological support, and weight reduction.

Management of atrophic vaginitis

Treatment with local oestrogen preparations in the form of pessaries or cream, or with hormone replacement therapy, is most successful in curing this complaint and the resulting urge incontinence.

Management of nocturnal enuresis

It is estimated that 10 per cent of the adult population have an unstable bladder, of whom 1–2 per cent of adult females will have nocturnal enuresis. The enuresis may be (1) primary—the patient has never consistently been dry at night, (2) secondary—the patient has relapsed after being dry for a least one year.

Before commencing treatment the following factors should be considered:

1. Has the patient a urinary tract infection?
2. Are physical or emotional problems involved—mobility, senility, neurological factors?
3. Is there obstruction or a fistula?

Patients with detrusor muscle instability can be helped by treatment with propantheline or oxybutynin. Antidepressants including imipramine are also effective. For patients who are occasionally incontinent at night, desmopressin, a synthetic analogue of antidiuretic hormone, may be administered nasally.

Referral to a consultant specializing in incontinence is advised if after a trial of three months drug treatment fails to be effective.

CONCLUSION

General practitioners are ideally placed to elicit and alleviate continence problems which are the cause of much human misery and embarrassment, and may affect and restrict family relationships. The majority of patients can be satisfactorily treated using non-invasive interventions which satisfy both cost-effective and cost-utility analysis criteria. It is important that general practitioners gain expertise in the management of incontinence, reserving referral for those patients with more complicated or serious problems. Furthermore, since patients are usually most grateful for management in the primary care setting, there is enhanced job satisfaction for the physician.

USEFUL ADDRESSES

Age Concern, 60 Pitcairn Road, Mitcham, Surrey. Advice on special problems of the elderly.

Association of Continence Advisers: c/o Disabled Living Foundation. List of continence advisers.

BACC (British Association of Continence Care), Prism International, Pinewood Studios, Iver Heath, Bucks SL0 0NH. Helpline Tel: 0753 656 716. Tape on incontinence giving advice and information on where to go to get help.

The Disabled Living Foundation, 380/384 Harrow Road, London W9 2HU. Tel: 071 289 6111. Leaflets on management, aids, and special clothing. Helpline: same telephone number—ask for Incontinence Advisory Service. Publications on incontinence available. Send s.a.e. to receive an order form.

Newcastle Council for the Disabled: continence advisory service. The Dene Centre, Castles Farm Road, Newcastle upon Tyne, NE3 1PH.

RADAR (Royal Association for Disability and Rehabilitation), 25 Mortimer Street, London W1N 8AB. Holidays for the disabled. Toilet-for-the-disabled keys.

SPOD (The Association to Aid the Sexual and Personal Relationships of People with a Disability), 286 Camden Road, London N7 0BJ.

Women's Royal Voluntary Service, 17 Old Park Lane, London W1Y 4AJ. Leaflet on adapting and making clothes suitable for the incontinent.

REFERENCES AND FURTHER READING

Brink, C. A., Wells, T. J., and Diokno, A. C. (1987). Urinary incontinence in women. *Public Health Nursing,* **4,** 114–19.
Brocklehurst, J. C., Fry, J., Griffiths, L. L., *et al.* (1972). Urinary infection and symptoms of dysuria in women aged 45–65 years: their relevance to similar findings in the elderly. *Age and Ageing,* **1,** 41–7.
Crist, T., Singleton, H. M., and Koch, G. G. (1972). Stress incontinence and the nulliparous patient. *Obstetrics and Gynaecology,* **40,** 13–17.
Giesy, J. D. (1986). Voiding problems in women. One physician's perspective on evaluation and therapy. *Postgraduate Medicine,* **79,(1),** 271–8.
Gosling, J. A. (1979). The structure of the bladder and urethra in relation to function. *Urology Clinic of North America,* **6,** 31–8.
Herzog, R. A., Fultz, N. H., Normolle, D. P., *et al.* (1989). Methods used to manage urinary incontinence by older adults in the community. *Journal of the American Geriatric Society,* **37,** 339–47.
Holding, U., Pedersen, K. H., Sidenius, K., *et al.* (1986). Urinary incontinence in 45 year old women—an epidemiological survey. *Scandinavian Journal of Urology,* **20,** 183–6.
Jarvis, G. J. (1980). An assessment of urodynamic assessment in incontinent women. *British Journal of Obstetrics and Gynaecology,* **87,** 893.
Jequier, A. M. (1976). Urinary symptoms and total hysterectomy. *British Journal of Urology,* **48,** 437–41.
Jeter, K. F. and Wagner, D. B. (1990). Incontinence in the American home. *Journal of the American Geriatric Society,* **38,** 379–83.

Jolleys, J. V. (1988). The reported prevalence of urinary incontinence in women in a general practice. *British Medical Journal, 296,* 1300–2.

Jolleys, J. V. (1989). Diagnosis and management of female urinary incontinence in general practice. *Journal of the Royal College of General Practitioners, 39,* 277–9.

Laycock, J. (1987). Graded exercises for the pelvic floor muscles in the treatment of urinary incontinence. *Physiotherapy,* **73,(7),** 371–3.

Mandelstam, D. (1986). *Incontinence and its management,* (2nd edn). Croom Helm, London.

McGrother, C., Castleden, C. M., Duffin, H., *et al.* (187*a*). A profile of disordered micturition in the elderly at home. *Age and Ageing,* **16,** 105–10.

McGrother, C., Clarke, M., Castleden, M., *et al.* (1987*b*). Do the elderly need better continence services? *Community Medicine,* **9,** 62–7.

Mohr, J. A., Rogers, J., Brown, T. N., *et al.* (1983). Stress incontinence: a simple and practical approach to diagnosis and treatment. *Journal of the American Geriatric Society,* **31,** 476–8.

Nemir, A. and Middleton, R. P. (1984). Stress incontinence in young nulliparous women. *American Journal of Obstetrics and Gynecology,* **68,** 1166–8.

Smith, N. and Clamp, M. (1991). *Continence promotion in general practice.* Oxford University Press, Oxford.

Stanton, S. and Cardoza, L. (1979). The colpo̥suspension operation for incontinence and prolapse: clinical aspects. *British Journal of Obstetrics and Gynaecology,* **86,** 693–7.

Thomas, T. N., Plymat, K. R., Blannin, J., *et al.* (1980). Prevalence of urinary incontinence. *British Medical Journal,* **281;** 1243–5.

Wolin, L. H. (1969). Stress incontinence in young healthy nulliparous female subjects. *Journal of Urology,* **102,** 545–9.

Yarnell, J. W. G., Voyle, G. J., Sweetnum, P. M., *et al.* (1982). Factors associated with urinary incontinence in women. *Journal of Epidemiology and Community Health,* **36,** 58–63.

Further reading for patients

Browne, B. (1978). *Management for incontinence.* Age Concern, Mitcham, Surrey.

Castleden, M. and Duffin, H. (1991). *Staying dry.* Quay, Lancaster.

Disabled Living Foundation. *Notes on incontinence.* (Obtainable from 380–384 Harrow Road, London W9 2HU.)

Feneley, R. C. L. and Blannin, J. P. (1984). *Incontinence.* Patient Handbook Series No. 18. Churchill Livingstone, Edinburgh.

Mandelstam, D. (1977). *Incontinence.* Heinemann Medical Books for The Disabled Living Foundation, London.

Millard, R. (1988). *Overcoming urinary incontinence.* Thorsons/Harper Collins, Glasgow.

Montgomery, E. (1974). *Regaining bladder control.* Wright, Bristol.

14. Sexual problems

Keith Hawton and Catherine Oppenheimer

This chapter is addressed in particular to those doctors who would like to offer help to their patients with sexual problems, but who feel they need further information in order to be able to help more effectively.

The main emphasis is on the sexual difficulties of women, but the difficulties of men are also discussed as it is almost invariable for a problem in one partner in a sexual relationship to be associated with some difficulty in the other partner, whether as a secondary effect or as a partial cause of the presenting problem. Most attention will be devoted to sexual dysfunction (such as reduced sexual desire, vaginismus, and erectile dysfunction) arising in a heterosexual relationship, but female homosexuality and male sexual variations are also mentioned because these may come to the attention of the general practitioner and can be related to sexual dysfunction.

HOW COMMON ARE SEXUAL PROBLEMS?

Relatively little is known about the incidence of sexual dysfunction in the general population. Masters and Johnson (1970) made the surprising claim that as many as 50 per cent of marriages in the USA are troubled by sexual dysfunction at some time, and their estimate received support in 1978 from a small interview survey carried out in the USA. A community survey in the UK of a random sample of women aged 35–59 years with partners indicated that approximately one-third reached criteria for a sexual dysfunction, the prevalence increasing markedly with age (Osborn *et al.* 1988). However, only one in ten of all the women regarded themselves as having a sexual problem (a similar figure to that found in most younger women attending family planning clinics) and less than half of these said they would like help if it were available.

Relatively little is known about the numbers of female homosexuals in the general population. It has been estimated that in England approximately one in 45 women will be exclusively homosexual, so that the average GP with a list size of 2500 patients can expect to have 20–30 women in the practice whose sexual interest is exclusively homosexual, and more who have experienced homosexual interest at some time. However, only a small proportion of these will regard their homosexuality as a problem.

THE EFFECTS OF SEXUAL PROBLEMS ON PEOPLE'S LIVES

All those, whatever their profession, who work with couples or families will know how often sexual problems are linked with marital disharmony, or with actual breakdown of a marriage, and will know also how in the absence of a happy sexual relationship one vital channel for the resolution of disharmony is removed from the partnership. Unfortunately, few statistics are available to confirm this clinical impression. It is impossible in a brief account to do justice either to the complexities of cause and effect between sexual difficulty and general tension in a relationship, or to the depth of unhappiness that such difficulties may cause. However, the following case illustrates some of the effects:

Mary and Arthur married when he was 24 and she was 20. They knew at the time that he had a problem with premature ejaculation, dating back to his first hasty intercourse at the age of 16 in the back of a car after a party. Mary had been involved in several unhappy relationships before she met Arthur, and found that she was very slow to become aroused during lovemaking. They hoped that the problems would resolve once they were married, but they did not, and by the second year of their marriage Margaret and Arthur were on the verge of separating. They tried to make a fresh start and Mary became pregnant. During the pregnancy Mary felt very keen on sex, but Arthur found her unattractive, and when after delivery his interest in her returned, she felt sore and began to be repelled by the idea of sex. On the few occasions that they did try to make love, Arthur ejaculated so quickly that he began to feel 'a complete failure', and acquiesced in Mary's avoidance of sex. By the time they went to their doctor they had not had sex for eight months, and the subject had become unmentionable. They were still determined to stay together for the sake of the child. Mary said, 'I want to sort things out but I feel it's impossible.'

Sexual dysfunction may also cause a woman to avoid forming further relationships, especially if a previous sexual encounter was unsuccessful. Such avoidance may lead to further unhappiness and lack of confidence, which in turn can add to the woman's conviction that she is 'sexually inadequate'.

HOW SEXUAL PROBLEMS MAY PRESENT TO DOCTORS

In spite of the drastic changes in public attitudes to sexuality that have occurred over recent years, many people still find it embarrassing to talk honestly about sexuality, especially their own. A very important part of the help that a doctor can give is in making it easier for patients to overcome this hurdle. Doctors need to be sensitive to clues that a patient has a problem that she (or he) wants to discuss, and be able to convey their willingness to enter into the discussion. Often patients have heard, through the press and elsewhere, of the availability and effectiveness of treatment of sexual problems, and such patients may come to the doctor with *direct requests for help*.

Other patients may be too shy to express their worry directly, or may not even realize that there is a sexual cause for the difficulty that they experience, and in these cases the doctor must be aware of the possible *covert presentation* of sexual problems. On the whole such covert presentations take the form either of emotional or psychological symptoms (such as depression, marital disharmony, poor sleep), or gynaecological complaints (such as requests for a change of contraceptive pill, or the report of a vaginal discharge). The following case illustrates such a presentation.

Alicia was 35 and had been married for nine years when she attended a cervical screening session at her doctor's surgery. The doctor found it almost impossible to take the smear and it then came to light that Alicia's marriage had never been consummated. For nine years she had allowed her husband to stroke her but not to approach her genitals, while she had masturbated him. She had been too ashamed of her inability to have sex ever to confide in anyone else. Her doctor referred her for sex therapy, but she cancelled the appointment; however, a few months later she asked to be re-referred.

A gynaecological examination can provide a surprisingly helpful setting in which to enquire into a patient's sexual anxieties, and in which reassurance (e.g. about the normality of the genitals) can be given. Another common presentation is for the patient to *complain of the partner's sexual dysfunction*. This sometimes may be because the partner is unwilling to attend, but often it is because the patient has not recognized that the problem is at least partly her or his own.

NORMAL SEXUAL FUNCTION

Understanding of the different types of sexual problems is facilitated by a knowledge of normal sexual behaviour, and particularly of the events that occur during the various stages of sexual desire and response. Only a brief summary of such information can be provided here. For further details the reader is referred to Masters and Johnson's (1966) book, *Human sexual response*, or Bancroft (1989).

Normal sexual behaviour can be divided into four phases:

1. *Interest or desire.* The background level of interest in sexuality, willingness to seek opportunities for sexual contact, and occurrence of sexual thoughts or fantasies outside as well as within times of actual sexual contact.

2. *Arousal or excitement.* The initial physiological responses to sexually stimulating activity or thought. This phase includes: (a) the *vascular* changes that produce genital engorgement and lubrication in the female, erection in the male, together with flushing of the face and body; (b) *neuromuscular* changes such as ballooning of the interior of the vagina and retraction of the clitoris in the female, elevation of the testes and tightening of the scrotum in the male. During this phase of arousal, thoughts and feelings also become increasingly focused on the sexual experience. It is normal for the subjective experience of arousal to intensify not gradually, but by a series of waves of arousal of increasing intensity.

3. *Orgasm.* This includes both the observable event of pubococcygeus muscle contractions in the female or ejaculation in the male, and the subjective experience of orgasm. The male response may be divided into two phases: the first in which seminal and prostatic fluid enters the urethral bulb, and the second, beginning from the point at which the process becomes inevitable and irreversible, in which the seminal fluid is ejected from the urethra.

4. *Resolution.* During this phase the physiological events of arousal are gradually reversed. Descent of the uterus and resolution of vascular engorgement occur in women. In men a moderate immediate loss of erection is followed by a slower complete reversal to the flaccid state. In both sexes these changes are accompanied by subjective sensations of relaxation and languor. For the male this phase includes a *refractory period* of variable length (from 15 to 30 minutes for a 15-year-old, to 24 hours or more for an 80-year-old) before full sexual arousal can recommence; for the female there may be no corresponding physiological refractory period, and some women experience a series of orgasms in close succession. However, degree of satisfaction is not necessarily a function of the number of orgasms.

These four phases normally follow each other in sequence. It is said however that for many women there seems to be less 'need for orgasm' than for many men: but whether this is physiologically or culturally determined is not clear. In any case, many women enjoy sexual arousal, intercourse, and the ebbing of arousal without necessarily experiencing an orgasm on each occasion, or regretting its absence (see Hawton (1985) for further discussion of this).

The role of hormones in sexual behaviour is not fully understood. Although *androgens* are essential for the development of full sexual functioning in men, their withdrawal, as occurs following castration, often does not cause loss of a man's ability to respond to sexual stimulation with erection, but sexual desire and the ability to ejaculate may be impaired. Androgens are important with respect to a woman's sexual interest or desire, although much lower levels of androgens are necessary in females than in males for this purpose. In women, *ostrogens* appear to be important in facilitating normal vaginal response to sexual stimulation, but have little or no direct effect on sexual interest. The role, if any, of *progesterone* in female sexual response is unknown.

TYPES OF SEXUAL PROBLEMS

Sexual dysfunctions

In general terms a sexual dysfunction refers to a failure or impairment of sexual interest or response. The types of sexual dysfunction of women and men are listed in Table 14.1. The classification is based on the first three phases of sexual response; that is, sexual interest or desire, arousal or excitement, and orgasm. However, vaginismus and sexual phobias do not usually correspond to a particular response phase.

Table 14.1 *Sexual dysfunctions of females and males*

Phase of sexual response	Sexual dysfunction	
	Female	Male
Interest or desire	Low sexual desire	Low sexual desire
Arousal or excitement	Impaired arousal	Erectile dysfunction
Orgasm	Orgasmic dysfunction	Premature ejaculation Retarded ejaculation Pain on ejaculation
Other types of dysfunction	Vaginismus Dyspareunia Sexual phobias	Sexual phobias

All the problems listed may be either *primary* or *secondary*. A *primary problem* is one that has been present since the onset of sexual activity. A *secondary problem* is one which occurs after a period of normal sexual function. The types of sexual dysfunction which occur in women and men will be described separately.

Sexual dysfunction in women

The general term 'frigidity' was in common use at one time to describe any female sexual dysfunction. The term is non-specific, incorrectly suggests a lack of emotional warmth, and is pejorative, so it should be avoided.

Low sexual desire

This is the most common sexual problem for which women seek help, although not always very willingly. Very often it is a woman's partner who insists on her obtaining help for this problem. The effect that low sexual desire will have on a woman's life will depend on the degree of the impairment and on other circumstances. Some women who experience no spontaneous interest in sex may choose to avoid sexual activity; but many others will choose to enter relationships in which they are expected to engage in sexual activity. In this latter category will be some women who also suffer from difficulties during the phases of arousal and orgasm, while others will find that, although they lack spontaneous sexual desire, they can respond to the partner's interest and experience orgasm during sexual activity. Primary sexual desire is often related to an upbringing in which sexuality was regarded as unmentionable, dirty, or wicked, while secondary low sexual desire is more usually related to general difficulties in the relationship, or to an important event such as childbirth, or to depression.

Impaired arousal

Problems of the excitement phase are characterized by failure of the normal physiological responses which occur during arousal, especially vaginal swelling and lubrication, and by lack of the sensations usually associated with sexual excitement. Such problems are relatively uncommon in women with unimpaired sexual drive, except during later life when hormonal changes may cause impairment of the normal vaginal response so that intercourse becomes uncomfortable and willingness to engage in it is reduced.

Orgasmic dysfunction

It has already been noted that enjoyment of sexual activity without reaching orgasm does not necessarily constitute a 'problem'; the extent to which a woman feels she has a problem concerning orgasm will depend in part on her or her partner's expectations. These can change with time and because of information obtained from a variety of sources, including novels and magazines. Sometimes this may be misleading and cause unreasonable expectations.

Orgasmic dysfunction can be *total*, which means that orgasm is never experienced during sexual activity of any kind, or it can be *situational*, which means that orgasm can be achieved under some circumstances but not others, such as during masturbation but not with a partner, or with one partner and not another. It is important to establish which type of orgasmic dysfunction is present, because the choice of treatment will depend on the nature of the problem.

Vaginismus

This refers to spasm of the pubococcygeus muscles surrounding the entrance to the vagina, which makes sexual intercourse impossible or difficult or painful. Vaginismus is usually due to a specific fear about penetration, the ability to enjoy other aspects of sexual behaviour being largely unimpaired. Occasionally, however, it is part of a more general sexual problem. Vaginismus is a major cause of non-consummation of marriage. It mostly presents as a primary problem although it can occur following vaginal trauma such as an episiotomy especially if this has not been satisfactorily repaired.

Dyspareunia

This refers to pain occurring during sexual intercourse. The pain may be localized to the entrance to the vagina (in which case it is usually related to mild vaginismus or a vaginal infection), or the pain may occur on deep penetration. This deep pain may result from lack of arousal and consequent absence of ballooning of the inner vagina, such that the cervix is buffeted during sexual intercourse. Deep dyspareunia may also be due to pelvic pathology, such as chronic salpingitis or endometriosis.

Sexual phobias

Some women are repelled by certain aspects of sexuality. These might be very specific, such as aversion to kissing, or to seminal fluid, or more generalized, such as aversion to foreplay. A sexual phobia need not necessarily inhibit a woman's enjoyment of the rest of sexual activity, but in many cases the phobia prevents arousal altogether. Sexual phobias are occasionally related to a past traumatic experience such as rape or incest.

Sexual dysfunction in men

Low sexual desire

It is common for most men to feel lessened sexual desire at some time. However, men are somewhat less likely than women to seek help because of long-standing low desire, although referrals of this problem to specialist services have increased in the past few years. Possibly the widely held myth that men are always ready and able to have sex makes it difficult for a man to acknowledge that his desire for sex is lacking. Also, men with low sexual desire often have associated erectile difficulties for which they are more likely to seek help. In some cases the problem presents in the context of a depressive disorder.

Erectile dysfunction

Whereas impairment of arousal in women is not a very common complaint, erectile dysfunction is the male sexual problem most commonly encountered in clinical practice. The erectile response is extremely vulnerable to psychological influences, especially anxiety, and may also be affected by organic disorders, such as diabetes and multiple sclerosis, and by several forms of medication, especially antihypertensive agents.

Erectile dysfunction is often a secondary phenomenon and is particularly likely to occur in middle-aged and older men. Where psychological factors contribute to the dysfunction it is usually situational, in that the man is able to get an erection on his own through masturbation or wakes with an erection at night, but fails to get an erection with his partner or easily loses it—especially when he wishes to penetrate. Sometimes the failure is complete, so that no erection occurs; in other cases a partial erection may be obtained.

Premature ejaculation

This is an extremely common problem among young men, and may be viewed as a relatively 'normal' phenomenon in many males having their first sexual relationships. There is no satisfactory definition of premature ejaculation. Probably the best guide is the extent to which a man himself feels that his ejaculatory control is sufficient to allow intercourse satisfactory to him and his partner. In its most severe form it includes failure to prevent ejaculation before vaginal penetration. More often the man ejaculates within a few seconds of the start of sexual intercourse or immediately he begins to thrust.

Retarded ejaculation

This disorder of ejaculation is relatively uncommon. It includes a total failure of ejaculation under any circumstances, partial failure where ejaculation is not possible with a partner but does occur through masturbation, and difficulty in ejaculating where sexual stimulation or intercourse must be continued for an excessively long time for ejaculation to occur. It is sometimes associated with a sexual variation such as fetishism when the man is unable to ejaculate unless the fetishistic object (e.g. female clothing) is present. Retarded or absent ejaculation can also be caused by some forms of medication, notably antidepressants, especially the recently introduced serotonergic drugs.

Pain on ejaculation

This is rarely encountered in clinical practice. However, some men do complain of acute pain in the perineum and penis during or following ejaculation. This is usually associated with an infection of the urethra or prostate, although in some cases it may be related to spasm of the perineal muscles.

Sexual phobias

Men rarely present complaining of aversion to specific aspects of sexual behaviour. However, phobias sometimes appear to be part of another sexual dysfunction. Thus among men with erectile dysfunction will be found some who experience aversion to extreme sexual excitement in their partners, and others who are particularly averse to vaginal penetration.

Sexual variations

The term 'sexual variation' refers to sexual interest or behaviour which varies from that experienced predominantly by the majority of the population, and in women it refers principally to homosexuality, transsexualism, and sado-masochism. 'Sexual variation' (or its alternative, 'sexual deviation') is a better term than the rather pejorative 'sexual perversion'.

Female homosexuality

Homosexual interest may range from simple feelings of attraction towards another woman, to full sexual activity with a female partner. Some women are exclusively homosexual, but many more experience sexual feelings towards both sexes, and some degree of attraction to other women among heterosexual women appears to be extremely common. Frank sexual feelings or fantasies are a more reliable guide to a woman's sexual orientation.

Occasionally, unacknowledged homosexuality turns out to underlie a complaint of sexual dysfunction such as low sexual desire (for a heterosexual partner). Therefore the doctor should routinely ask an appropriate question about homosexual interest during the course of a full assessment of a sexual problem, and be receptive to any sign that the patient wishes to discuss the issue further.

Other sexual variations

A *transsexual* is a person who feels that his or her gender is really that of the opposite sex. This leads in many cases to a wish to adopt the style of dress of the opposite sex and to undergo hormonal and surgical treatments in order to bring about appropriate anatomical changes. The greater general acceptance of masculine styles of dress for women than feminine styles for men may allow many female transsexuals to go relatively unnoticed. Occasionally a female transsexual will seek specialist help to obtain hormonal treatment and surgery. The latter can include mastectomy, hysterectomy, and genital reconstruction, although the last of these is unlikely to be successful.

Sado-masochism is the only other sexual variation likely to be found in women. Sadistic behaviour includes infliction of pain or restriction of the partner's mobility ('bondage'), while 'masochism' refers to the wish to be the recipient of such activities. It has been argued that a mild degree of sado-masochistic behaviour should be regarded as abnormal only when it consistently provides the main focus of a sexual relationship, and where sex cannot be enjoyed in its absence. It is unequivocally a problem either when one partner does not wish to take part, or where the sadistic or masochistic activities become dangerous.

Male sexual variations

Not uncommonly a woman will present to her doctor complaining directly or indirectly about her partner's sexual behaviour or desires because in her opinion these are abnormal. The behaviour may be of a kind which many couples ordinarily include in their lovemaking, such as orogenital sex, or anal intercourse, but sometimes the source of concern will be a sexual variation such as fetishism, sado-masochism, or homosexuality. Sometimes couples may only need reassurance that they can continue with a practice that they both enjoy, but usually the problem arises from the unwillingness of one partner to engage in a practice that the other wants. Where this is so, the doctor should try to see the partner and discuss this with him, not moralistically, but with the intention of helping the couple come to an arrangement that suits them both. Sometimes the woman can be helped, if she wishes, to accept the practice; in other cases it may be possible to encourage the man to restrict his interest in the variation to masturbatory activity or to fantasy alone. Sometimes the sexual variation seems to be maintained because of a sexual dysfunction in one or other partner and therefore this should be the focus of treatment.

CAUSES OF SEXUAL DYSFUNCTION

In many cases there are multiple causes for sexual dysfunction. The range of possible causes is very wide but may be separated into *psychological* and *physical factors*.

Psychological factors

Factors which may lead to sexual dysfunction can usefully be divided into: (1) *predisposing factors*; (2) *precipitants*; and (3) *maintaining factors*. These will be considered separately and some of the more important are summarized in Table 14.2.

Predisposing factors

Often these are factors arising out of experiences early in life which either made a person vulnerable to developing a sexual problem at a later date or actually caused a sexual dysfunction to develop at that stage. Such factors typically occur in three areas of early experience: family attitudes to sexuality, sex education, and traumatic sexual experiences.

Family attitudes to sexuality. The attitudes to which a person is exposed during early development can have a profound effect on later sexual adjustment. In many families, sex is never discussed and to the children

Table 14.2   *Some psychological causes of sexual dysfunction*

1. *Predisposing factors*
   Family attidudes to sexuality
   Inadequate sex education
   Traumatic sexual experiences
2. *Precipitants*
   Psychiatric illness
   Childbirth
   Infidelity
   Dysfunction in the partner
   Problem in the general relationship
3. *Maintaining factors*
   Anxiety
   Poor communication
   Lack of foreplay
   Depression
   Dysfunction in the partner
   Poor sexual information
   Problem in the general relationship

this can imply that sex is a taboo subject and must be in some way wrong or shameful. In other families, negative attitudes towards sex may be expressed openly. For example, a mother may tell her daughter that sex is a chore that must be undertaken in order to please her partner. Either type of experience is likely to make a young woman feel guilty about her sexual desires or enjoyment, and may contribute to the development of sexual dysfunction. Attitudes which suggest that sex is dirty or shameful are likely to lead to difficulties in arousal or orgasm difficulties. Those which suggest that lovemaking is painful may contribute to the deveopment of vaginismus.

The following case is an example of a mother's adverse attitudes that may have been important in causing a subsequent problem for her daughter:

Helen's parents had frequent rows and separated when she was in her early teens. She lived with her mother, a tense, nagging woman who had instructed Helen carefully from an early age in the 'facts of life', while conveying an idea of sex as something joyless and mechanical. When Helen began to go out with boys she repeatedly warned her to 'be careful', and when a few years later Helen got engaged and allowed her fiancé to persuade her to make love, it was her mother who first detected Helen's pregnancy. Helen had enjoyed lovemaking before marriage, but after the baby was born (after a difficult delivery), she enjoyed it no longer; she came easily to climax but was overcome by guilt afterwards. She enjoyed foreplay with her husband but would rarely agree to go on to intercourse.

Inadequate sex education.   Inadequate or poor information about sexuality is a very important factor in the development of sexual dysfunction. For many people, especially those now of middle or older age, sex education has been either woefully inadequate or entirely lacking. Such information as they possess is likely to be based instead on 'dirty' jokes heard during childhood and adolescence, or on discussion with other children whose information may have been equally inadequate. This can lead to serious misinformation, and particularly to those incorrect beliefs which have been termed *sexual myths*. Some examples of these are given in Table 14.3. Belief in such myths can lead to false expectations concerning sexuality and therefore may cause dysfunction because of the anxiety that results. Lack of knowledge about sexual anatomy (e.g. the position of the clitoris, or even that it exists) can likewise lead to sexual dysfunction. Knowledge of sexuality is likely to be particularly poor with regard to that of the opposite sex. This may mean that a person does not know how to provide a partner with adequate stimulation.

Table 14.3   *Some common sexual myths*

---

1. A man always wants and is always ready to have sex
2. Sex must only occur at the instigation of the man
3. Any woman who initiates sex is immoral
4. Masturbation by either sex is dirty or harmful
5. Sex equals intercourse: anything else does not really count
6. When a man gets an erection it is bad for him not to use it to get an orgasm very soon
7. Sex should always be natural and spontaneous: thinking or talking about it spoils it
8. All physical contact must lead to intercourse
9. Men should not express their feelings
10. Any man ought to know how to give pleasure to any woman
11. Sex is really good only when partners have orgasms simultaneously
12. If people love each other they will know how to enjoy sex together
13. Partners in a sexual relationship instinctively know what the other partner thinks or wants
14. Married partners with a good sexual relationship never masturbate
15. If a man loses his erection it means he does not find his partner attractive
16. It is wrong to have fantasies during intercourse

Traumatic sexual experiences.   It is now clear that the number of women who have had traumatic sexual experiences earlier in their lives, especially childhood sexual abuse (see p. 368), is considerable (Jehu 1988). Such a history is common in women with sexual dysfunction, especially low sexual desire, problems concerning sexual arousal, and specific sexual phobias. Traumatic experiences most likely to lead to problems are those that involved threat, force, or pain, which took place repeatedly, and which involved someone considerably older than the woman herself. Sexual assaults and rape (see p. 366) may cause sexual difficulties, especially if the woman has not received support following the trauma. The consequences of sexual traumas are often related to their damaging effects on the victim's self-esteem and to confused feelings of guilt and anger about the experience.

As with the other remote factors, the extent to which such experiences lead to sexual dysfunction will often depend upon events which occur later, and particularly upon the type of relationships which are established. Some women have very adverse early experiences in terms of family attitudes, sex education, or early sexual relations, yet enjoy highly satisfactory sexual relationships in adulthood.

Precipitants

These are numerous and only some of the more common ones (listed in Table 14.2) will be dealt with here. Psychiatric disorder, as well as physical illness and medication, which can be particularly important precipitants, are discussed later.

Chidlbirth.   Sexual problems in women are especially likely to develop after childbirth, particularly after the birth of a second or subsequent baby. Most women experience a decline in sexual interest and activity in the later stages of pregnancy and during the early puerperium. A number of factors may then inhibit the return of sexual interest which normally occurs during the three months after childbirth (see p. 369).

Infidelity.   Discovery of her partner's infidelity may cause a woman to lose interest in continuing a sexual relationship with him, or infidelity on her own part may cause loss of interest because of anxiety resulting from guilt, or simply because her other sexual relationship is more rewarding. Sometimes a woman first discovers that she has a sexual problem, or that she has one only with her current partner, when she encounters a new partner who is perhaps more knowledgeable or sensitive than her regular one. This is illustrated in the following case example:

Sally and George had difficulties from the beginning of their marriage, mainly because of his premature ejaculation and her lack of enjoyment of sex. In the fourth year of the marriage they began to attend an infertility clinic where it was discovered that George had a moderately low sperm count. The sexual difficulty was not picked up then, nor when Sally became depressed and went into a psychiatric hospital for a month. After this they separated, and Sally had an affair with an older man. With him she discovered that she enjoyed sex and was orgasmic. A year later she and George decided to live together again, and at this point she came to her doctor to ask for help with their sexual difficulties.

Dysfunction in the partner.   Where the male partner either already has, or develops, a sexual problem this may cause the woman herself to suffer sexual dysfunction. For example, orgasmic dysfunction or reduced sexual desire in a woman are often associated with premature ejaculation or erectile dysfunction in her partner. In such cases it is important to determine which dysfunction developed first because that should usually be the initial focus of treatment.

Problems in the general relationship. Deterioration in the general relationship between a woman and man often, although by no means always, leads to problems in their sexual relationship. Where the partners' affection for each other has declined or disappeared then the sexual relationship is almost certain to be disrupted. Distinguishing between a sexual dysfunction which has *resulted* in general relationship difficulties and one which is *symptomatic* of problems in the general relationship is one of the most important tasks in the assessment of sexual dysfunction.

Maintaining factors

It is the factors perpetuating a sexual problem which are most important for treatment purposes because only these perpetuating or maintaining factors are directly amenable to modification. Recognition of the predisposing factors and precipitants can provide the doctor with an understanding of the disorder, and explanations to the patient on this basis may be therapeutic in the sense of helping the patient see that the problem is explicable. However, one cannot change events that have already occurred; one can only try to deal with the consequences of such events. The following are some of the more common maintaining factors (listed in Table 14.2).

Anxiety. This is the main factor underlying most sexual problems. Anxiety may be due to a wide range of causes, including sexual inhibitions, poor self-image, fear of failure, fear of pain, a specific phobia concerning vaginal penetration, and ignorance. Whatever the cause of the anxiety, it can affect sexual function by leading to avoidance, by causing lack of drive, by inhibiting arousal, or by preventing orgasm. Some women clearly recognize that they become anxious during sex. Others may notice a sense of detachment from the sexual activity, amost as if the woman had become an uninvolved observer. This experience has been termed 'spectatoring' by Masters and Johnson (1970).

Poor communication. If a woman fails to let her partner know about her sexual needs and anxieties it is very likely that difficulties will result. In addition, partners often become less communicative about sex once a problem begins, thus making the situation very much worse. This is illustrated in the following case example:

Andrew and Jackie were in their 50s when they came for help. They had married in their 20s, having known each other for a while before that. Sex was always enjoyable for Andrew; for Jackie it was less good at first, but improved as the years went by. Neither had ever read any books about sex, or discussed sex at all with friends, and their lovemaking was simple. Four years before they presented, Andrew came under a lot of stress at work. He became very tired, and on a couple of occasions he lost his erection. Jackie was upset but did not know how to help him, and Andrew refused to talk about it. On holiday things improved a little, but gradually Andrew's interest in sex declined and he found his erections becoming more transient. He became irritable if Jackie made tentative advances to him, and began to cut off all affectionate physical contact with her. Jackie felt very hurt and rejected, and dealt with this, as she had done with similar feelings in her rather neglected childhood, by withdrawing into silence.

When communication is impaired there is a danger that each partner will try to guess what the other is thinking, and this is likely to lead to further problems due to incorrect guesses. Two 'sexual myths' are likely to aggravate this situation. The first myth assumes that men should know all about sex and especially should know 'how to handle a woman', the implication being that if the man does not he is not a proper man. The second myth assumes that people who love each other, instinctively know what the other thinks and feels. On the basis of this myth, where communication is already hampered, people may begin to think 'He (or she) doesn't understand what I feel, he doesn't say what I need to hear; it must be because he doesn't want to, because he doesn't love me.'

Lack of foreplay.   A sexual problem, such as impaired sexual arousal, orgasmic dysfunction, or vaginismus, may well be caused and also persist because there is little or no foreplay. This may of course be due to ignorance on the partner's part, especially about the longer amount of foreplay required by many women (although not at all times) in order to become aroused compared with men. In addition, where a problem has developed it is very common for the amount of foreplay to decline because one or other partner encourages this. Thus a woman who has lost interest in sex may hurry her partner through the sexual act because she knows it is not going to be enjoyable for her and so she would prefer to get it over with quickly. A man with erectile dysfunction may try to have sexual intercourse as soon as he gets an erection, for fear of losing the erection.

Depression.   Loss of interest in sex is usually found in patients who develop depression, and may bring additional distress to the patient through the guilt she feels over the loss of affectionate feelings towards her partner. It is important to reassure such a patient that these are normal symptoms of depression, and that her interest in sex will return as her depression lifts, although sexual desire is often one of the last things to be restored to normal.

An episode of depression may have an important aetiological role in persistent low sexual desire, even though the psychiatric disorder may have resolved. Thus a much higher proportion of people (mostly women) with low sexual desire but not currently depressed were found to have a history of depression than were people with unimpaired sexual desire, the onset of the sexual dysfunction always following or accompanying the depressive disorder (Schreiner-Engel and Schiavi 1986). Furthermore, all the subjects with primary low sexual desire had a history of depression during adolescence. The nature of this association between low sexual desire and depression is unclear. It could reflect persistent psychological disturbance (e.g. with regard to self-esteem and/or self-image) or a biological factor (e.g. neurotransmitter abnormality).

Other factors mentioned already, as predisposing factors or precipitants, can also, if they persist, help to maintain the dysfunction.

Physical factors

Physical disorders and medication can have very profound effects on sexual function. They may directly interfere with physiological or anatomical mechanisms involved in sexual response, or cause secondary psychological reactions leading to sexual dysfunction, or, and not uncommonly, they may disrupt sexual function due to a combination of direct and psychological effects. Thus a woman who initially finds sexual intercourse very uncomfortable after a gynaecological operation may subsequently lack interest in sex because of secondary fear, in spite of complete healing at the surgical site.

The physical disorders and surgical procedures which may lead to sexual problems are listed in Table 14.4 and briefly discussed in the text. The reader who wishes to obtain more detailed information is referred to Bancroft (1989) and Hawton (1985).

Medical disorders

Endocrine. In men, *diabetes* very often causes erectile dysfunction. The sexual effects of diabetes in women are less clear. It appears that whereas Type I diabetes may have relatively little effect, many women with Type II diabetes experience reduced sexual desire, ability to experience orgasm, vaginal lubrication, and sexual satisfaction (Schreiner-Engel *et al.* 1987). In addition to physical effects of diabetes, the psychological impact of the disorder on the women and on their relationship with their partner may also be an important determinant of any negative sexual consequences.

Both *hyperthyroidism* and *myxoedema* may affect sexual function, the former because of anxiety and irritability, and the latter because of tiredness and menorrhagia. Reduced activity of the *adrenal glands*, as in Addison's disease, often affects sexual interest and performance, presumably due to impairment of androgen production.

Table 14.4   *Some medical disorders and surgical procedures which may cause sexual dysfunction*

(a) *Medical disorders*

Endocrine	Diabetes
	Hyperthyroidism; myxoedema
	Addison's disease
Cardiovascular	Myocardial infarction
	Angina pectoris
Respiratory	Chronic obstructive airways disease; asthma
Arthritic	Osteoarthritis
	Rheumatoid arthritis
	Sjögren's syndrome
Neurological	Pelvic autonomic neuropathy
	Spinal cord disease or trauma
Renal	Dialysis
Gynaecological	Vaginitis
	Pelvic infections
	Endometriosis

(b) *Surgical procedures*

Mastectomy	
Colostomy and ileostomy	
Gynaecological	Oophorectomy
	Episiotomy
	Vaginal repair of prolapse
Amputation	

Cardiovascular.   At present there is a scarcity of information about the effects of *myocardial infarction* on female sexuality. However, it seems that many women reduce the frequency of their sexual activity after a heart attack. As with men who have had heart attacks, this may be because of an unfounded fear of precipitating further attacks. Depression, poor self-esteem, and medication may be other factors. Sexual difficulties, including erectile dysfunction or fear of resuming sexual activity, commonly occur in men after heart attacks. This is likely to cause sexual problems for their partners, who in addition may feel guilty about continuing to experience sexual desire. *Angina pectoris* may also limit sexual enjoyment if chest pain or palpitations occur during sexual activity. Prophylactic use of a nitrate preparation or a beta-blocking agent can help prevent these symptoms.

Respiratory.   *Severe chronic respiratory disease* is likely to inhibit sexual activity because of limitations on sexual positions which can be tolerated, especially the 'missionary' position. Occasionally patients with *asthma* repeatedly experience asthmatic episodes during sex.

Arthritis. Joint pain, especially if this arises in the hip joints, may severely limit a woman's ability to enjoy or even participate in sexual activity. Chronic pain is likely to lead to tiredness and loss of interest in sex. In *Sjögren's syndrome* there may be impairment of vaginal lubrication.

Neurological. As sexual response is mediated largely through neural pathways it is obvious that disruption of such pathways will affect sexual performance. Thus damage to the pelvic autonomic nerves (e.g. through neuropathy, malignant disease, or surgery), or the spinal cord, is likely to interfere with genital swelling and lubrication and orgasm. Further discussion of the effects of spinal cord damage occurs later (p. 372).

Renal. Low sexual desire and difficulties in becoming sexually aroused are found in some women on *renal dialysis*. This may in part be due to tiredness and depression, and also to electrolyte and hormonal disturbances.

Gynaecological. Obviously many gynaecological disorders may be associated with sexual problems. Examples include *vaginitis*, due to infection (e.g. thrush) or oestrogen deficiency, which may cause soreness during sexual intercourse, and *pelvic inflammatory disease* or *endometriosis*, which can cause pain on deep penile thrusting.

Surgical procedures

Several surgical procedures in women are likely to affect sexual function (Table 14.4); some because they interfere directly with organs and structures involved in sexual activity and response; others because of their psychological effects.

Examples of surgical procedures which may cause organic damage are gynaecological operations such as *oophorectomy*, following which reduction in circulating oestrogens is likely to impair vaginal lubrication, *episiotomy*, which if poorly sutured may cause tenderness or tightness of the introitus, and *vaginal repair of prolapse*, which may have a similar effect if the repair is unsatisfactory. Finally, *amputation*, especially if a leg has been removed, can cause considerable mechanical difficulties during sexual activity.

Several surgical procedures are likely to have psychological consequences which may profoundly affect a woman's ability to enjoy her sex life. A common psychological sequel is an altered self-image leading to a decreased sense of sexual attractiveness. This is particularly likely after mastectomy. At least one-third of women who have had a breast removed suffer severe long-standing deterioration in their sexual relationships, and in many cases sex is abandoned altogether. Part of the problem may be revulsion experienced by the woman's partner. Similar impairment of self-image may occur following amputation, or after colostomy or ileostomy, where, in addition, concern about possible odour or fear that discomfort or damage might result from sexual intercourse are likely to complicate the picture. Although hysterectomy has been regarded as being associated with a high incidence of sexual problems, in a systematic prospective study this was not found to be so (Gath *et al.* 1982). Indeed, some of the women studied experienced an improvement in their sexual relations. Depression, which commonly occurs following some operations (e.g. mastectomy), is likely to be an added factor contributing to impairment of sexual function following surgery.

Effects of medication

Unfortunately there is a paucity of information concerning the effects of medication on female sexuality. Largely by extrapolation from what is known about the effects in men, it seems that several types of medication may have important consequences for sexual interest and performance in women and that one should always enquire about medication when a woman presents complaining of impaired sexual desire or arousal, or difficulty in achieving orgasm.

The drugs which may affect female sexuality are listed in Table 14.5.

Table 14.5   *Some drugs which may affect female sexuality*

Anticholinergics (e.g. probanthine)
Anticonvulsants (phenytoin; carbamazepine; phenobarbitone)
Antihypertensives and diuretics (beta-blockers; bendrofluazide)
Anti-inflammatory drugs (indomethacin)
Hormones (oral contraception; steroids)
Hypnotics and sedatives (benzodiazepines)
Antidepressants (especially serotonergic agents)
Major tranquillizers (especially thioridazine)
Alcohol
Opiates

Anticholinergic agents may interfere with vaginal engorgement and lubrication. It is possible that *anticonvulsants* may in some cases have an adverse effect on a woman's sexual desire because of their induction of hormone-binding globulin which binds testosterone and therefore leads to a reduction in circulating free testosterone. It is worth considering as a cause of impaired libido where the decline in interest has developed after a long period of anticonvulsant therapy. Drugs used to treat hypertension, such as beta-blockers (e.g. propranolol) and diuretics (bendrofluazide), are known to have erectile dysfunction as a major side-effect (*Lancet* 1981), and can cause reduced sexual desire.

Controversy has surrounded the possible role of *oral contraception* in causing sexual dysfunction. A higher incidence of reduced sexual desire was found in contraceptive pill-users than non-users in the Royal College of General Practitioners' (1974) study, an effect possibly related to mood disturbance. With the modern low-dose oral contraceptives most women experience no significant changes in their libido, and some report enhancement of their enjoyment of sex.

Some *antidepressants* (notably the mono-amine oxidase inhibitors and the new serotonergic agents) can cause delay or absence of orgasm in both sexes). Because the *major tranquillizers*, especially thioridazine, can have profound effects on male sexual performance, this suggests that they may also interfere with female sexual response. Although *benzodiazepines* (e.g. diazepam) are occasionally prescribed as treatment for sexual problems related to anxiety, it seems likely that they have an adverse effect in some patients because of their tendency to cause drowsiness. While *alcohol* is likely to enhance sexual desire and reduce inhibitions when used in moderation, chronic alcohol abuse often leads to loss of interest in sex because of its depressant effects, and to erectile difficulties associated with autonomic neuropathy, liver disease, and testicular failure. *Opiate* abuse often causes sexual dysfunction, especially reduced sexual desire, in both men and women.

If it is thought that a particular drug is having a deleterious effect on a woman's sexual interest then it will be necessary to weigh up the pros and cons of stopping or changing the medication and the likely effect on the physical or psychological condition for which the drug has been prescribed. Where an effective alternative drug is available this might be tried. However, it is important to be alert to the fact that changes in sexual interest or enjoyment are often blamed on medication when other factors, especially those of an interpersonal nature, are the real cause.

Some forms of medication can improve sexuality. *Androgens* administered for medical conditions can enhance sexual interest, and some attempt has been made to incorporate these drugs in the treatment of women with impaired sexual desire, though results of most studies suggest little or no effect. However, they are beneficial for many women who experience postmenopausal reduction in sexual desire (Sherwin *et al.* 1985). *Oestrogens* administered for menopausal symptoms may improve sexual arousability because of their beneficial effects on the postmenopausal vaginal mucosa.

HOW TO ASSESS PATIENTS WITH SEXUAL PROBLEMS

Help or advice should *never* be offered to anyone presenting with a sexual problem without first making a careful assessment and coming to a clear understanding about what the problem is. Often the problem is very different from that suggested by the initial complaint. Sometimes the woman may believe that it is she who has the problem when in fact it is primarily her partner's, so that, for example, a woman whose husband has premature ejaculation may complain to her doctor of inability to achieve orgasm during intercourse.

Assessment of a sexual problem has in itself a very important therapeutic function:

1. It can begin to clarify and make intelligible a problem that, in the patient's mind, is obscure and associated with shame, bewilderment, and suffering.
2. It demonstrates that it is both respectable and feasible to talk effectively about sex, and that it may therefore be possible for the woman to talk to her partner about it too.
3. It demonstrates that sexual difficulty is regarded by doctors as a legitimate worry, and one that they are trained to deal with. The doctor can make it clear that the problem is neither extraordinary nor blameworthy, and that it can be helped.
4. It offers an opportunity for mistaken fears and beliefs to be dispelled. Much anxiety and self-blame is based on half-truths, muddled information, and 'sexual myths' (see Table 14.3).

Unfortunately many doctors have not received training in taking a sexual history. Two general points are important here. First, it is essential for the doctor to feel comfortable about the procedure, in order to concentrate on dispelling the patient's embarrassment and anxiety, and also so that accurate information can be obtained without the doctor feeling obliged to side-step any issues because of her or his own embarrassment. Secondly, there is a difficulty about the words used to discuss the problem. Doctors feel comfortable using medical terminology, but many patients will not comprehend words like lubrication, ejaculation, and so on; on the other hand, colloquial words do not always have a precise enough meaning, and also they may seem shocking or inappropriate to the patient when spoken in medical consultation. Often the only remedy to this problem is to discuss the difficulty openly with the patient, and then to come to a gradual agreement on the terms to be used in the interview, by translating frequently between the technical and the colloquial terms, and allowing the patient to select and to become accustomed to using the words that she prefers. For example, the doctor might say, 'Ejaculation is the technical word for the moment when the seminal fluid comes out of the end of the penis. In ordinary speech people often call that "coming", and they may call the seminal fluid "spunk". Do you know what I mean by that? Which words would you like to use?. . . All right, now you were telling me that when your husband ejaculates, he. . . .'

There are other considerations, applicable to interviewing in general, that can help to make the interview less stressful for the patient, and more productive of information. Thus it is often a good idea to proceed from 'less painful' to 'more painful' topics, and to switch temporarily to less painful topics if the patient needs to recover herself at any time later in the interview. Examples of 'less painful' areas are: simple factual information (times, places, events); information about other people; and happy or successful aspects of the patient's life. Examples of 'more painful' areas may be: details of the sexual difficulty; the patient's own feelings; and any discussion of marital or family tension. It is worth trying to use a judicious mixture of 'open-ended' questions that allow the patient to tell her story in her own words, contaminated by the doctor's presuppositions, and more 'closed', detailed questions that allow precise information to be established while relieving the patient of some of the burden of naming embarrassing things. Examples of open-ended questions are: 'Tell me more about the problem' and 'How did you feel when that happened?' A closed question might be: 'I think you are telling me that you feel that your vagina doesn't become wet enough, so that it feels uncomfortable when your husband wants to put his penis in. Is that what you mean? Or did you mean something different?'

It is particularly helpful to ask the patient to recall a *specific* occasion, as recent as possible, on which the sexual difficulty arose. If the patient can describe such an occasion, she can be asked to give a minute-by-minute account, which should include an idea of how her partner responded to anything she did, of her response to his actions, of her thoughts and what she imagined he was thinking at the time. Such a detailed account of a single episode, which is probably best obtained later in the interview when the patient is more relaxed, is much more informative than any general statements about the nature of the problem that the patient may have worked out for herself. Having established a picture of one occasion, the doctor should then ask whether other occasions have followed the same pattern, or, if not, how they have differed.

When a patient appears embarrassed it can be helpful if the doctor acknowledges this and then explains that she will get more confident with time. It is crucial not to side-step issues because they are embarrassing; they may be central to the problem.

If the woman has a partner and he is relevant to her difficulty it is important to try to see him. Apart from the possible necessity of involving him in subsequent treatment, the information obtained from him may cast a very different light on the problem. When a woman says she doubts if her husband will attend, the doctor might consider dropping him a note to encourage him, provided the patient gives her permission.

History taking

The main points to be covered in carrying out a detailed assessment of a patient with a sexual problem are contained in the Appendix to this chapter (p. 374). A systematic assessment of this kind will take at least half an hour and therefore might be spread over two or three interviews. Certainly a detailed assessment is required if the doctor is considering treating the patient with some form of sex therapy. For other purposes a briefer assessment might be sufficient. If the doctor is short of time on the day when a woman first mentions that she has a sexual problem, she could be asked to return for a longer and more leisurely interview later. However, every effort should be made to ensure that at the *first* interview she has said enough and has received enough encouragement for her to want to attend for a second longer interview.

In making a *brief assessment* the doctor should cover the following points: (1) what is the precise nature of the problem?; (2) what is the effect of the problem on the woman and her partner?; (3) is there a major problem in the couple's general relationship?; (4) has the patient had a satisfactory sexual relationship in the past?; (5) is the patient adequately informed about sex?; (6) is there any medical or psychiatric condition which might contribute to, or cause the problem?; (7) is the patient on any medication and what is her level of alcohol consumption?; (8) what changes would the patient like to achieve in her sexual adjustment?

It will be clear that even a brief assessment must be far from cursory if the doctor is to obtain sufficient information to decide what help to provide, including whether or not to refer for specialist treatment.

MANAGEMENT OF SEXUAL PROBLEMS

The variety of approaches available for dealing with sexual problems can be separated conveniently into two categories, distinguished by the intensity and scope of the treatment. These are (1) *brief counselling*, and (2) *sex therapy*. The first category, which includes the provision of simple advice and information, should be within the scope of all GPs. Some GPs will also want to practise sex therapy, in which a detailed step-by-step programme is used to help an individual or couple. However, this requires special training and is fairly time-consuming so that the majority of GPs may not wish to carry this out themselves.

The important therapeutic function of the assessment interview must be re-emphasized here. Often a patient or couple will experience a great deal of relief from simply having the opportunity to talk about the problem and from the reassurance that the doctor can provide during the assessment. It is not always necessary to provide advice at this stage; often it is better to ask the patient(s) to return a few days later, when the doctor will have had time to think further about the problem and the best means of tackling it, and the patient(s) will have had time to discover whether they need any further help.

In this section the two categories of management in relation to couples with sexual dysfunction are considered. Then treatment of the individual woman without a partner, the management of problems related to sexual variations, and the referral of patients for specialist treatment are discussed. Finally, management of problems associated with rape and childhood sexual abuse are described.

Treatment of couples with sexual dysfunction

Brief counselling

This is most appropriate for those problems that arise from inadequate or muddled information, and for those which involve anxieties about sexual behaviour of a particular kind (e.g. oral sex) or at a particular time (e.g. pregnancy; after the manopause). Usually such problems can be managed over the course of only a few consultations. Sometimes only one consultation will be necessary, although the doctor should always try to assess subsequently whether the counselling has been effective.

Brief counselling can include the following strategies:

Provision of information. As ignorance or misinformation are often shared by a couple, both partners should, if possible, be present when information is to be given by the doctor, so that they can both question it at the time, and discuss it together afterwards. The doctors can provide accurate information on sexual anatomy (especially using pictures), can describe what happens during sexual arousal in either sex, can convey an idea of the range of normal biological variation in anatomy and physiology, and the frequency (and therefore 'normality') of different types of sexual behaviour, such as oral sex or homosexual contacts during adolescence. The patient might also be recommended suitable reading material (David Delvin's (1974) *Book of love* being an excellent example).

Advice. For example, the doctor may give advice on the following: how to engage in more enjoyable foreplay, suitable positions for sexual intercourse during pregnancy or recovery from a physical illness, and means whereby a couple can come to a compromise over their differing levels of sexual desire. Advice should be given only after careful appraisal of what is likely to be acceptable for the couple.

Permission-giving. Sometimes a patient feels needlessly guilty about some aspect of sexual behaviour (such as masturbation or the occurrence of sexual fantasy). Where such feelings are the legacy of repressive parental attitudes, they can be countered by the doctor adopting a different parental role, helping the patient to accept that the activity in question is not harmful or wicked and is shared by most other ordinary people. However, this must be done with caution and respect, to avoid putting pressure on patients to accept a value system that is alien to them.

Sex therapy

Masters and Johnson (1970) revolutionized the treatment of couples with sexual problems when they introduced their relatively brief but intensive therapeutic approach. This is based on the rationale that although sexual problems may arise from a wide range of causes, some of which are rooted in the past, nevertheless the problems are maintained by factors which operate in the present, and therefore are amenable to modification by techniques focused on present occurrences, feelings, and thoughts.

The methods of Masters and Johnson have proved very effective, with some modifications, within the setting of the National Health Service. This modified approach will be summarized here; anyone wishing to use the method will need to consult a fuller account (e.g. Hawton 1985) and obtain appropriate training.

After full assessment of each partner individually, the couple is pre-sented with a *formulation* of the problem, setting out its nature, and the likely predisposing factors, precipitants, and maintaining factors that have contributed to it. The purpose of the formulation is to provide the couple with a better understanding of their problem and to provide a rationale for the treatment approach. The principal components of the treatment are (1) homework assignments; (2) counselling; (3) education.

Homework assignments.   These have two purposes. The first is to provide a method by means of which couples can establish or re-establish the con-fidence and freedom in their sexual contact with each other that will allow unhindered sexual response to occur. The second is to assist the therapist and the couple to identify precisely the factors that are contributing to maintenance of the problem. In essence the programme of assignments consists of a graduated series of clearly defined tasks in touching and being touched by each other in specific ways, so that the difficulty is broken down into manageable steps, in which room is made for discussion of obstacles arising at any stage. Where appropriate, additional specific techniques are used to tackle particular kinds of dysfunction.

The couple is first asked to agree to undertake the programme which includes an initial ban both on sexual intercourse and on touching of the genital areas and the woman's breasts. Instructions for *sensate focus* are then provided. The partners are asked to find a suitable time when they can concentrate on this exercise in a relaxed fashion. The exercise consists of each partner taking turns at caressing the other over all areas of the body, apart from the 'no-go' areas already mentioned. The purpose of this is for each to learn to accept pleasure from the other, for each to find out how and where the partner likes being caressed, and to help the partners feel relaxed and comfortable with each other without striving towards arousal. Through this they can begin to learn to communicate on sexual matters, and advice specifically addressed to this issue will also be given by the therapist.

When this stage is satisfactorily established, the couple is asked to progress to *genital sensate focus*, during which both the genitals and breasts are included in caressing, but the emphasis is still on discovery of each other and on improving communication. Subsequently the couple moves from individual caressing, turn and turn about, to simultaneous mutual pleasuring. The next stage is a gradual progression to sexual intercourse via an intermediate stage of *vaginal containment* in which penetration occurs but there is no movement.

Specific techniques are used for particular types of dysfunction, only some of which can be mentioned here. Finger exploration of the vagina in a series of graded steps by both partners is suggested where the woman has vaginismus. Masturbation exercises are often advised where the woman is unable to achieve orgasm. Kegel's vaginal muscle exercises (as advised for women following childbirth) are useful for both vaginismus and orgasmic dysfunction. The 'stop-start' or 'squeeze' techniques may be suggested where the man has premature ejaculation. In both of these the woman provides her partner with intermittent penile stimulation according to his level of sexual arousal. In the squeeze technique she also applies firm pressure with her fingers to the base of the glans penis when her partner feels he is near to ejaculation. Masturbation exercises are also suggested in the treatment of ejaculatory failure.

Counselling. As the couple moves through the graduated programme, discussion at each stage enables both the therapist and the couple to get a clearer idea of the factors maintaining the problem. In addition, at some stage almost every couple encounters a block to progress, which yields further valuable information. In order to help modify the factors maintaining the sexual problem and particularly to overcome blocks to progress, a considerable amount of counselling will be necessary. The components of such counselling include the following:

1. Helping the partners reconsider *attitudes* they hold and perhaps have never questioned (e.g. that sexual activity should always be the responsibility of the male partner, with the woman playing a passive role). As discussed in relation to brief counselling, the therapist should avoid imposing values on patients, but should help them to look at attitudes which clearly obstruct their progress towards the goals they have chosen for themselves.

2. *Confronting* patients when there appears to be a discrepancy between their stated aims and what they are actually doing in practice. Quite

often partners say that they are keen to improve their sexual relationship but in fact fail to carry out the therapist's instructions.

3. Identifying and discussing *feelings* originating from other areas of the relationship but finding expression through the sexual relationship.

4. *Permission-giving,* as when a therapist encourages the partners to carry out sexual activity which they had not thought of, or regarded as taboo (such as masturbation) but which is likely to help overcome their problem.

5. Providing *reassurance*.

Some of the techniques employed in cognitive therapy for a variety of emotional problems are useful in sex therapy (see Hawton 1989), especially when trying to help a couple (and the doctor) understand the reasons why particular reactions and feelings occur in sexual situations and attempting to modify such factors.

Education. The educational aspects of sex therapy are similar to those involved in brief counselling. It is often advisable to devote part of an early treatment session to providing simple information about sexual anatomy and response.

The duration of sex therapy will vary from couple to couple but between eight and 16 sessions of treatment are usually required. Although Masters and Johnson use male and female co-therapists to treat couples, it seems that one therapist is just as effective and that the gender of the therapist is usually not important, except in some cases where there may be obvious benefits for the therapist to be of the same gender as the dysfunctional partner (e.g. a very timid woman with vaginismus).

The results of sex therapy originally reported by Masters and Johnson (1970) have proved to be far superior to those obtained by other workers. However, results obtained elsewhere are far from disappointing. Thus, in clinical practice in this country (Bancroft and Coles 1976; Hawton and Catalan 1986) it appears that two-thirds of couples derive considerable benefits from treatment. Vaginismus and premature ejaculation respond particularly well. Results are less good for low sexual desire, partly because this problem often reflects general relationship difficulties. The long-term outcome of sex therapy suggests that while progress is maintained for many couples, especially those who originally presented with vaginismus, a considerable proportion will experience relapses, although the attitudes of partners to their problems may be more tolerant (Hawton *et al.* 1986).

Treatment of women without partners

It may happen that a woman will present asking for help, but have no partner, or be unwilling to involve her current partner in treatment. Fortunately there is much that can be done to help such women, especially those with vaginismus or orgasmic dysfunction. For some women brief advice can be given, e.g. concerning the use of a vibrator. For others, more detailed graduated programmes will be necessary.

A woman with vaginismus may first be asked to become familiar with her vaginal anatomy, perhaps while in the bath. Subsequently, after a vaginal examination by the doctor, the woman will be encouraged to explore her vagina with a finger in order to become more comfortable with vaginal penetration. She can also be taught the Kegel exercises.

In orgasmic dysfunction, the woman will be encouraged to learn to masturbate. During the course of such treatment she may require help to modify her attitudes to masturbation. She will also need advice on ways of subsequently showing a partner how to stimulate her appropriately. The results of such treatment of orgasmic problems are usually very good.

Treatment of problems related to sexual variations

It will be rare for the GP to be called upon to counsel a woman with established homosexual interest. Most such women do not feel they need help. However, a GP who is asked for help by a homosexual woman who wishes to come to terms with her sexual interest might be best advised to refer her to an organization such as Friend (p. 375) which provides a counselling service.

The female transsexual who asks for help will almost invariably require referral to a specialist.

When a woman complains about her husband's deviant sexual interest it will be most important to try to see the husband and to find out whether he is concerned about his sexual interest and whether he wishes to do anything about it. If he does, specialist referral will usually be necessary.

Referral of patients for specialist treatment

Only a rough guide can be given as to which patients with sexual problems should be referred for specialist attention. This will depend in part on how well equipped the GP feels to deal with the problem. Assuming the GP does not wish to undertake sex therapy, referral will be indicated for women who present with a sexual problem that appears to be the result of significant early experiences and where simple advice and reassurance do not have any effect. This applies to any type of sexual dysfunction. It is also particularly worth trying to arrange treatment where the man has erectile dysfunction, because a variety of effective treatments are now available.

Before initiating referral the partner should be seen if possible to assess his attitudes to the problem and particularly whether he is willing to do anything about it. A brief assessment, along the lines suggested earlier, should be made for both partners before making the referral. A physical examination should be carried out where indicated. This applies particularly to vaginismus and erectile dysfunction. Advice on what is likely to happen when the couple see the specialist may help to reassure them.

Sometimes a couple may say they would prefer not to be referred at present. They may already have been helped by their discussion of the problem with their doctor and therefore referral might be delayed a while to see whether this was enough to allow them to make further progress unaided.

The GP will need to know who runs the nearest sexual dysfunction clinic. Unfortunately the availability of such clinics varies greatly from area to area. Many Relate (formerly Marriage Guidance) counsellors are now specially trained in sex therapy; likewise a number of family planning doctors undertake such training; and some sex therapy clinics are based in psychiatric hospitals. The doctor might enquire from any of these agencies locally.

Rape

'Rape is not a sexual encounter in the usual sense. Instead, it is an event in which one person hurts another *by means of sex*.' (Everstine and Everstine 1983.) Rape represents many different kinds of assault simultaneously: on a person's sense of control over her own life, on her trustful assumptions about other people and her safety in the world, as well as a devastating invasion of her personal space. The victim's responses and her needs for help follow the same patterns as those of victims of other kinds of life-threatening trauma, especially those involving sudden overwhelming loss. Like them, she will experience an immediate period of *shock*, in which ordinary patterns of behaviour are wholly disrupted (in ways she may afterwards find difficult to understand or to accept), followed by a variable *post-traumatic phase* in which severe anxiety, depression, guilt, anger, somatic symptoms, sleep disturbance, sexual difficulty, feelings of isolation and worthlessness may all play their part.

These emotional consequences need to be kept in mind from the earliest moments in the aftermath of a rape, but the practical aspects must also not be overlooked. If the woman consents to report the rape to the police, the GP can give useful advice about what to do. She should expect to be seen by a police surgeon and examined if medical evidence is needed in court. She should not wash or change her clothing, nor have a drink nor take any medication, until she has been seen by a police surgeon. As she may be asked to leave her clothes behind at the police station she should take a change of clothing with her. She may be helped if she is accompanied by a supportive friend, especially if this friend saw her soon after the incidence and can give evidence to the police. Finally, she should be advised to make a note of details of the sequence of events associated with the rape to help her in making her statement to the police.

The main possible *physical* after-effects of rape are damage to pelvic organs and the rest of the body, venereal infection (including HIV), and pregnancy. Examination of a raped woman by a police surgeon for forensic purposes may not necessarily deal with these aspects, and the GP's help may be vital here. The psychological violation experienced by a raped woman can unfortunately be compounded by attitudes of suspicion or contempt encountered from doctors, lawyers, or police, or even from those closest to her. These attitudes arise partly as defences to the very powerful feelings provoked by the occurrence of a rape, and partly from the many myths that surround the subject. Such myths include the belief that a woman can always resist rape if she really wants to, that women lead men on and falsely cry rape afterwards, that respectable girls do not get raped, that a woman with sexual experience is not harmed by being raped, and that rape is subconsciously enjoyable. The feelings of guilt and self-questioning ('why me?') that are part of the woman's normal psychological response to acute trauma may further increase the impact of these attitudes on her and cause her to believe the myths to be true in her case.

The most immediate need of a raped woman is for sympathetic, informed, and gentle handling. Early support is thought to be very important in preventing long-term psychological damage, and it should be offered in a way that fosters the woman's sense of autonomy and her freedom to choose what help she wishes, so as to counter the feelings of enforced helplessness induced by rape. She should be encouraged but never pressurized to talk about the details of what occurred, and she may need to tell the story many times to the same listener before she gains the strength to recount its most distressing or humiliating aspects. The doctor has an important role in meeting the need, both of the victim and her family, to understand what has happened to them and the feelings they are experiencing. Simple explanations about the mechanism of shock, or of psychological defences (such as denial or projection), refutation of damaging assumptions based on myths, reassurance about the normality of feelings they may experience (including paradoxical and rapidly changing feelings) so as to dispel fears of insanity, and joint decisions about the kinds of support the family can most usefully give, will all form part of the psychological first aid that a general practitioner can appropriately provide.

The woman is likely to have to cope with the feelings of those close to her, especially of her sexual partner. He may succeed in being supportive, or may instead be overwhelmed by his own feelings of rage, helplessness, or revulsion, which can in turn lead to sexual difficulties for him (especially erectile dysfunction). For her part, the victim may find it hard to accept her partner's support, because of her feelings (however irrational she knows them to be) of anger or despair at his failure to protect her when she most needed his help. It is advisable for the doctor to give time separately therefore to the family, and especially the partner, so that they can be free to say things which they might otherwise conceal for fear of hurting the victim further. It is useful, too, if at an early stage a suitable person close to the victim or a fellow professional (e.g. a social worker) can be identified who will be able to continue the support through the weeks that follows.

Research on the long-term consequences of rape indicates that the commonest enduring consequences are probably depression and sexual dysfunction (especially fear of sex, lessened enjoyment, and arousal difficulties). The risk of long-term consequences seems to be greatest where the rape was associated with much violence, where the woman had pre-existing difficulties, either psychological or social, where early support was lacking or inadequate, and (perhaps) where an apparently rapid return to normal adjustment concealed a denial of feelings, or guilt, which prevented the acceptance of help. Where such risk factors exist, and in other cases as necessary, referral for specialist help should be considered.

Rape crisis centres are available in most areas. In some places, self-help groups for the victims of rape have been formed, with the object of providing emotional support, information on medical and legal matters, companionship at court hearings or other stressful times, and often with the additional and wider aim of educating the general public and encouraging a change in attitudes.

Sexual abuse

Increasing numbers of women are seeking help for the long-term consequences of being abused in childhood. Characteristics of sexual abuse likely to have long-term effects include prolonged experience of abuse, early age at onset and at cessation, abuse by the father rather than a non-relative, actual physical sexual contact, and the use of force. The main negative consequences of childhood sexual abuse are mood disturbances, often linked to chronic low self-esteem, interpersonal difficulties, especially with partners, and sexual dysfunction, particularly low sexual desire, sexual phobias, and problems of arousal. Sexual promiscuity is also sometimes found in victims of abuse.

Many factors may contribute to sexual abuse of daughters by their father (this being the most common form of childhood sexual abuse), including personality disorder and alcohol abuse in the father, marital disharmony between the parents, and collusion of the girl's mother. Often a girl is drawn into an incestuous relationship when she is too young to appreciate its implications. Only when older might she come to experience guilt and remorse about the relationship, this then being likely to have implications for her subsequent sexual adjustment.

It is common for a woman not to disclose childhood sexual abuse at initial presentation to a doctor, for fear of not being believed or because she feels guilty or ashamed about it (Hobbs 1990). When a history of abuse is revealed, the doctor's reaction is going to be an important initial step in any therapeutic process. An accepting and understanding attitude is essential and can do much to reduce the woman's sense of abnormality. Referral for specialist help from either a psychiatrist, clinical psychologist, or counsellor will usually be necessary because considerable time and expertise are often required to help women overcome the effects of sexual abuse (Jehu 1988).

SEXUALITY AND SEXUAL PROBLEMS AT SPECIAL TIMES IN A WOMAN'S LIFE

There are certain times in a woman's life when sexuality is particularly likely to undergo change and these are times when sexual problems commonly occur. The most significant of these times are pregnancy and childbirth, the menopause, and older age.

Pregnancy and childbirth

Although there is some variation in the findings from different studies of the changes in sexual activity during pregnancy, all studies agree that most women's sexual interest declines during the third trimester, with a consequent decline in the frequency of sexual intercourse. Reduced frequency of intercourse may also be due to physical discomfort, awkwardness, sense of loss of attractiveness, and recommendations from doctors to avoid sex.

Although only limited information is available about the effects of intercourse during pregnancy, it appears that there are no specific complications of, or contraindications to, intercourse at any stage in normal pregnancy. Thus there is no evidence that coitus will cause physical damage to the fetus, or rupture the membranes, nor that orgasm might induce premature labour. Some clinicians may advise against sexual intercourse if there is a history of miscarriage, ante-partum bleeding, or pain during intercourse. Under such circumstances the doctor might recommend non-coital sex but female orgasm need not be avoided. However, orgasm should probably be avoided where there is either a history of premature deliveries or any evidence of premature labour.

Apart from providing reassurance to the woman who is concerned about her loss of sexual interest during pregnancy, the doctor might also advise a woman about positions for sexual intercourse that are likely to be comfortable for her. These include side-by-side and rear-entry positions.

Following childbirth, most women experience a reduction in their interest in sex, which may last for up to three months or even longer. In addition, soreness of an episiotomy scar and post-partum vaginal dryness associated with reduced levels of circulating oestrogens, particularly in breast-feeding mothers, may make intercourse uncomfortable and therefore lead to avoidance or reduced interest. The stress for both partners in adapting to their new roles as parents, the husband's possible sense of partial exclusion, and puerperal depression may all contribute to sexual difficulties. In addition, a nursing mother may feel guilty about sexual arousal that can occur with breast-feeding. Finally, previous sexual maladjustment often manifests itself as frank sexual dysfunction following childbirth.

The GP can forewarn women about some of these problems and give appropriate advice if they actually occur. If post-partum vaginal dryness occurs the patient can be given an explanation and recommended to use a lubricant (such as KY jelly) during intercourse. Where soreness of an episiotomy scar prevents intercourse, a gradual return to non-coital sexual activity might first be recommended. It is important to reassure both women and their partners that loss of interest in sex is normal after childbirth and that it will gradually return. It is especially important to encourage the partners to maintain physical contact with each other over this period. Some couples may only want a loving cuddle; in other partnerships, the wife may wish to continue caressing her husband, though not yet wishing to be caressed by him.

Menopause

The onset of the menopause can provide a profound sense of liberation for some women and this may lead to enhanced interest in sex. However, in others there is a decline in sexual desire. A number of factors are likely to be influential at this time. Reduction in circulating oestrogens will often cause decreased sexual arousability and may make sexual intercourse painful. Decline in androgen levels may have specific effects on sexual interest or desire. Other factors include, for example, children being about to leave home, a woman worrying that she is unattractive (especially by comparison with an attractive daughter), the increased risk of developing depression, and the partner possibly experiencing a decline in sexual performance.

Hormone replacement therapy, or vaginal application of hormonal cream, will benefit any vaginal dryness. While reduced sexual desire following the menopause is little affected by oestrogen or progestogen therapy, androgens will usually help restore sexual desire, especially when the menopause has been precipitated by oophorectomy. In addition to hormone administration the GP may be able to provide counselling, along the lines suggested earlier, which will assist the woman who is experiencing sexual difficulties. Whenever possible the partner should be included in such consultation. The management of problems of the menopause is discussed in more detail in Chapter 7.

Older age

Several studies have demonstrated that the majority of women and men remain sexually active beyond the age of 60, and, depending on the availability of a partner, as many as one in five are active at 80. For women in particular, it is very often the loss or disability of the spouse that determines the end of sexual activity.

'Sexual myths' affect the attitudes of both young and old towards sexuality in later life. These myths include the following: (1) because procreation is not possible after the menopause sexual activity should therefore cease; (2) sex is the prerogative of the young and attractive person; (3) sexual performance declines rapidly after middle age; (4) the problems associated with ageing preclude any interest in sexual activity. Belief in such myths may cause guilt in people who find that their sexual interest does not suddenly decline after middle age, and may contribute directly to problems such as loss of interest and impaired performance.

A number of physical and psychological difficulties may affect the sexual life of older women. First, the physical changes which occur with normal ageing, such as atrophic vaginitis, a decline in the vaginal response during sexual arousal, sagging breasts, impaired mobility, and weight gain, may impair the sexual interest and performance of both the woman and her partner. In addition, those physical illnesses which are likely to impair sexual function become more common in old age. These include cerebrovascular disease, especially strokes, degenerative joint disorders, maturity-onset diabetes, thyroid dysfunction. Parkinsonism, malignant disease, especially of the breast and bowel, and amputations. In parallel with the increase in physical disorders, the numbers of women receiving medication, and the range of medication used, steadily increase with age. Some of the drugs used may have profound effects on sexuality (p. 356). Finally, psychiatric disorders, especially depression, anxiety, and dementia become more common, and all three, together with drugs used to treat them, are likely to be associated with impaired sexual interest and function.

Some of the difficulties will be amenable to brief counselling, particularly if the doctor has an understanding of sexuality during older age and is able to discuss the topic without embarrassment. Sexual dysfunction in older persons is often very amenable to sex therapy, provided the therapist is sensitive to the sexual value systems of older patients, which may be considerably more restricted than those of some younger people. On the other hand, some couples welcome the change in social attitudes and the opportunity it gives them to discuss problems they may have uncomplainingly accepted for years. Particular attention should be paid to physical aspects of therapy, including hormone replacement and the use of physical aids.

SEXUAL PROBLEMS ASSOCIATED WITH DISABLEMENT

Only in recent years have the sexual problems encountered by physically and mentally handicapped people begun to receive appropriate attention. Several factors seem to have contributed to this neglect. Some people responsible for the care of the disabled have maintained the illusion that disabled persons somehow lack sexuality. Not only is this obviously untrue but it is also apparent that as many as three-quarters of persons who are disabled encounter problems in fulfilling their sexuality. Probably this attitude stems partly from the fact that both disablement and sex are found by many people to be sensitive and difficult topics; the combination of the two therefore tends to provoke extreme discomfort which is dealt with by denial. This is reinforced by a general notion that to be sexy one must be able-bodied and attractive.

We can consider the problems of disablement in terms of (1) the woman who is disabled; (2) the woman with a disabled partner; and (3) management of sexual problems associated with disablement.

Sexual problems of the disabled woman

Although most of our information about sexual problems and physical disability concerns men, it is clear that disabled women are likely to suffer just as many problems as disabled men. Several aspects of a woman's sexuality can be affected. First, her image of herself as a physically desirable individual is likely to be precarious. Secondly, her awareness of the stigma attached to sexuality of the disabled may limit her interest in sex. Thirdly, the debilitating effects of the disorder from which she suffers, or of the medication she receives for it, may impair her drive. This particularly applies to chronic painful conditions. Fourthly, the condition may interfere with her mobility; thus, for example, severe arthritis or a spinal cord lesion may make coitus difficult or impossible. Fifthly, her capacity to receive the sensory input necessary for sexual satisfaction may be limited: this is particularly likely with neurological disorders. Finally, if she is being cared for by others (whether by relatives or in an institution) it is their attitude which will determine whether she has any opportunities for sexual activity, alone or with a partner.

Some of the conditions which may cause disability and affect sexuality have already been considered (see pp. 353–6). Others deserve mention in this context. Many neurological conditions, such as multiple sclerosis and cerebral palsy, are associated with sexual problems. The woman with a complete spinal cord transection will be unable to achieve an orgasm through genital stimulation, though she may well still be capable of pregnancy. She is also likely to have problems of urinary and bowel control. Often the woman with a spinal cord lesion develops new erogenous zones, especially at the level of the lesion. A woman who is blind may face taboos concerning learning about sexuality through touch, may be concerned about odour associated with sexual activity, embarrassed about nudity, frustrated due to the extra dependency she must have on her partner, and will lack completely the visual components of sexuality. Social isolation and difficulties in communication are likely to lead to poor sexual information for the woman who is deaf. Finally, mental retardation is associated with a whole range of further problems, particularly those arising from the attitudes of staff responsible for the woman's care, and especially from their concern about the woman's vulnerability to sexual exploitation and risk of pregnancy.

Sexual problems for the spouse of the disabled man

The woman whose partner is physically disabled is likely to face numerous difficulties concerning their sexual relationship. First and foremost there are the problems that arise because other people are often unable to accept a sexual relationship between an able-bodied woman and a disabled man. In addition, there are the problems arising out of role reversals that may be necessary in the general relationship, the concern the woman may have about hurting her partner, impairment of fertility (especially when the partner has a spinal cord lesion), difficulties the man may have in accepting his wife in a more sexually active role, and the attitude both partners have to non-coital sexual activity where sexual intercourse is impossible. The man may suffer considerable jealousy about the wife's ability to enjoy sex more than he does, and about the risk that she may develop another relationship. Furthermore, the woman may have great difficulty in accepting a role that combines the tasks of nurse (especially where excretory functions need to be looked after) and the feelings of a sexual partner.

Management of sexual problems of the disabled

Many of the sexual difficulties discussed here are straightforward and ideally should be dealt with by those who care for the disabled in the course of their everyday work. However, carers need education and support in order to do this. Many other sexual problems associated with disability are of a special nature, and will need referral for expert counselling. Until recently there were few people experienced in this type of work, but in some areas in the UK special clinics offering expert counselling have now been established and should receive every encouragement. The voluntary organization called SPOD (Sexual Problems of the Disabled) can offer advice and assistance to the disabled themselves, their partners and families, and also to those who care for the disabled. The address of this organization is supplied at the end of this chapter (p. 376). The general practitioner who wishes to learn more about sexual problems of the disabled and their management is recommended to read Heslinga's (1974) book, *Not made of stone*.

CONCLUSION

General practitioners are in the front line for presentation of most of the sexual difficulties discussed in this chapter. They should be able both to detect and assess patients with sexual difficulties, and provide counselling for at least the most straightforward cases. Teaching of human sexuality in medical schools should provide the necessary background knowledge for such work, but this needs to be supplemented by opportunities through general practice training schemes of experience in managing sexual problems. Most sexual dysfunction clinics can arrange further training for those who wish to improve their counselling skills in this area and some may be able to offer supervision to those who wish to treat their own patients with difficult or complicated sexual problems. Relate offers specific training courses for those wishing to learn how to do therapy. For the patient the most critical moment is when she first hints to her GP that she has a problem, and it is the GP's response which will determine whether she ever discusses this fully and receives appropriate help.

APPENDIX

ASSESSMENT OF A PATIENT WITH A SEXUAL PROBLEM: MAIN POINTS TO BE COVERED

1. *The problem.* Clarify in detail the nature of the sexual problem, its duration, any precipitants, and the way it has developed including any factors that have made it worse and any that have led to improvement.

2. *Partner's response.* What has been the partner's response to the problem? Does he/she have a sexual problem? Are the couple able to discuss the problem, or talk about sex in general?

3. *Family history.* Parents' ages and occupations; nature of their relationship; nature of patient's relationships with both parents and siblings; was sex discussed in the home?—if so, in what context and what impression did this have on the patient? Is there any important family history of physical or psychiatric disorders?

4. *Early development.* Was patient happy during childhood? Did she encounter any problems in developing her sense of femaleness? What age did menarche occur, whether informed beforehand, and what was her reaction. What age did puberty (development of breasts, pubic hair, etc.) occur and what was patient's reaction?

5. *Sexual information.* How did patient acquire her knowledge about sex; does she feel she has adequate knowledge? (One should check on the patient's knowledge about sexuality throughout the interview.)

6. *Early sexual experiences.* Age at which sexual interest developed; masturbation (ask 'when did you find out about masturbation?') and reactions to it if she has masturbated; nature of early relationships with boyfriends including sexual experience; any homosexual interests or behaviour; any traumatic sexual experiences, including sexual abuse or rape?

7. *Current relationship.* Duration; how relationship developed; nature of general relationship, especially interests, friends, communication and friction; nature of sexual relationship; (if married) effect of marriage on sexual and general relationships; effect of pregnancy and childbirth on sexual relationship; relationships with children and attitudes to their sexuality.

8. *Schooling and occupations.*

9. *Religious beliefs.*

10. *Medical history.* Including menstruation, contraception, and medication.

11. *Psychiatric history.* Including medication.

12. *Use of alcohol and drugs.*

13. *Mental state examination.* In particular is the patient suffering from depression or anxiety?

14. *Physical examination and investigations.* If appropriate (e.g. vaginal examination should be carried out, with care, if a woman complains of vaginismus).

15. *Goals of treatment.* What would the patient consider a satisfactory sexual relationship, and what would she like to change in her relationship? (i.e. what might be the aim of treatment?)

USEFUL ADDRESSES

Association of Sexual and Marital Therapists, PO Box 62, Sheffield S10 3TS. Will give advice on sex therapists available in different parts of UK.

London Friend, 86 Caledonian Road, London N1. Tel: 071 837 3337. Monday to Sunday from 7.30 pm–10.00 pm; Monday and Tuesday 2.00 pm–6.00 pm. Women's Helpline: Tel: 071 837 2782. Tuesday and Thursday 7.30 pm–10.00 pm.

SPOD (Sexual Problems of the Disabled), 286 Campden Road, London N7 0BJ. Tel: 071 607 8851. The association to aid the sexual and personal relationships of people with a disability.

Relate (Marriage Guidance), Herbert Gray College, Little Church Street, Rugby, Warwickshire, CV21 3AP. Tel: 0788 573241.

REFERENCES AND FURTHER READING

Bancroft, J. (1989). *Human sexuality and its problems* (2nd edn). Churchill Livingstone, Edinburgh. (Excellent authoritative account of all the major aspects of human sexuality.)

Bancroft, J. and Coles, L. (1976). Three years' experience in a sexual problems clinic. *British Medical Journal,* **i,** 1575–7.

Catalan, J., Hawton, K., and Day, A. (1990). Couples referred to a sexual dysfunction clinic: psychological and physical morbidity. *British Journal of Psychiatry,* **156,** 61–7.

Everstine, D. S. and Everstine, L. (1983). The adult woman victim of rape. In *People in crisis: strategic therapeutic interventions,* pp. 177–200. Brunner/Mazel, New York. (Detailed guidance on the psychological effects of rape and its management.)

Gath, D., Cooper, P., and Day, A. (1982). Hysterectomy and psychiatric disorder: I Levels of psychiatric morbidity before and after hysterectomy. *British Journal of Psychiatry,* **140,** 335–50.

Greengross, W. (1976). *Entitled to love: the sexual and emotional needs of the handicapped.* Mallaby Press and National Marriage Guidance Council, in association with National Fund for Research into Crippling Diseases. (For patients and professionals: sensitive account with more emphasis on emotional and social aspects than on practical details of sex.)

Hawton, K. (1985). *Sex therapy: a practical guide.* Oxford University Press. (A detailed acount of how to help people with sexual problems by sex therapy or counselling.)

Hawton, K. (1989). Sexual dysfunctions. In *Cognitive behaviour therapy for psychiatric problems: a practical guide,* pp. 370–405. Oxford University Press. (Focuses especially on the psychological components of sex therapy.)

Hawton, K. and Catalan, J. (1986). Prognostic factors in sex therapy. *Behaviour Therapy and Research,* **24,** 377–85.

Hawton, K., Catalan, J., Martin, P., *et al.* (1986). Long-term outcome of sex therapy. *Behaviour Therapy and Research,* **24,** 665–75.

Heslinga, K. (1974). *Not made of stone.* Charles Thomas, Springfield, Illinois. (A clinical approach to the management of sexual problems of the disabled.)

Hobbs, M. (1990). Childhood sexual abuse: how can women be helped to overcome its long-term effects? In *Difficulties and dilemmas in the management of psychiatric patients* (ed. K. Hawton and P. Cowen), pp. 183–96. Oxford University Press.

Jehu, D. (1988). *Beyond sexual abuse: therapy with women who were childhood victims.* Wiley, Chichester. (A detailed account of a psychological treatment approach for women experiencing various negative consequences of sexual abuse.)

Kaplan, H. S. (1974). *The new sex therapy*. Ballière Tindall, London. (A detailed account of an eclectic approach to sex therapy, with more attention to emotional aspects than Masters and Johnson provide.)

Lancet (1981). Adverse reactions to bendrofluazide and propranolol for the treatment of mild hypertension. *Lancet*, **ii**, 539–43.

Masters, W. H. and Johnson, V. E. (1966). *Human sexual response*. Little Brown, Boston. (A very detailed account of research concerning physiological and anatomical aspects of sexual response.)

Masters, W. H. and Johnson, V. E. (1970). *Human sexual inadequacy*. Churchill, London. (The original description of intensive sex therapy.)

Mezey, G. C. (1985). Rape—victiminological and psychiatric aspects. *British Journal of Hospital Medicine*, March, 152–8. (A survey of the literature on rape.)

Osborn, M., Hawton, K., and Gath, D. (1988). Sexual dysfunction among middle aged women in the community. *British Medical Journal*, **296**, 959–62.

Royal College of General Practitioners (1974). *Oral contraceptives and health*. Pitman Medical, London.

Schreiner-Engel, P. and Schiavi, R. C. (1986). Lifetime psychopathology in individuals with low sexual desire. *Journal of Nervous Mental Disorders*, **174**, 646–51.

Schreiner-Engel, P., Schiavi, R. C., Vietorisz, D., *et al.* (1987). Diabetes type and female sexuality. *Journal of Psychosomatic Research*, **31**, 23–33.

Sherwin, B. B., Gelfand, M. M., and Brender, W. (1985). Androgens enhance sexual motivation in females: a prospective, crossover study of sex steroid administration in the surgical menopause. *Psychosomatic Medicine*, **47**, 339–51.

Steketee, G. and Foa, E. (1987). Rape victims: post-traumatic stress responses and their treatment. A review of the literature. *Journal of Anxiety Disorders*, **1**, 69–88.

Further reading for patients

Brown, P. and Faulder, C. (1979). *Treat yourself to sex: a guide for good loving*. Penguin, London. (A useful self-help guide for couples who wish to try and overcome their sexual difficulties themselves.)

Castleman, M. (1988). *Making love: a guide to sexual fulfilment for men—and women*. Penguin, London. (A fairly detailed and wide-ranging book on sexual relationships and sexual problems.)

Coope, J. (1984). *The menopause: coping with change*. Pergamon, Oxford.

Delvin, D. (1974). *The book of love*. New English Library, London. (A very useful general book covering many aspects of sexuality and sexual relationships in a pleasantly simple and direct manner.)

Greengross, W. and Greengross, S. (1989). *Living, loving and ageing*. Age Concern, Mitcham. (An easily read, pleasant, and short book.)

Heiman, J. and LoPiccolo, J. (1988). *Becoming orgasmic: a sexual and personal growth program for women*. Piatkus, London. (An excellent self-help book for women with orgasmic problems, but also has a wider focus on female sexuality.)

Kitzinger, S. (1985). *Women's experience of sex*. Penguin, London. (An excellent account of female sexuality and the experience of being a woman, from many angles. Useful for women who may be inhibited, of low self-esteem, or feel they are 'different' from others. Fairly sophisticated.)

Lacroix, N. (1989). *Sensual massage.* Dorling Kindersely, London. (A tasteful practical guide to caressing. A good self-help book and also useful in the context of sex therapy.)

London Rape Crisis Centre (1984). *Sexual violence: the reality for women.* Women's Press, London. (Good practical guide for rape victims.)

Yaffe, M. and Fenwick, E. (1986). *Sexual happiness for men and sexual happiness for women.* Dorling Kindersley, London. (Fairly sophisticated self-help books for more liberal readers. Covers a variety of sexual problems.)

Books on sex education for young people

Claesson, B. H. (1971). *Boy, girl, man, woman.* Penguin, London.

Hemming, J. (1986). *Teenage living and loving.* BMA Publications, Family Doctor Booklets.

Trimmer, E. (1986). *Knowing about sex.* BMA Publications, Family Doctor Booklets. (Questions and answers for teenagers.)

15. Emotional problems

Susanna Graham-Jones

THE RANGE OF EMOTIONAL DISORDERS

It is now well-known that GPs fail to detect and act upon a large proportion of the psychosocial problems of their patients (Goldberg and Blackwell 1970; Blacker and Clare 1987). In some consultations the patient makes a direct 'offer' of a psychological symptom ('It's my nerves, doctor'; or 'I just feel so tired, I feel like crying all the time, nothing gets done around the house'); here the doctor is likely to recognize the psychological agenda. However, doctors tend to ignore more subtle messages about emotional problems. Campion *et al.* (in press) have shown that even when a clear emotional cue is given by the patient, it is frequently ignored by the doctor.

There is not space in this chapter to describe the whole range of emotional and psychiatric disorders. However, an attempt will be made to outline the principles of an appropriate approach for general practice for the most common ones. Increasing availability of training in communication and counselling skills, as well as psychiatry trainee posts, is gradually increasing the repertoire of skills of successive generations of general practitioners; not many psychiatric diagnoses represent 'no-go areas' for adequately trained GPs. As psychiatric admissions to hospital continue to decline in the future, GPs will be expected to help to manage a proportion of major psychiatric illness in the community.

Nevertheless, this chapter is mostly about 'minor psychiatric morbidity', much of which can be classified as anxiety or depression. Other topics such as major affective disorders, including manic-depressive illness, schizophrenia, organic psychoses, and dementia, as seen in general practice, are covered in a parallel volume (Marcus and Murray-Parkes 1989).

Classification of emotional disorders

The general practitioner may not be concerned with the niceties of formal psychiatric diagnosis. Goldberg (1982) made a pragmatic, three-way classification of psychological disorders based on the level of intervention which might be made in the general practice setting. The appropriate focus, in general practice, is usually on the understanding of symptoms in the context of the woman's life, and the formulation of a coping strategy which the woman feels is appropriate. Goldberg's three levels were:

(1) major illness such as psychoses, for which accepted medical treatment, for example with phenothiazines, would be suitable;

(2) psychological distress syndromes not requiring specific treatment, but which might, if detected, be relieved by discussion in a single consultation;

(3) psychological distress syndromes which do call for intervention with psychological, social, or drug treatment.

The main 'syndromes' of psychological morbidity commonly encountered in general practice can be described as follows. Any of these conditions may merge into or coincide with others in individual women; and symptoms can fluctuate in intensity over time.

- *Anxiety*: 'free-floating', phobic, or in the form of panic attacks; these may include feelings of lightheadedness, palpitations, depersonalization, de-realization, poor concentration and memory, and faintness.

- *Depression*: a spectrum ranging from mild frustration, irritability, and feeling 'low' and 'tired all the time' to severe suicidal or retarded depression accompanied by 'biological' symptoms such as lethargy, loss of libido and appetite, and early morning wakening.

- Problems of *dependence*: on alcohol, nicotine, opiates, or benzodiazepines.

- *Adjustment reactions*: following life events at work or in the family, including the effects of job loss, marital breakdown, bereavement reactions, and other important losses which affect the patient and the entire family.

- *Relationship* and *psychosexual* problems: including the aftermath of child sexual abuse and domestic violence; behaviour difficulties in children; anorexia nervosa.

- *Premenstrual tension, dysmenorrhoea, and menopausal symptoms*: when accompanied by significant psychological distress (see below).

- *Parasuicide* (attempted suicide, often by drug and alcohol overdose): often an impulsive action in the context of relationship difficulties. Commoner in young women than in men. Not necessarily accompanied by other symptoms, but carries a significant recurrence rate and risk of successful suicide.

- The many and various 'medical' manifestations of stress and arousal that come under a *'psychosomatic'* heading, such as: tension headaches, migraine, psychogenic chest or back pain, nervous gastritis, dermatitis, 'nervous diarrhoea', irritable bowel or bladder syndromes, exacerbations of asthma, etc.

All the physiological systems of the body react to stress in characteristic ways, and individuals may be helped to recognize a personal set of symptoms which seem to be triggered by stress. These symptoms may precede, and accompany, the development of overtly psychological symptomatology. A general practice study of functional disorders showed, for example, that sufferers from irritable bowel symptoms had scores on the General Health Questionnaire (GHQ) which did not usually reach 'significant psychiatric morbidity' levels, whereas those recognized as having depressive symptoms had high scores on the GHQ, but also scored unexpectedly highly on 'irritable bowel' ratings (Graham-Jones 1983).

The 'periodic syndrome' (also called 'abdominal migraine') in young girls is another example from the gastrointestinal system; the recurrent bouts of abdominal pain (often misdiagnosed as appendicitis if a full history is not taken) often bear some relation to excitement or stresses (such as birthdays or exams).

SEX DIFFERENCES IN SYMPTOMATOLOGY

Social determinants

Women certainly have no monopoly on psychological distress. Several studies confirm that 'when rates of all types of mental disorders are examined, including alcoholism, drug abuse, and sustained patterns of anti-social behaviours in addition to disorders characterized by subjective distress, women and men evidence similar disorder rates' (Dohrenwend and Dohrenwend 1976; Robins *et al.* 1984).

Women do, however, present symptoms of anxiety and depression to general practitioners and to psychiatrists more commonly than do men (Briscoe 1982). Why is this? Schwartz (1991) believes that this disproportionate representation of women in the psychological statistics is not attributable only to 'role stress' (Parry 1987); nor to the necessity for women to play several different roles serially and in parallel (housewife, mother, carer, spouse, factory worker, etc.) as compared to the more limited repertoire of roles generally demanded of men.

It seems likely that when subjected to the same degree of stress or conflict or loss, men and women react in different ways which correspond to the way they have been socialized, or brought up. The socially sanctioned way for women to react to intolerable strains is to carry on with their burdens but to manifest psychological or psychosomatic symptoms which are the unconscious expression of their inability to cope. When these symptoms become too severe for them to carry on normally at home or in work, many women come (via their own advice networks) to expect that their symptoms can be to some extent relieved with help from doctors, health care teams, and medication. Women (and men) vary in their inclination subsequently to take up psychological treatments or counselling. This variation too is likely to be culturally determined to some extent (cf.

trans-Atlantic differences in the acceptability of counselling and psychotherapy).

Brown and Harris (1978) studied women in a London borough and were
able to pick out from their analysis several characteristics of women who
were likely to be vulnerable to depression. These included: death of
mother before the age of 11 years; lack of a confiding, intimate relationship; having more than two children under the age of 14; unemployment;
poor housing and overcrowding. Vulnerable women were more likely than
others to become depressed in response to major life events, disruptions of
relationships, or other losses.

Boys and men are socialized in a different way from women, and this is
reflected in their expectations and behaviour. A minority of men will
follow the above pathway to medical/psychological care. A more typical
scenario for men when the going gets tough is an increase in their alcohol
intake; they may also deal with conflict by 'acting out' in physical ways
which follow well-trodden paths in different communities. The combination of alcohol and domestic violence is a well-known and distressing
example. Men are less likely than women to come to doctors for help, even
if they consciously feel 'stressed'. The 'macho image' does not sanction
such help-seeking; the problem is not perceived as an illness, and doctors
are not therefore sought out as helpers.

These gender differences are of course not absolute. Particularly under
conditions of extreme social stress in deprived inner-city areas, women too
may resort to release of intolerable tension—through violent acts towards
themselves or others, or through alcohol-induced oblivion, other drugs, or
attempted suicide. These women may find it hard to trust anyone to help.
The current emerging awareness of the high but hidden prevalence of
sexual abuse may help health workers to understand the extreme tensions
such people have suffered, and their difficulty in making 'cries for help'
which are acceptable and coherent and which meet the high standards
expected by the medical profession.

Hormonal causes of emotional symptoms

Premenstrual tension, dysmenorrhoea, and pregnancy can be accompanied,
in some women, by emotional distress indistinguishable from manifestations of anxiety and depression described here; and some of this ground is
covered elsewhere in this volume. The relationship between serum hormone
levels and psychological symptomatology is far from clear, as yet, though
postnatal depression seems a likely candidate for a hormonally-triggered
state (O'Hara 1986).

Premenstrual tension (PMT), on the other hand, may incorporate anxiety
or depressive symptomatology which initially fluctuates with the menstrual
cycle. Worsening PMT over several months may merge into a depressive

state which lasts for several months continuously, and may need anti-depressant medication as well as hormonal manipulation (Jacobs and Charles 1970; Watson and Studd 1990). Worsening PMT may also be accompanied by exacerbations of other psychosomatic disorders such as migraine or irritable bowel syndrome.

Oestrogen deficiency at the menopause may well contribute to depressive symptomatology, including irritability and weepiness as well as insomnia; increased use of hormone replacement therapy in general practice may reduce the need for antidepressants in menopausal women.

HOW COMMON ARE EMOTIONAL DISORDERS?

Community studies, using self-report questionnaires to screen the general population for psychiatric symptoms (whether or not they were reported to a doctor) have shown that between 14 and 30 per cent of various populations sampled experienced symptoms in the space of a year. Females report rates twice as high as those for men, and there were also increased rates for older and unemployed patients and those not married (Goldberg and Huxley 1980; Finlay-Jones and Burvill 1978).

A majority of people with new psychological symptoms do go to their GP, but the psychological element is missed in one-third of these cases, according to Goldberg and Huxley (1980). Taken together, emotional disorders of all kinds are detected as significant in up to 40 per cent of consultations in inner-city practices (1985 figures from the National Morbidity Survey attribute 65 million consultations during 1985 to 'neurotic disorders'). Prevalence and detection rates would be expected to be lower in more stable, middle-class areas. Table 15.1 offers a simple method for classifying consultations in practice.

Such apparent-prevalence figures obviously reflect the 'detection threshold' of the doctors concerned, as well as the 'help-seeking threshold' of the patients. Both these factors are culturally determined and may indeed interact. Psychologically-minded doctors will attract patients who see their problems in psychological terms, and vice versa. Women are more likely to experience psychiatric symptoms, and present them to the GP; but given the same symptoms, men are more likely to be referred to hospital. The GP therefore seems to expect to 'absorb' much of the psychiatric symptomatology of women.

SKILLS FOR MANAGING EMOTIONAL DISORDERS

Most vocational training schemes for general practice now explicitly aim to equip trainees with the skills to detect and manage common psychosocial problems.

Table 15.1   *Classifying your consultations*

It is always an interesting exercise to classify a series of consultations in a group practice, using either your own classification of symptoms, or a tally under the headings:

1. physical complaints only
2. purely psychological presentation
3. mixture of psychiatric and physical symptoms
4. other reasons for consultation, e.g. preventive medicine

Doctor's name and sex, and patient's sex and age can also be recorded. Having done this, it is possible to compare and discuss the results for different doctors in the practice. There are many factors which will influence the 'case-mix' described by different partners and trainees; threshold for detection of psychosocial problems is one of them.

Many of the training programmes focus on consultation and interview skills (Neighbour 1987; Pendleton *et al.* 1984); and Gask and McGrath (1989) point out the close relationship between these skills, which are easily learned by GPs and trainees, and the elements of counselling and psychotherapy. The characteristics of the 'good therapist' in the counselling literature (Truax and Carkhuff 1965) are those of genuineness, empathy, and warmth, with a capacity for 'unconditional positive regard'. These characteristics are arguably as important for good general practice as they are for psychotherapists. Doctors can learn to be good listeners, and to respond to the emotional needs of their patients, without letting go of their skills in diagnosing and managing organic disease.

THE FIRST CONSULTATION

There is no 'right way' to conduct a general practice consultation; each one is a private encounter between two individuals and cannot be legislated for. Nevertheless, practitioners can be trained to pay attention to features of the outcome of their own consultations, and thereby to work towards modifications in technique aimed at improvements in perceived outcome. This kind of work can be done in small groups, and video-feedback from consultations recorded on video-camera is an increasingly popular and powerful training tool. Video workshops can focus on specific topics such as 'breaking bad news', or 'difficult patients', or 'detecting depression'; or they can be used simply for random case analysis.

Stott and Davis's 1979 model (see Fig. 15.1) points to the wide-ranging potential of the consultation as an encounter. If all four areas are borne in mind during a consultation, the chances of detecting a psychosocial

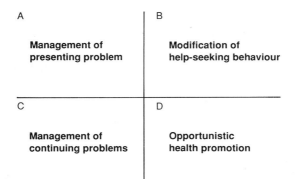

Fig. 15.1 The exceptional potential of the general practice consultation. (From Stott and Davis 1979.)

problem are maximized. Attention to the patient's 'help-seeking be-haviour' and its consequences is particularly helpful in addressing the questions 'Why has the patient come to me for help?' and 'Why has the patient come now?' Consultations which do not clarify these points often feel uncomfortable; the discomfort may be a sign that a significant psycho-social problem remains unexplored.

New methods of analysing the content of consultations should be com-plementary to the standard clinical method as taught in hospital. The chronological sequence of history taking, examination, followed by clari-fication and management, has obvious logic, fits the patient's expecta-tions, and serves its purpose. Indeed, we deviate from it at our peril, no matter what the patient's problem. *History taking*, for example, deserves to be completed before the doctor moves on to physical examination. This ideal is not always achieved; but it is undoubtedly best to have taken a thorough history before management issues are addressed. The 'door-handle' utterance is a classic example of unfinished business. As the patient goes out, she turns around: 'Oh, by the way, doctor, I just thought I'd mention I've been having this pain . . .'

The patient will give and receive clues which are relevant to diagnosis right from the very begining of a consultation; hence the emphasis by GP trainers on eye-contact and attention to non-verbal signals. In contrast to the barrage of direct questions which used to pass for history taking in some hospital clinics, most patients can be trusted to set the agenda themselves, or at least provide significant clues to the main problems, within the first two or three minutes, provided they are not deviated off course by interruptions.

The clues patients offer will of course require expansion. 'You said you weren't sleeping well?'—interpretation: 'Might the rows you're having be part of feeling anxious and irritable?'—and clarification: 'What exactly goes through your mind when you feel really low? . . . have you ever thought about doing away with yourself?' This will be achieved ideally by the doctor's careful use of 'open' questions. Later in the consultation, the doctor may wish to use direct, and sometimes closed, questions to cover important areas like sexual relationships, suicide risk, or alcohol consumption; and occasionally the doctor may need to 'hold the floor' firmly in order to explain a finding or suggest a course of action. Following this, the patient's views should be monitored stage by stage to check her involvement. 'Before we go on, I would like to know what you think about this?' gives a clear signal to the patient that her views matter.

Clinical examination is, at the very least, a 'laying-on of hands' which has great significance to most patients. The baleful complaint, 'The doctor never even examined me', often follows a dysfunctional consultation. Even when the doctor expects no abnormal physical sign, it may be worth fulfilling the patient's hope and going ahead with a physical examination. Tuckett (1985) showed the importance of fully addressing the patient's 'agenda'. The patient's co-operation is vital to the diagnostic and therapeutic process and if the doctor seems dismissive about the patient's symptoms, or her theories about the aetiology, this co-operation may be lost. The patient may appear to agree passively with the doctor's conclusions, but may well be angry and contemptuous, or confused, underneath a passive exterior. She will then be unlikely to comply with a management plan in which her own theories have not been acknowledged.

This is especially important in patients inclined to somatize, that is, to present and emphasize exclusively physical symptoms in contexts where the doctor believes a psychological problem is at the root of the trouble. The correct goal of the doctor may well be the re-attribution of the symptoms to a 'psychogenic' category, rather than further emphasis on detailed physical investigation of a symptom; but the proper examination of the 'affected part' should not be neglected. Indeed the normal findings, and explanation of them, may help to reinforce the 'non-organic' diagnosis, and the confidence of the patient in her doctor.

After history and examination there should be time for the *clarification* of findings and *diagnosis*. Modern consultation technique emphasizes the exploration of the patient's view of the aetiological factors and diagnosis, as well as the doctor's view. It is often helpful to point out to patients puzzled by their symptoms that the pain threshold, and indeed any perceptual threshold, may be lowered by tension or unhappiness. People in distress are therefore likely to have more sensations which reach the level of significant symptoms than other people; they are, so to speak, receiving 'bodily messages' about their mental state. Some anxiety- or stress-management groups use this interpretation to help patients consider lifestyle changes as a means of tackling the underlying problem as well as the symptoms.

Skilled negotiation is often required before a diagnosis is accepted, especially in psychosomatic disorders. The difficulty may lie in the patient's use of a physical-illness explanation as an unconscious defence against the emergence of distressing anxiety (Bloch 1979). It may take some time and trouble before the patient perceives this for herself; 'chronic somatizers' may never reach this point (see 'Difficult patients', p. 399).

The need for negotiating may be new to hospital doctors who are used to patients playing a passive role in the diagnostic process. Other professions incorporate training in negotiating skills as a matter of course; it remains to be seen whether this will happen in medical education too.

PLANNING THE FOLLOW-UP CARE OF THE PATIENT

Make a management plan at the end of the first interview

If an emotionally-laden consultation has had to be squeezed into an ordinary 5- or 10-minute appointment, the management plan at this point may simply take the form of a formal acknowledgement of the patient's distress, a very brief summary of what has been revealed, and the assurance of a proper and prompt response by the doctor. A further appointment with the same doctor will usually be required, and should be offered sooner rather than later. This will emphasize the doctor's commitment to 'getting to the bottom of the problem'. Although an inexperienced doctor may feel confused and unconfident at this point, being unsure what she or he has to offer, the patient is likely to feel both unburdened and supported.

Don't rush into referrals

Unless there is clear evidence of an immediate need for inpatient care, questions of referral and indeed investigation can often be best dealt with at a subsequent, planned consultation. A short interval allows the interested doctor to digest the new information and perhaps ask advice from colleagues; and the patient needs time to pursue whatever avenue seems appropriate in the new patient–therapist relationship she has initiated. To announce, after a first encounter with a new patient who may have had to screw up her courage to reveal significant emotional problems, that the problem requires referral to a specialist is, in a sense, a rejection of the therapist role. The patient may not feel able to start all over again with someone else. Furthermore, although the doctor may lack self-confidence about the skilled management of a distressing problem, it is worth bearing in mind that the patient has by the end of the first interview exercised a choice to reveal this significant information, and is likely to be experiencing some new hope in relation to the investment made. This hope will be reinforced by the offer of further time with the same doctor in a few days. If possible, sufficient time should be allowed for in the second appointment; perhaps 20 or 30 minutes. Referral may indeed be valuable and provide further hope when more is known and shared about the extent of the problem.

Follow-up appointments with the general practitioner

Some patients do not, of course, come back. When a patient does attend for a follow-up appointment, her thoughts since the first consultation are of great importance. She should be given time to air them before the doctor proceeds with further plans. The patient may demonstrate an increase or a decrease in symptoms; she may have been consciously preoccupied with the problem as described in the first interview; she may have reformulated or 'buried' it; or she may be feeling a lot better.

Her motivation is a key factor at this stage. Missed appointments may testify to patients' misgivings about having revealed too much about themselves too early. Many doctors will leave it up to the patient to re-book a further appointment if so wished; sometimes, on the other hand, it feels appropriate to send an invitation for a further appointment.

Consider the family background

The first interview is unlikely to have included a full family history, and this can be covered at a second or subsequent consultation, or on a home visit. Various methods can be used to help a patient to focus on the relevant parts of a complex family tree. Depending on the history, themes such as sibling rivalry, parenting, or reactions to losses or deaths in the family could be explored. Another tool, which is quicker and easier to use than the full family tree, is the family circle. Figure 15.2 shows a 24-year-old's feeling of distance from her parents. She became quite upset explaining how her younger sister was, in contrast, very close to her mother. This family circle was used as a tool to explore a repetitive pattern of under-achievement: she was a graduate but had only ever worked in unskilled, low-paid jobs. Her presenting symptom had been a feeling of lethargy and tearfulness 'for no reason'. She returned, as planned, two weeks after drawing the family circle, saying that she had been 'in a daze' after thinking about it all day: 'It really made me think!' She was subsequently offered counselling to help unravel her personal problems with relationships and work situations. Drawing the 'family circle' seemed to have unlocked her motivation to take herself seriously. It also spared her from undertaking a conventional but usually unhelpful series of investigations 'to exclude

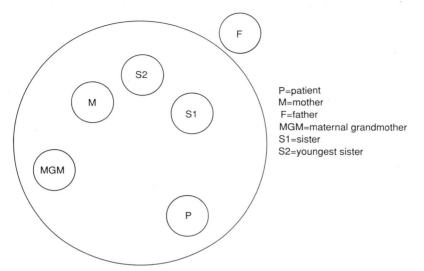

Fig. 15.2 Family circle. (From Nelki, personal communication.)

organic causes' for her malaise. She continues to have symptoms, but regards them now as part of the 'pleasure and pain' of therapy.

Other investigations

Before considering therapeutic options more thoroughly, there are some further investigations which may be worth pursuing.

Investigations of psychological morbidity, in the form of standardized questionnaires, may be useful

Although not routinely used in general practice, there are a number of questionnaires which have been validated for use by patients in general practice settings. Goldberg and colleagues have used various versions of the well-known 'General Health Questionnaire', which has been validated against a standardized Present State Examination to look at the detection of minor psychiatric morbidity in general practice (see Fig. 15.3). The Beck Depression Inventory and other well-established research instruments (see Wilkinson 1986) can be used for screening, to detect unmet need for care; for assessment of individuals before and after treatment, using the initial score as a baseline against which to measure change over time; or as a one-off measure of severity or risk, to help to target scarce resources appropriately.

Psychometric methods will presumably develop under academic roofs initially; but psychosocial aspects of chronic or recurrent disease monitoring

Anxiety scale
(*Score one point for each 'Yes'*)
1. Have you felt keyed up, on edge?
2. Have you been worrying a lot?
3. Have you been irritable?
4. Have you had difficulty relaxing?

(*If 'yes' to two of the above, go on to ask*)
5. Have you been sleeping poorly?
6. Have you had headaches or neck aches?
7. Have you had any of the following: trembling, tingling, dizzy spells, sweating, frequency, diarrhoea?

Depression scale
(*Score one point for each 'Yes'*)
1. Have you had low energy?
2. Have you had loss of interests?
3. Have you lost confidence in yourself?
4. Have you felt hopeless?

(*If 'Yes' to ANY question, go on to ask*)
5. Have you had difficulty concentrating?
6. Have you lost weight (due to poor appetite)?
7. Have you been waking up early?
8. Have you felt slowed up?
9. Have you felt worse in the mornings?

Interpretation:
Add anxiety score, add depression score. Patients with anxiety scores of five or depression scores of two have a 50% chance of having a clinically important disturbance; above these scores the probability rises sharply.

Fig. 15.3   Short version of the General Health Questionnaire.

are of increasing interest in routine assessment of outcome, to inform decisions about allocation of resources. Indicators of psychosocial functioning will need to be set alongside other clinical indicators and instruments for medical audit, in general practice as elsewhere.

Laboratory investigations

Laboratory investigations may be needed to aid differential diagnosis. Thyroid function tests can be used to exclude myxoedema or hyperthyroidism in women with lethargy and depression on the one hand, or overactivity, palpitations, and tension on the other. A full blood count will detect anaemia as a cause for fatigue; blood levels of some anticonvulsants are worth knowing in case of behavioural side-effects in people with epilepsy; screening of urine for opiates and other street drugs is useful for monitoring compliance of dependent drug users.

Consider non-drug treatments

Patients who can see the connection between their symptoms and anxiety or stress may be able to use direct advice about stress reduction, exercise or relaxation routines, and lifestyle changes such as cutting down tea and coffee (which exacerbate tension symptoms such as heartburn, diarrhoea, and tremor). If they feel able to embark on a self-help routine straight-away, so much the better. Relaxation audio-tapes and stress-management booklets are available commercially, can be distributed by staff in the health centre, and can help patients motivated enough to use them regularly.

If the patient herself expresses a desire to work through the problem, or 'to sort myself out', then the GP may consider offering a limited number of sessions to explore the problem, thus initiating the counselling process. In preparation for this, the patient may be asked to write something about her problem and to state some aims of the work for herself. If she can be helped to explore the problem, relax enough to set feasible goals, and work in a step-by-step way towards them, her self-esteem will rise and she may shortly start to feel better and be less tense or depressed. The GP will be able to treat a few patients in this way, booking long appointments or setting aside separate sessions for this kind of work. Other patients will be referred elsewhere for counselling or therapy (see below).

Consider advantages and disadvantages of medication

See section on psychotropic drugs below.

REFERRALS: THE NETWORKING ROLE OF THE GP

The general practitioner has access to a network of statutory, voluntary, hospital-based, and private-sector agencies with expertise in handling psychosocial problems. It takes time to build up knowledge of the resources available and personal relationships with the agencies; this 'networking' aspect varies enormously between practices and between individual GPs. A GP who is aware of all that is going on locally in the mental health field will have a wide range of options to offer an individual patient (e.g. family therapy, psychosexual counselling, tranquillizer withdrawal groups, day centre provision). Conversely, a GP who is not aware of specialist resources may leave needy patients feeling dissatisfied, or even guilty about 'having bothered the doctor'.

Referral decisions are complex. Table 15.2 shows some of the factors which affect the decision as to whether to refer.

Table 15.2   *Factors affecting referral decisions*

- the nature of the problem (symptoms, diagnosis)
- positive or negative attitude of patient to referral, and underlying reasons
- knowledge of patient's previous history, access to family support, previous uptake or non-uptake of referral offers, etc.
- GP's awareness of local resources appropriate to the problem, community groups, self-help groups, etc., as well as NHS resources
- urgency of the problem, crises foreseen
- GP's awareness of waiting times for different agencies
- GP's confidence and time available for handling the problem without referral.

The *purpose* of a referral should be made clear to both specialist and patient. It is helpful to review both referral letters and discharge or out-patient clinic letters to check whether clear requests have been made and responded to. The quality of these communications varies widely at present. In general, the maximum benefit for patients will derive from a rapid referral for a straightforward problem for which a reliable treatment is known to be available. The more common reasons for referring to a specialist (e.g. a psychiatrist) are shown in Table 15.3.

Except in the case of emergency admissions, there will be a significant delay before the specialist sees the patient, which may be a matter of months. The GP's management plan must therefore include a strategy for this 'holding' period, and must take account of the possibility that the specialist may not feel that she or he can contribute usefully, in which case the patient will be returned to GP care after a single assessment interview. (Referrals to other mental health professionals within the NHS are discussed under 'Community Mental Health Teams', page 396.) Many emotional crises are followed by rapid resolution, so a referral at a time of crisis may turn out later to be unnecessary. Unfortunately it is still difficult to predict which patients will rapidly recover spontaneously.

Referral, especially in situations of urgency, can be extremely time-consuming, involving telephone calls, letters, and suspense for both doctor and patient. A practice folder containing details not only of addresses, telephone numbers, and contact people at local agencies, but also response times and outcomes, is useful and time-saving. Different practices have evolved their own mechanisms for expediting referrals, and some of the different possibilities are outlined below.

As emotional problems gain increasing recognition in both lay and professional domains, networking and communication between different agencies concerned with mental health become ever more important for the GP and the practice as a whole. Ideally the 'resources folder' would be

Table 15.3 *Purposes of referral to a hospital specialist*

- to make a firm diagnosis
- to learn more about the condition from the specialist
- to obtain treatment or advice which is not available in general practice because of lack of skills, personnel, or other resources
- at patient's request, for a second opinion
- for reassurance of doctor or patient
- to obtain alternative treatment if the GP's first-line treatment has been unsuccessful
- to gain access to hospital facilities: occupational therapy, nursing staff, clinical psychologists
- to provide respite for the doctor in a difficult situation
- to obtain emergency admission to hospital if the patient is severely ill and either a danger to themselves or to others; this could be a voluntary admission, or more rarely admission under one of the sections of the Mental Health Act.

shared by GPs, practice nurses, counsellors, social workers, and health visitors as well as reception and administrative staff. Comments might also be added by patients who have used the resources.

COMMUNITY RESOURCES

A list of some of the groups which may be active in the community can be found in Table 15.4. Others are referred to in the chapters on alcohol, psychosexual problems, and other relevant topics. Community and voluntary resources are being used more and more as waiting lists lengthen for hospital and district health authority care.

Voluntary agencies may be contracted by local health authorities or social services departments to provide certain services to a particular area or group of patients. Self-help groups in the voluntary and the statutory sector may provide first aid and continuing care to some patients. Above all, they can reduce the sense of isolation which many patients suffer.

Many patients will initially have an understandable reluctance to joining a group, and if a first interview can be arranged on a one-to-one basis this may help. Group functioning obviously depends on the members of a group, and from time to time social workers or GPs will hear of a group which is going through a bad patch, and will be reluctant to make referrals to such a group. One resource for checking such rumours, or asking about

Table 15.4   *Community resources (examples)*

Age Concern support and befriending for the elderly

Alcoholics Anonymous

British Association For Counselling can provide list of local affiliated counsellors with recognized training

Citizens Advice Bureau trained volunteers backed up by information resources

Community volunteer services (may have directory of local resources)

Council for Involuntary Tranquilliser Addiction. Also *Tranx* groups

CRUSE support groups and individual help for the bereaved

Depressives Anonymous self-help for depressed patients

Gingerbread support for single-parent families

MENCAP help for people with learning disorders

MIND support and information for people with mental illness (National Association for Mental Health)

Rape Crisis support for women who have been sexually abused

RELATE (previously known as Marriage Guidance Council) for relationship and psychosexual problems (*not* just for married couples)

SAFE for victims of sexual abuse

Samaritans Samaritans and Nightline, telephone help lines

SANDS (Stillbirth and Neonatal Death Society), support for bereaved parents

Schizophrenia Fellowship for patients and families

Victim support groups (inner cities)

---

such community resources, might be the local social services district office, or a social worker specializing in mental health work.

REFERRALS WITHIN THE PRACTICE TEAM

Practices which employ or have definite 'attached' relationships with counsellors, social workers, community psychiatric nurses, or psychologists have made a decision to share the psychosocial workload with a group of other professionals. Other practices may have regular visits from psychiatrists or other members of the district Community Mental Health Team.

Such 'liaison' arrangements have generally implied that the referrer expects the specialist professional to make an assessment and then probably see a patient for a number of consultations, in much the same way as would have occurred in the context of an outpatient referral to a hospital. Feedback may be rather informal and minimal in the context of the patient being seen under the same roof with the same notes set available to all parties; or it may be in the form of a letter. These 'shifted outpatients' arrangements, while providing easy access to some forms of specialist care for a few patients, are easily overtaken by demand, and the waiting list for a practice counsellor may not be any shorter than that for an outpatient psychiatry appointment, for example.

A different 'skill-sharing' model is being explored by some practices and local teams, with the aim of using the specialists who come into the practice as teachers and facilitators for the practice team, rather than as outsiders who have minimal input into the activities of the team members (Mitchell 1985; Wilson and Wilson 1985). Thus, a visiting psychologist or psychiatrist might come to the practice on a regular basis, but instead of running her own consulting session in parallel with the GPs, the main activity would be a group meeting of GPs and health visitors to discuss, and possibly interview, one or more families with particular problems. The outcome would be a management plan which the practice team would try to implement, with support from the specialist as necessary, and an increase in the confidence of the individuals in the team in dealing with similar problems. The specialist might never see the family discussed; s/he would certainly not 'take over' their care.

Similarly, counsellors, psychologists, community psychiatric nurses, and social workers may be invited to work with groups of staff to develop the skills of the group members as well as doing work with individual patients or groups of patients.

Given the framework of general practice and the recurring need for expertise in managing complex psychosocial situations, the 'skill-sharing' model clearly has a lot to offer. As the practice team acquires expertise, referrals for 'expert advice' might be expected to decline. Practitioners' job satisfaction and health centre services to patients might improve. However, the skill-sharing model requires commitment to group meetings, and ideally commitment to practising new skills with patients in surgery and to evaluating the results. Time for these new activities must be found, and this is the major constraint for most practices. Many practices continue to run a mixture of conventional referral patterns and skill-sharing attempts, but cannot expect to reduce their referral rates once the available counselling hours are filled. There is as yet only equivocal evidence to suggest that consultation rates or other indices of workload are reduced by such attempts to provide for the psychological needs of patients (Trepka and Griffiths 1987). On the contrary; queues may increase wherever support is to be found.

Stress management within the practice

Practices aware of a high burden of psychosocial ills must organize to cope with a potentially ever-increasing workload. This means that stress among staff needs to be anticipated. This is predictably more of a problem in inner-city deprived areas than in rural areas and market towns. Indicators of stress, such as staff time off sick, or the frequency of confrontations between patients and reception staff, may be worth monitoring. Some practices run 'away-days' for team members in work time, sometimes facilitated by outsiders, to help the team to put their work in perspective and prevent them from being overwhelmed by such 'front-line' work. All members of a practice team will benefit from having a clear job description, and from involvement in setting goals and objectives for the work of the team. Other practices use an attached psychologist to help the health team function as well as possible.

These strategies are well established in industrial and other professional settings. Health professionals have been slow to undertake self-care and to practise what they preach.

REFERRALS OUTSIDE THE PRACTICE TEAM

Which problems should be referred as priority cases?

In general, the advantages of early referral in psychological medicine are those of damage-limitation. Suicidal patients may need psychiatric referral for immediate care and/or admission which may be life-saving; but it is also true that the success rate for treatment of (for example) phobic states by clinical psychologists or community psychiatric nurses is highest if treatment is initiated promptly when symptoms are of recent onset and mild degree. People left untreated are rather more likely to progress to having chronic disabilities and sometimes to the stigmatized status of a 'difficult patient' (see below).

Counselling and psychotherapy outcome studies have also shown that symptoms of recent onset are the easiest to resolve through treatment. Clearly, the sooner a problem is tackled definitively and with confidence, the better. Life-threatening emergencies will naturally take priority; other distinctions will be much more difficult to argue. Priorities for scarce resources will continue to have to be determined by service providers at health district level, by practice teams, and by patients too.

Referral to Community Mental Health Teams

General practitioners are increasingly being asked to refer patients to multidisciplinary Community Mental Health Teams (CMHT) serving a defined area within a health district. On intake, referrals may be allocated directly to different professionals working within the team as key-workers.

This avoids the bottleneck of the uniform waiting list for psychiatry out-patient clinics.

GPs will need to keep themselves informed about the work of these teams, and may then be able to influence the treatment of their patients through explicit requests in the referral letter. Referral letters which do not make the reason for referral clear, nor state an objective for the referral (see above), are very difficult for the specialist team to respond to. The patient may gain little benefit from an unfocused long assessment interview with a stranger; she might in fact gain much more from spending this amount of time with her own GP (Balint 1957).

The CMHT will include psychiatrists, clinical psychologists, occupational therapists, social workers with specialist experience in mental health, and community psychiatric nurses. It may operate from a base in a hospital or from a Community Mental Health Centre, and may include day-care provision or even drop-in facilities. There may be group therapy with behavioural or interpretive techniques, social skills, and occupational therapy, as well as individual casework with patients. There may be considerable overlap between the roles of the different professionals, who may act as 'key-workers' for patients with widely differing problems.

Referrals for psychotherapy

Much of what is offered by general psychiatrists and the CMHT amounts to supportive, and sometimes psychodynamic, psychotherapy. However, specialist psychotherapy services for individuals and groups have now been set up in a number of centres; they were previously almost unknown outside London. These services may be separate from the CMHT (and may therefore require separate referrals). Referral to scarce NHS psychotherapy resources may involve intensive individual assessment of patients: GPs should be prepared to deal with feelings of rejection in patients who are refused therapy. Criteria for acceptance of patients for individual or group psychotherapy vary, but may include evidence of motivation and real potential for understanding long-established relationship problems and for changing severely disturbed behaviour patterns.

ARE WOMEN'S NEEDS BEING MET?

Attempts are being made, in the new NHS, to make closer links between consumer needs and service provision. For example, resources are being mobilized to cut waiting times for out-patient appointments. Long waits have always been a bugbear of the NHS and not enough priority has been given to this important aspect of care.

It remains to be seen, however, whether factors which are particularly important to women patients can be better acknowledged in the new provisions in the health service. For example, women are more likely than men to express a preference for a female or male therapist, and with good reason (Meeuwesen *et al.* 1991). They may also be very anxious about disclosure of important but sensitive material such as a history of childhood sexual abuse or a drink problem, so they may need reassurance about confidentiality, and they may take longer to 'engage' in therapy than men. Ashurst and Hall (1989) have reviewed 'the special ingredients of women's distress'.

Feminist psychotherapy has developed from a sense that classical psychoanalysis and the post-Freudian and counselling traditions of male-dominated societies often miss, or distort, the conscious and unconscious material brought by women patients (Chesler 1972). Women mental health workers and doctors have expressed discomfort about having to collude in the 'normalization' of women who, through their psychiatric symptoms, seem to be rebelling against oppression in their family or work situation (Women in Medicine 1991).

Feminist therapists working both alongside and separately from established psychotherapeutic practice, are attempting to offer women more choice. For example, a woman may be helped in therapy to reinterpret her individual struggle to develop as a daughter, as a woman in a patriarchal society, and as a mother, through understanding that 'mothering is not simply an individual relationship, it is a social institution' (Eichenbaum and Orbach 1985). The Women's Therapy Centre in London is one such group which offers individual and group therapy and also runs a series of weekend workshops which introduce women to the scope of feminist thought and therapy (Ernst and Maguire 1987).

Clearly, national health service facilities can offer only a limited range of psychotherapeutic options for women at present. Not all health authorities have departments of psychotherapy. But there are other, and very pragmatic, requirements to be met before women can be said to have equal access to NHS facilities. Women with young children, at high risk for depression, may have great difficulty making time to attend for appointments unless childcare is available in hospitals and community clinics. Crèches are still few and far between.

Service provision is being monitored in such a way as to provide accessible data on, for example, waiting times. GPs as 'purchasers' of services will have opportunities to press for appropriate services, and will need to be well informed on what is offered by different teams. The changes in the health service will encourage the evaluation and audit of different methods of treatment in general practice settings as well as in specialist services. These are not easy tasks and there are few satisfactory studies of a definitive nature so far (see Trepka and Griffiths (1987) and Wilkinson (1986) for reviews of therapeutic outcomes); but information gathering is improving and audit is welcomed as a challenge in some centres.

'DIFFICULT PATIENTS': THE NON-RESPONDERS

Approximately one-third of patients referred for psychiatric care make no progress and return, dissatisfied, to the GP. Psychological and somatic symptomatology ('somatic fixation') may result in successive demands for referral; the patient appears contemptuous of what medicine has to offer, and yet demands more.

Ungrateful patients get short shrift at many interfaces with health and welfare services. They can usually continue to get access to a GP, however. If we accept that there are no easy answers for these patients, we can as GPs acknowledge the challenge they provide, and look further into the problem. Using the Stott and Davis (1979) framework (Fig. 15.1), it is the *help-seeking behaviour* which may provide a useful starting point, since it is precisely this which is the issue for the GP. The patient behaves 'unreasonably', in a 'juvenile' manner, even a 'babyish' manner, complete with metaphorical tantrums, as if she has rights over the doctor's time which other patients do not. It may be useful to consider the origins of these behaviours, along with the resulting negative feelings generated in the doctor. This is the kind of work often done in Balint groups, and in seminars which focus on the 'difficult patient'.

The patient's unreasonable and demanding behaviour may be an unconscious cry for help, which the doctor tries to respond to; but the nature of the message is unclear, and the doctor–patient relationship gets 'stuck', with anger and frustration predominant on both sides. In psychodynamic terms, the patient's problems are manifested in the 'transference' with the doctor. In 'consultation analysis' terms, there will be signs of a problematic doctor–patient relationship.

Outsiders attuned to such behaviour patterns may be able to help the doctor to understand some of the messages which the patient is trying to convey. The infantile behaviour may be a sign that the patient's emotional development may have been stunted because of some long-standing deprivation. Perhaps it will be necessary to re-examine the history for anything which suggests this?

Further, is there anything to explain the onset of the unreasonable behaviour in the context of the doctor–patient relationship; for example, has there been a bereavement or other event which has destabilized an already precarious emotional life? The doctor may need the group's help to work out a new management plan which will use these insights. The result will not always be a transformation of the patient's life; but many doctors can attest to the value of such work in demystifying unsatisfactory consultations (Balint 1957; RCGP 1988; Elden and Samuel 1987).

PSYCHOTROPIC DRUGS IN GENERAL PRACTICE

Hard lessons have been learned from the excessive prescribing of barbiturates in the 1950s and then benzodiazepines in the 1970s to patients in search of a 'magic bullet' cure for distress (£38 million was spent in the UK on anxiolytics and antidepressants in 1985). Large numbers of women have become addicted to these drugs and many have had extreme difficulty in withdrawing successfully from them. As with patients institutionalized for years in mental hospitals, their iatrogenic suffering has been acknowledged by the medical profession, but they are still living with the consequences (Priest and Montgomery 1988).

The therapeutic window of these tranquillizing drugs seems to be narrow, as is that of the tricyclic antidepressants. Many well-informed patients are therefore very wary of all psychotropic medication. Others still see medication or 'a tonic' as a much-desired escape from the predicament in which they find themselves, and resent the relative unwillingness of general practitioners to prescribe pills for depression, insomnia, and anxiety. The danger of dependence in the future is a relatively weak deterrent to someone who wants immediate relief from disabling and frightening symptoms; and although some practices have started successful programmes to wean long-term tranquillizer patients off all or most of their medication, this often requires several months of one-to-one or group work. Skilled GPs can successfully manage many patients without prescribing tranquillizers (Catalan and Gath 1985).

The common uses of psychotropic drugs in general practice are outlined below:

- *Hypnotics*: (sleeping tablets) There is still a high level of demand for the benzodiazepines. When a prescription is deemed necessary, temazepam 10–20 mg is an effective short-term hypnotic. It can safely be used for crises when night sedation is needed. Its use should be restricted to 5–7 consecutive nights if possible, as longer courses will result in a degree of dependence. People who have become dependent on nitrazepam can be changed over to temazepam without much trouble once the patient is motivated.

  However, temazepam is much sought after by street drug-users and it is sold on the black market. The drug is often prepared for intravenous injection from capsules and tablets and even from the syrup. Chloral hydrate 500 mg is another effective hypnotic and may be of help as an alternative to benzodiazepines. Barbiturates are best avoided, both because of the dangers of tolerance and dependence, and because they are dangerous in overdose.

- *Minor tranquillizers*: Despite the problems of addiction, there is still a role for occasional new prescriptions of a benzodiazepine for stress reactions, fuelled by requests from those who have previously had benzodiazepines. However, a further problem which may arise is an *increase* in aggressive and impulsive behaviour (probably mediated by an alcohol-like behavioural disinhibition). This is a risk in many patients and families, and may increase the risk of suicidal behaviours.

Diazepam is a commonly used benzodiazepine, the dose range being 2–30 mg per day. Advice to women withdrawing from other benzodiazepines (such as the now notorious lorazepam) may include a change to diazepam in equivalent doses (see Fig. 15.4) prior to cutting down. The longer half-life of diazepam should provide for a smoother withdrawal.

Alternatives to benzodiazepines include other hypnotics (see above) where indicated; antidepressants, many of which have equal anxiolytic effect; and beta-blockers (atenolol, propranolol) which can effectively control peripheral signs of arousal and thereby alleviate distress.

- *Antipsychotic drugs*: mostly phenothiazines (chlorpromazine, trifluoperazine, flupenthixol, etc.) which control 'voices' and other symptoms of thought disorder, and have brought about the change to largely outpatient treatment for schizophrenic patients. General practitioners will occasionally need to start phenothiazine treatment for acutely psychotic patients. It is also worth bearing in mind the anxiolytic effect of, say, flupenthixol or trifluoperazine as a substitute for benzodiazepines in patients with severe anxiety. Most of the phenothiazines are sedative. The need for additional anticholinergic medication to control extrapyramidal side-effects varies widely between individuals.

- *Drugs to alleviate withdrawal symptoms*: nowadays chlodiazepoxide and diazepam are preferred to chlormethiazole for alcohol withdrawal (if drug substitution is really necessary). Methadone mixture is used for detoxification or maintenance in opiate addiction. Clonidine is occasionally used for these purposes and by people trying to give up smoking.

Since chlormethiazole, the benzodiazepines, and methadone mixture

Other benzodiazepines		Diazepam
Lorazepam	1 mg =	10 mg
Temazepam	1 mg =	1 mg
Nitrazepam	1 mg =	2 mg
Oxazepam	1 mg =	1 mg
Chlordiazepoxide	1 mg =	1 mg
Triazolam	1 mg =	20 mg
Loprazolam	1 mg =	10 mg
Lormetazepam	1 mg =	10 mg

Fig. 15.4 Equivalent doses of benzodiazepines.

all induce dependence, and since clonidine causes a rebound increase in blood pressure when stopped suddenly, none of these are ideal treatments. Benzodiazepines such as diazepam may therefore be chosen as the 'best of a bad lot'. Individual management plans are needed in all cases, and should be clearly recorded in the notes for the benefit of other doctors who may see the patient. (See also chapter on drink problems, p. 448.)

- *Antidepressants*: Major depression is disabling and carries a real risk of suicide. Tricyclic antidepressants (TCA) have proved their worth, despite their slow onset of action. Drugs such as imipramine and amitryptiline have some disabling anticholinergic side-effects such as dry mouth, blurring of vision, sedation, and urinary retention, and they are dangerous in overdose. This has led to poor compliance despite the convenient single-evening-dose regime (two-thirds of patients in one study had stopped taking them within a month (Johnson 1981)) and reluctance to prescribe full doses. Dothiepin, also commonly used, is often prescribed at doses of less than 75 mg daily, which may be 'sub-therapeutic'. It is possible that the placebo and sedative effects are then as important as the anti-depressant effect.

  The implication is that patients prescribed tricyclics need careful and intensive supervision and support through the several weeks before the therapeutic benefit is apparent. The dose should be gradually increased in the expectation that higher doses are more effective, and patients should be encouraged to continue treatment for at least four months *after remission* of depressive symptoms. The distinction between benzodiazepines, where short-term or intermittent treatment is advisable, and antidepressants which are best continued for six months, must be made clear to the patient.

- *Newer antidepressant drugs*: 5-hydroxytryptamine uptake inhibitors such as fluvoxamine and fluoxetine are reported to have fewer side-effects, less sedation, and less toxicity than the older tricyclics (Montgomery 1990). In terms of efficacy and delay in therapeutic effect, however, they are similar to the older TCAs. These 5-HT uptake inhibitors are also being used for obsessive-compulsive disorders.

- *Monamine oxidase inibitors*: Tranylcypromine, phenelzine, and isocarboxacid, and a new selective MAOI, moclobemide, may be useful in treating brief recurrent depression and patients with a mixed picture of depression and anxiety. They may also be useful for women with migraine, premenstrual tension, and irritable bowel. The fears of hypertensive crises induced by a combination of MAOIs and amine-rich food and wine have been exaggerated, and have prevented wider exploration of the role of MAOIs.

Practice formularies

It is not difficult to draw up a practice formulary for those psychotropic drugs considered essential for the practice. This would need revision every year or two, but it would include two or three drugs in each of the above categories, and could also give guide-lines about drugs which the practice had decided to avoid, or to use only in exceptional circumstances. GPs treating large numbers of people with psychological problems are obvious targets for advertising and pressure from the pharmaceutical industry as well as from patients. It is important to weigh the risks and benefits of new drugs very carefully, and many practices are content with a 'wait and see' policy on new products, and to let others experiment with new drugs until their limitations are exposed.

Using a formulary might reduce the number of different drugs in use. PACT data could be used as a next step, to generate feedback for the practice about prescribing patterns. This information can be set alongside morbidity data and whatever information is routinely collected about each doctor's workload and visits for audit purposes.

A written practice policy is particularly useful for doctors who are being pressured to prescribe. Many doctors have experienced unpleasant confrontations with patients demanding a particular drug which they have been given by a previous doctor. Patients who are made aware of a practice policy on, say, sleeping tablets or appetite suppressants, will realize that 'shopping around the practice' is unlikely to result in a prescription for the medication they have already been refused by one partner. Such a situation calls for careful management if the doctor–patient relationship is to remain a therapeutic alliance. The patient needs to know that her frustration is understood. She may need to rehearse an elaborate series of arguments before 'letting go' of her attachment to the idea of the particular prescription. It is important to understand fully what the much-valued drug represents for this patient. Once this is clear, the focus can often be shifted, with the aim of achieving the patient's goals by other means.

Helping drug-dependent women

Patients using opiates may present as 'demanding' patients (although many addicts keep their drug habit entirely secret from their GP for years). Often the request is for 'something to help me come off', i.e. the patient is asking for a detoxification withdrawal. This may not always be the real intention, but it is an understandable ploy; requests for methadone maintenance as such are often refused outright by GPs who are anxious about 'getting involved with addicts'. Illicit drug-users can occasionally get very upset if their demands are not met. They may be very frightened of the insomnia and shakes, diarrhoea, dry mouth, and irritability which may occur during opiate withdrawal. GPs who are regularly treating a few drug-users from among their practice lists report that this type of aggressive reaction is rare, if a contract has been worked out and agreed with the patients. These patients are those who would rather accept dependency on the GP than the uncertain lifestyle of relying on street drugs. From the family health point of view, it is to be hoped that more GPs will consider treatment of drug-using mothers as a priority, involving health visitors to help provide stability in these homes.

Just as with other patients, doctors need to know their drug-using patients as people, before classifying them as addicts with no future. It is probably unwise to prescribe opiates at all to patients not registered with the practice. For a new patient, the outcome of the first consultation need not include a prescription; indeed the necessity for informing the Home Office Drugs Unit may preclude the possibility of a prescription at this stage. Instead the time can be used to assess the patient's background and general health needs, which may have been neglected; the patient, however, may take some time to trust the GP and reveal the full extent of her difficulties. It is worth remembering that pregnant opiate-users and prostitutes will be priority groups for specialist workers in drug dependency, partly because of the danger of HIV infection. Others may have to wait to be seen at specialist clinics and may rely on GPs or have to resort to street drugs. Guidelines for helping illicit drug-users are available from drug dependency clinics and from the Home Office.

CONCLUSION

I hope I have shown that it is possible to work at a number of different levels in general practice. Doctors may take different approaches with different patients who present with superficially similar problems. Women suffering from depression and concerned about their weight, for example: should endocrine disorders be excluded before any other help is offered? Might they be helped most with a step-by-step behavioural programme to aid their self-control and self-esteem? Or do they have 'controlling mothers' lurking in the background who need to be dealt with in psychotherapy before the patient can stop eating? These approaches all seem to require quite different behaviour on the part of the doctor. All of them require exploration within the conventional framework of medical practice: history taking, physical examination, investigation, and clarification. Only then can a management plan be negotiated; and at this stage each doctor will probably be able to offer a range of options. The range can be extended; general practitioners can learn new skills and can evaluate their own and others' work.

Patients exercise their choice of doctor on the basis of experience. Doctors in turn can choose and negotiate different approaches to many common problems, or they can stick to previously tried and tested methods. Unfortunately, progress in comparing different therapies is constrained by the difficulty of collecting samples of similar 'cases' for comparison purposes. No two GPs are likely to have the same case-mix. Nevertheless, the work of evaluating treatment outcomes for emotional disorders (with both drug- and no-drug strategies, and looking at outcomes in terms of families as well as for individuals) is vital for teaching and training. There is enough work on risk factors for depression in women, for example, to suggest new patterns of *anticipatory care* for women at risk.

REFERENCES AND FURTHER READING

Ashurst, P. and Hall, Z. (1989). *Understanding women in distress.* Tavistock/Routledge, London and New York.

Balint, M. (1957). *The doctor, his patient and the illness.* Pitman, London.

Blacker, R. and Clare, A. (1987). Depressive disorder in primary care. *British Journal of Psychiatry,* **150,** 737–51.

Bloch, S. (ed.) (1979). *An introduction to the psychotherapies.* Oxford University Press.

Briscoe, M. (1982). Sex differences in psychological wellbeing. *Psychological Medicine,* Monograph Supplement No. 1, Cambridge.

Brown,G. W. and Harris, T. (1978). *Social origins of depression: a study of psychiatric disorder in women.* Tavistock, London.

Campion, P. D., Butler, N. M., and Cox, A. D. (in press).

Catalan, J. and Gath, D. H. (1985). Benzodiazepines in general practice. *British Medical Journal,* **290,** 1374–6.

Chesler, P. (1972). *Women and madness.* Avon Publishers, New York.

Dohrenwend, B. D. and Dohrenwend, B. P. (1976). Sex differences and psychiatric disorders. *American Journal of Sociology,* **81,** 1447.

Eichenbaum, L. and Orbach, S. (1985). *Understanding women.* Penguin Books, London.

Elder, A. and Samuel, O. (1987). *'While I'm here, doctor.' A study of change in the doctor–patient relationship.* Tavistock, London.

Ernst, S. and Maguire, M. (ed.) (1987). *Living with the Sphinx: papers from the Women's Therapy Centre.* The Women's Press, London.

Finlay-Jones, R. A. and Burvill, P. W. (1978). Contrasting demographic patterns of minor psychiatric morbidity in general practice and the community. *Psychological Medicine,* **8,** 455–66.

Gask, L. and McGrath, G. (1989). Psychotherapy and general practice: a review. *British Journal of Psychiatry,* **154,** 445–53.

Goldberg, D. (1982). The concept of a psychiatric 'case' in practice. *Social Psychiatry,* **17,** 61–5.

Goldberg, D. and Blackwell, B. (1970). Psychiatric illness in general practice. *British Medical Journal,* **2,** 439–43.

Goldberg, D. and Huxley, P. (1980). *Mental illness in the community.* Tavistock, London.

Graham-Jones, S. (1983). *The functional disorders: diagnosis and symptomatology.* Royal College of General Practitioners, Occasional Paper No. 29, 21–31.

Hibbard, J. H. and Pope, C. R. (1991). Effect of domestic and occupational roles on morbidity and mortality. *Social Science and Medicine,* **32,** (7), 805–11.

Howell, E. and Bayes, M. (ed.) (1981). *Women and mental health.* Basic Books, New York.

Jacobs, T. and Charles, E. (1970). Correlation of psychiatric symptomatology and the menstrual cycle in an outpatient population. *American Journal of Psychiatry,* **126,** 10.

Johnson, D. A. W. (1981). Depression: treatment compliance in general practice. *Acta Psychiatrica Scandinavica,* **63,** (suppl. 290), 447–53.

Marcus, A. and Murray-Parkes, C. (1989). *Psychological problems in general practice.* Oxford University Press.

Meeuwesen, L., Schaap, C., and Van der Staak, C. (1991). Verbal analysis of doctor–patient communication. *Social Science and Medicine,* **32,** 1143–50.

Mitchell, A. R. K. (1985). Psychiatrists in primary health care settings. *British Journal of Psychiatry,* **147,** 371–9.

Montgomery, S. A. (1990). *Anxiety and depression.* Wrightson Biomedical Publishing, Petersfield.

Najman, J. M., Morrison, J., Williams, G., *et al.* (1991). The mental health of women 6 months after they give birth to an unwanted baby: a longitudinal study. *Social Science and Medicine,* **32,** 241–7.

Neighbour, R. (1987). *The inner consultation.* MTP Press, Lancaster.

O'Hara, M. W. (1986). Social support, life events and depression during pregnancy and the puerperium. *Archivs General Psychiatrie,* **43,** 569–73.

Parry, G. (1987). Sex-role beliefs, work attitudes and mental health in employed and non-employed mothers. *British Journal of Social Psychology,* **26,** 47–58.

Pendleton, D., Schofield, T., Tate, P., *et al.* (1984). *The consultation: an approach to learning and teaching.* Oxford University Press.

Priest, R. G. and Montgomery, S. A. (1988). Benzodiazepines and dependence. *Royal College of Psychiatrists Bulletin,* **12,** 107–9.

RCGP (Royal College of General Practitioners) (1981). *Prevention of psychiatric disorders in general practice.* Report No. 20. RCGP, London.

RCGP (1988). *To heal or to harm: the prevention of somatic fixation in general practice* (ed. R. Grol). RCGP, London.

Riessman, C. K. and Gerstel, N. (1985). Marital dissolution and health: do males or females have greater risk? *Social Science and Medicine,* **20,** (6), 627–35.

Robins, L., Helzer, J., Weissman, M., *et al.* (1984). Lifetime prevalence of specific psychiatric disorders in 3 sites. *Archivs General Psychiatrie,* **41,** 949.

Ross, M. and Scott, M. (1985). An evaluation of the effectiveness of individual and group cognitive therapy in the treatment of depressed patients in an inner city health centre. *Journal of the Royal College of General Practitioners,* **35,** 239–42.

Schilling, R. F., Schinke, S. P., and Kirkham, M. A. (1985). Coping with a handicapped child: differences between mothers and fathers. *Social Science and Medicine,* **21,** (28), 857–63.

Schwartz, S. (1991). Women and depression: a Durkheimian perspective. *Social Science and Medicine,* **32,** 127–40.

Stott, N. C. H. and Davis, R. H. (1979). The exceptional potential in each primary care consultation. *Journal of the Royal College of General Practitioners,* **29,** 201–5.

Trepka, C. and Griffiths, T. (1987). Evaluation of psychological treatment in primary care. *Journal of the Royal College of General Practitioners,* **37,** 215–17.

Truax, C. and Carkhuff, R. (1965). *Towards effective counselling and psychotherapy.* Aldine Press, Chicago.

Tuckett, D., Boulton, M., Olson, C., *et al.* (1985). *Meetings between experts. An approach to sharing ideas in medical consultation.* Tavistock, London.

Watson, N. R. and Studd, J. W. W. (1990). The premenstrual syndrome. *British Journal of Hospital Medicine,* **44,** 286–92.

Weissman, M. and Klerman, G. L. (1977). Sex differences and the epidemiology of depression. *Archivs General Psychiatrie,* **34,** 98–111.

Wilkinson, G. (1986). *Overview of mental health practices in primary care settings.* National Institute of Mental Health, Series DN 7. DHHS Pub. No. (ADM) 86–1467. Washington, D.C.

Wilson, S. and Wilson, K. (1985). Close encounters in general practice: experiences of a psychotherapy liaison team. *British Journal of Psychiatry,* **146,** 277–81.

WIM (Women in Medicine) (1991). *Women and mental health.* January Newsletter.

16. Health promotion

Jenny Griffiths

A wide range of issues relevant to women's health promotion are discussed extensively elsewhere in this book, in particular, family planning, breast and cervical screening, emotional problems, diet, alcohol use, and smoking. The aim of this chapter is to provide a framework of ideas to support primary health care teams (for health promotion is quintessentially a team activity, and not only the province of doctors) in the development of an overall strategy which will be both generic and holistic, but will also ensure that women's special needs are addressed.

The chapter initially presents an overview of 'Health for All by the Year 2000' and the range of current approaches to health promotion. A review of groups of women who may have particular health promotion needs is followed by a discussion of the opportunities and problems presented by the 1990 GP Contract. The chapter concludes with an overview of the national and local resources available to primary care teams.

HEALTH FOR ALL

The European Regional Office of the World Health Organization published in 1992 a revised list of targets for its member countries in pursuit of 'Health for All by the Year 2000' (WHO 1992). This strategy forms a robust framework for health promotion in primary care, because it emphasizes:

1. Primary care itself, encompassing all forms of community-based care and services, as the most important and most appropriate level of service activity.

2. A broad and positive view of health which includes emotional and social well-being and a safe environment, as well as lack of illness. (This approach is consistent with women's own views: the Health and Lifestyle Survey (HPRT 1987) found that 60 per cent of women defined health as a feeling of psychological well-being; only 11 per cent described it as never being ill, the absence of illness, or never having to see a doctor.)

3. The importance of ensuring that effective mechanisms exist for people to participate in decisions that affect their health.

4. The need for an effective coalition and partnership among the various health and social service professionals, voluntary organizations, indi-

viduals, families, and communities to devise strategies for the attainment of local targets.

5. The key principle of equity, that is, the need to focus on the reduction of inequalities in health between different social groups, by giving priority to those with particular problems caused by age, gender, disability, or social circumstances.

Much of the resource invested in this country in health promotion is wasted, because it fails to change the circumstances and behaviour of those people who are most at risk through environment and lifestyle. Health education is often 'by the middle class for the middle class'. This point is particularly important in the context of the evidence that the gap between the health experiences of the more and less disadvantaged groups in society in fact widened, not reduced, in the 1980s (Smith *et al.* 1990).

The more disadvantaged groups are less healthy partly because of the environment in which they live and partly because they follow less health-promoting lifestyles (Whitehead 1987). Such people need support to exert more control over their lives, which will assist both in improving their social circumstances and demonstrating the value to them of reducing risky behaviour. This approach implies targeting resources on vulnerable groups in ways sensitive to their needs. The logic of this social chain of causation is very important in any disease prevention or health promotion strategy. Programmes that put all the responsibility on the individual while ignoring the social, economic, and other environmental causes of ill-health are doomed to failure.

If the Health For All principle of equity is accepted, services to target more deprived groups will require outreach and community-based work. The concept of Health Action Areas is an important way forward, focusing action on the locality served by the practice. By definition such an endeavour involves the extended primary health care team, including not only doctors and practice nurses, but health visitors, social workers, counsellors, environmental health officers from the local district council, community workers, schools, leisure and recreation services, local employers, voluntary organizations, self-help groups, and any other resources that can be mustered. This approach can be conceptualized as a planned convergence of primary and community care.

If an outreach philosophy is adopted, priorities will have to be negotiated with local communities. To communicate effectively, professionals and the public will have to meet in the middle: health promotion is a process of negotiation. The outcome could include adding a wide range of issues to the conventional list of smoking, diet, exercise, hypertension, stress, etc.; for example, debt counselling, neighbourhood action to prevent violence, or work with homeless people may well emerge as local priorities.

Practitioners need to be careful that health promotion does in fact reduce stress in the individual, for it can increase guilt about 'wrong' behaviour because of a perceived gap between healthy and actual lifestyle. They should work within a 'holistic' model, promoting a sense of balance and well-being, rather than fear over matters of relative unimportance to the individual at that point in time (Griffiths and Adams 1991). The encouragement of participation and of a sense of belonging are important: health education can unfortunately have the unintended consequence of contributing to social isolation for particular groups, such as smokers or HIV-positive people.

DEFINITIONS OF HEALTH PROMOTION

Health promotion is generally agreed to include three main kinds of activity, which often overlap (Tannahill 1985), and general practitioners clearly have a role in all three:

1. *Health education*—the provision of readily available information on healthier lifestyles, and how to make the best use of health services, with the intention of enabling rational health choices, and of ensuring awareness of the factors determining the health of the community.

2. *Prevention of ill-health*—measures to reduce the risk of disease, illness, disability, or any other unwanted state of health, for example, screening for breast and cervical problems.

3. *Health protection*—which is derived from the tradition of public health and includes legal, fiscal, and political measures and regulations to prevent ill-health, for example, seat-belt laws, tax on cigarettes and alcohol, fluoridation of water. Doctors have an important role in influencing the development of healthy public policy because they hold positions of influence at local, regional, and national levels.

CHALLENGING STEREOTYPES: WOMEN AS HEALTH-KEEPERS

The previous paragraphs have described the range of concepts and activities involved in health promotion as opposed to health education. The next sections focus specifically on women's health needs.

In designing a health promotion programme for a practice population, it is as well to remember that what mothers do in the home is not so much housework as health-work (Graham 1987). The domestic tasks of shopping and cooking, washing, ironing, and cleaning all serve to promote health. In looking after their family's needs, mothers are also engaged in teaching about health. Messages are conveyed indirectly through the way mothers deal with everyday concerns. The encouragement of exercise and provision of a healthy diet are obvious examples. Health-keeping is related also to local and public policy: the availability of safe play space and of adequate income for a healthy diet, for example.

It is important to challenge the stereotype of an economically inactive wife (with two dependent children), whose time may seem to be less constrained and life generally easier than that of the wage-earning husband. In 1981, only 5 per cent of all households conformed to this pattern. Women generally combine domestic work with paid employment and therefore have multiple commitments (Women's National Commission 1984).

Sociological literature of the 1960s and 1970s suggested that doctors often feel frustrated and bored by women's vague complaints (headache, fatigue, or unhappiness) and view them as trivial. Historically GPs may have seen as troublesome patients neurotic females with small children in tow (Pollock and West 1987).

It is to be hoped that such obvious gender bias is now a thing of the past. But it is important for GPs—and their patients—to think through how far they can incorporate the challenges posed by feminist outlook into health promotion services. The hallmark of the feminist approach is encouragement of change and coping in women rather than merely adjustment and adaptation. In other words, an attempt is made to change the circumstances surrounding the problem rather than simply coming to terms with it. Feminist approaches also address political and social problems such as battered women and rape. It needs to be realized, therefore, that the health-promoting message 'take care of yourself', and the provision of counselling and support groups, will foster increased independence and egalitarianism among women in their attitudes to their general practitioners.

THE NEEDS OF PARTICULAR GROUPS OF WOMEN

The many women with dependents to care for have particular health promotion needs. The two main groups of dependents are obviously children and older relatives. To take children first:

Women in our society are generally expected to play the major nurturing role, performing daily the essential household tasks and being primarily responsible for the care of children, spouses and aged relatives. As a consequence in most living arrangements women will find it more difficult than men to adopt completely the sick role and there are demands from others which are excessive and tend to impair their ability to rest and relax. As a further result they tend to become run down . . . this bears on both real illness through higher acquired risk and self-reported illness (Gove and Hughes 1981).

The experience described in this quotation may (although it is a hypothetical explanation difficult to prove) explain the consistently higher rates of short-term illness among women. In any event, practitioners need to be sensitive to the particular stresses experienced by women when offering health promotion advice. These stresses are experienced by all women regardless of socio-economic status, but are naturally felt most by single parents. Lone mothers have a higher rate of self-reported illness (32 per cent) than either men or women in couple households (26 per cent and 23 per cent). The poorest health is reported by lone mothers in the manual occupational class (Popay and Jones 1987).

Turning to the caring role for older relatives, it is pertinent that the 1990 GP Contract requires doctors to make a written offer of an annual visit and consultation for all patients aged 75 and over on their list. The consultation can be combined with the home visit. The Terms of Service highlight that the purpose of this assessment is as much social as medical, including mobility, sensory functions, mental condition, physical condition, the social and caring environment, and use of medicines. These visits and consultations are an important opportunity to address women's health issues. The majority of the patients will be women, for example, seven out of ten of those aged 80 or over are females and mass diseases of old age such as dementia and arthritis are thus largely women's diseases. Secondly, most of their informal carers will, of course, be women themselves.

The assessment of those aged over 75 is linked to the implementation of the Community Care White Paper *Caring for people*, which developed multi-disciplinary assessment procedures to support more effective planning and co-ordination of community care. For those elderly people for whom substantial home care, day care, or admission to residential/nursing home facilities are caring options, a duty was placed on social services departments to develop these procedures in association with other agencies. Many health authorities have developed common documentation and procedures with social services departments, thus emphasizing the holistic nature of the process and the essential need for team-work in this, as in all, areas of health promotion. GPs are urged to regard the assessment of the over-75s as an opportunity and not a burden.

STRESS, SOCIAL ISOLATION, AND WELL-BEING

The common theme running through the needs of particular groups of women described above is the need to promote psychological well-being, to control the worst effects of stress, and to break down social isolation. For example, Charlton (1990) has shown that some women smoke for 'affect control'. Smokers are more likely to suffer from stress and feel out of control of their lives. Smoking is perceived as a means of controlling stress. In an urban study, 47 per cent of mothers with partners smoked, but 58 per cent of single mothers smoked. Women whose lives are difficult, perhaps because of poverty, lone parenthood, or stressful jobs, may smoke as a means of escape.

Similarly, social stress and lack of social support is crucial in the excess experience of depression by women documented by many studies. It is suggested that women have more chronic social stress than men (Jenkins 1990): the unremitting responsibilities of caring, fewer leisure activities, less overall status in society, are some illustrations. The 1990 GP Contract offers [depending on the local Family Health Services Authority's (FHSA's) policy] the possibility of remuneration for counselling clinics and self-help groups to provide social support that can help act as a buffer against the effects of stress. Primary care teams can plan an invaluable role for support networks of friends, family, neighbours, churches, and clubs.

Another buffer can be provided by drugs. Benzodiazepines were introduced in the early 1960s and have been among the most widely prescribed drugs in the world. The existence of tranquillizer dependency has been well known since the early 1980s and the blame for this should not be directed solely at doctors, who have had to respond to an explosion in the need for treatment of stress-induced disorders. Twice as many women as men have taken tranquillizers at some time in their lives.

Many practitioners are pressurized by their patients to prescribe these drugs. There is a correlation between the use of prescribed drugs and the circumstances of women with dependent children or other relatives and/or lacking social and emotional support. The average doctor may expect women to be more likely than men to need such drugs, because of the popular concept of women's need for emotional props (that old label, 'the weaker sex', dies hard). This view is reinforced by the tranquillizer advertisements in medical journals which depict women patients rather than men (Women's National Commission 1988). Once again, the GP needs to ask him/herself whether it is appropriate to expect women to adapt continually to the demands made on them.

One alternative to prescriptions is counselling which, of course, requires time. The availability of time in general practice is a key issue for women's health. Quality of care is often correlated with length of consultation. Howie *et al.* (1991) showed that a consultation time of ten minutes was associated with more health promotion, increased patient satisfaction, and more attention to underlying social and psychological issues. Simple arithmetic demonstrates that a personal list size of more than 2250 patients is likely to generate a workload that is incompatible with consultations of this length.

The other option for creating time for counselling is to delegate it to practice nurses, who must be adequately trained, or to experienced counsellors paid by the practice; or to organize self-help groups, which will need some professional support if they are to be successful. Most FHSAs will give substantial reimbursement against the employment of counsellors by GPs. Doctors setting up such a service should contact their local district mental health services (community psychiatric nurse, psychiatrist, psychologist) for advice at the planning stage, to ensure that new provision reflects the best of current professional practice.

1990 GP CONTRACT

The 1990 GP Contract includes health promotion explicitly for the first time in GPs' Terms of Service, a welcome recognition of the importance of positive health within primary care. The new Contract also includes specific payments for the following activities:

- Health promotion clinics.
- Health checks for defined groups in the population, specifically for people aged over 75 years, people newly registered with a GP, and those who have not consulted their GP during the last three years.

The merits or otherwise of these specific provisions are complex and beyond the scope of this chapter, particularly as the Statement of Fees and Allowances is subject to continuing revision, through negotiations between the General Medical Services Council and the Department of Health. However, in general it can be said that the revised Contract encourages only one major approach, namely the health check carried out within the health promotion clinic.

Tudor Hart (1990) made the following trenchant comments about health promotion clinics in the context of the prevention of coronary heart disease:

However, clinics do not necessarily prevent heart disease. The great danger of paying for means rather than ends is that the means become the end. Health promotion clinics . . . attract people who need them least and repel those who need them most. At best, they are a means to an end, at worst they become yet another profitable but irrelevant ritual.

People in affluent (and healthier) social classes are most likely to take up invitations for health checks, thus exacerbating inequalities in health between social groups. Research in one general practice, involving over 2000 men and women, after five years of offering health checks, showed that those most likely to attend were those with the lowest risk of cardiovascular disease (Waller *et al.* 1990).

Practitioners should therefore endeavour to develop the following complementary approaches to the health promotion clinic, which should go some way towards ensuring that advice is targeted towards those groups and individuals who need it most.

Opportunistic health promotion

This can be carried out by the doctor or nurse while the patient is attending the surgery for another reason. Opportunistic advice has several advantages: it is convenient for the patient (preventing a return visit to a health promotion clinic); it is the best way of ensuring that hard-to-reach individuals are seen (more disadvantaged groups have the most risk factors but are less likely to come forward for health checks by appointment); advice is often most effective when the patient is ill, for example, the smoker is most likely to be motivated to quit when she has bronchitis than when she has recovered a fortnight later.

GPs' Terms of Service include the provision of health promotion advice within the consultation. In a consultation with an average length of seven to eight minutes, it should normally be the case that (say) two minutes are spent on: routine, regular reinforcement of advice on smoking, alcohol, exercise, or diet; and on routine regular checks for previously abnormal weight or blood pressure.

In addition, however, GPs should endeavour to make available longer slots of (say) 10–15 minutes for selected patients who consult for other reasons, but who would benefit from more comprehensive advice at that time, perhaps for smoking or alcohol. Some practices structure their appointment books to allow time for two or three of these longer health promotion consultations during a surgery session. In other words, this system allows some time within a surgery for responding to identified need rather than patient demand.

Outreach or community-based health promotion

Innovative methods of taking health promotion into the community should be sought, in partnership with other primary health care teams, health visitors, local authorities, and voluntary groups. Health promotion is inextricably linked to the well-being of communities as a whole, as well as individuals. It is also important to take services to people as well as expecting people to come to the surgery, if the objectives are to be met of encouraging participation and reaching those who need the most support. Examples might include 'mobile' clinics in local community centres, and talks/discussions with voluntary groups (the Women's Institute, Mothers and Toddlers Groups, and so on). Women are likely to be particularly interested in stress management, but this is not irrelevant as the subject allows professionals to introduce other 'risk factors' into the discussion.

Health advice

Nevertheless, it is likely that the majority of the health advice given to women in primary care will be focused around the health check and the health promotion clinic. The following paragraphs give some general guidance on how to set up the highest quality service. These guide-lines are equally applicable to assessment and advice offered under the GP Contract to newly-registered patients, to patients who have not been seen for three years, and to people aged 75 years and over.

General points to consider are, first, that it is unlikely that good quality health advice can be given without allowing at least 15 minutes per patient.

Second, there is evidence that advice from the general practitioner is likely to be more effective than advice from the practice nurse, because of the respect with which patients view their doctors (Sanders *et al.* 1989). In any case, it is important to remember that the Terms of Service specify that delegation should take place only to appropriately trained and supervised staff, with the GP retaining overall responsibility.

Third, it is all too easy to conduct an excellent check or assessment but to give poor quality advice thereafter. Yet it is the communication of advice, not the carrying out of a check, that may result in change in the woman's knowledge, attitudes, or behaviour and therefore make the whole process worthwhile. Attention needs to be paid both to the content of the messages that are given and to the communication skills of practice staff. Effective communication is an art that is more often acquired than innate, and sophisticated training may be necessary.

Fourth, careful consideration should be given to the merits of contracting in a health visitor to undertake one or more clinic sessions, as they receive particularly thorough training in this field. Clinics can be made self-financing on the basis of paying a health visitor for a sessional commitment.

In addition to the other issues set out below, particular attention should also be given to the invitation letter, the wording of which can do much to achieve a high uptake of the service; and any patient questionnaires used to collect a basic health profile. Local facilitators (see section below on local resources) will have models of questionnaires and letters.

GUIDELINES FOR A HEALTH PROMOTION CLINIC PROTOCOL

Management

1. What are the objectives of the clinic? Have the needs of the local population been identified and taken into account?
2. Have all relevant members of the primary care team been consulted at the planning stage, e.g. non-clinical practice staff, attached staff, other practice teams, patient representatives, and local specialists such as facilitators?

3. What are the call and recall arrangements for inviting patients? Are they appropriate and acceptable for the particular groups targeted?

4. How frequently will a full assessment be carried out on individual patients?

5. How will non-respondents be identified and followed up? Those who do not respond to an invitation may well be the group that it is most important to reach. Phone calls may be worthwhile.

6. What format will be used, e.g. structured clinic, opportunistic consultations, group sessions?

Implementation

7. Which personnel will be involved in the delivery of the service? Are they all agreed on the protocol and fully informed about their role? Is the staffing adequate?

8. What information will be collected from the patient and how? For example, what patient questionnaires, record cards, or computer data screens will be used?

9. In planning the sessions, have safety, security, privacy, size, and accessibility all been considered?

10. How will attendance and outcome be recorded to allow audit later on?

Intervention

11. Has consideration been given to the health care model upon which the intervention will be based? Alternatives include the medical or disease-based model, or a patient health beliefs model which takes as its starting point the woman's own concepts of health.

12. Is there agreement among all staff involved on the standard health advice to be given?

13. What is the protocol for follow-up and referral within the practice?

14. What is the protocol for referral to other agencies? Does it reflect the local policies of those agencies (e.g. district health authority, social services, voluntary groups). This can be very important with such services as cholesterol measurement which vary from area to area.

15. What support material (e.g. leaflets, videos) will be used? The quality of available resources varies enormously in terms of both content and presentation.

Quality assurance

16. What relevant training or education is needed for the practitioners and other staff involved?

17. What are the arrangements for internal audit of the service (e.g. audit of risk factor modification through checks of patient notes, uptake of service among target groups, surveys of consumer satisfaction, etc.)?

18. What are the arrangements for external audit of the service (e.g. participation in practice visiting programmes, meetings with hospital consultants)?

19. How frequently will the service be evaluated as a whole?

20. How will the service be described in the annual report and practice leaflet which provide both publicity and accountability to the local population?

WHAT IS A HEALTH CHECK?

The Wycombe Primary Care Prevention Project has developed material for health checks which has been widely disseminated. They define a health check as having three aims:

1. To screen patients for the presence of factors which put them at risk, particularly from arterial disease and cancer.

2. To promote the adoption of a healthier lifestyle.

3. To enable patients to make choices about their lifestyle and to take control of their own health.

It is helpful to structure the health check into three phases:

Agreeing the agenda.   Why has the woman come for a health check? Does she have any particular concerns she wishes to discuss?

Information collection.   A health check record card (facilitators will have examples) is a useful aid to enable the interview to be structured systematically. The phrasing of the questions on the guide-lines accompanying the commonly used health record cards has been carefully considered to elicit accurate information and to use time efficiently. It is important to keep to the same general wording as far as feasible.

Negotiation and counselling.   Having established the woman's initial concerns and elicited any risk factors, a decision has to be taken on which areas to discuss. Areas should be chosen which the patient recognizes as a problem and in which she is most willing and able to achieve early changes. Smoking is, of course, the biggest single risk to the patient's health: it may or may not be possible to tackle this at the first session.

The four stages in effective counselling for lifestyle changes are:

1. *Exploration* of the nature of the patient's health problems and her ideas and concerns about her health.

2. *Explanation* by reacting to the patient's ideas and achieving a shared understanding.

3. *Negotiation* by exploring the possibilities for change, selecting and agreeing appropriate goals, and involving the patient in the management.

4. *Support* by providing positive reinforcement, using available resources, and arranging appropriate follow-up.

Follow-up.   Agreed goals and the follow-up date should be noted on the record card. Further follow-up for tests, immunizations, cholesterol or blood pressure measurement should be recorded.

WELL WOMAN CLINICS

Both general and specialized health promotion clinics (the latter for smoking, diet, or exercise, for example) can be appropriate for both men and women. Similarly, most elements of health checks and health record cards do not need necessarily to be gender specific.

Nevertheless, it is strongly recommended that primary health care teams also set up Well Woman Clinics or Centres as a focus for women's health promotion. The terms are undefined and services offered vary from clinical check-ups to counselling and support groups. The concept is to take a positive attitude to the health and well-being of women. Staffed by women, Centres should encourage self-responsibility for maintaining good health and should offer a full check-up service. The best centres provide counselling and self-support groups for premenstrual symptoms, the menopause, miscarriage, stillbirth and bereavement, sexual relationships, stress, and problems with smoking, drugs, or alcohol—many of the issues discussed in this book.

Well Woman Clinics are intended to attract women from all backgrounds. They should be run informally, and should encourage discussions and questions which women may be diffident to raise with their own doctor, perhaps feeling that their GP is too busy or that their problem is too trivial. The timing of Clinics, their location and friendliness, are key factors in attracting women (Women's National Commission 1984), and should be researched in each particular locality.

Women have been shown to respond better in single-sex group therapy sessions and this option should be available to them if possible. All treatment and counselling services for stress or substance abuse should have access to childcare facilities. Where provision of gender-specific facilities would make the difference between ethnic minority women feeling able to come forward or not, effort should be made to meet this need.

HEALTH EDUCATION AUTHORITY: LOOK AFTER YOUR HEART

In planning their health promotion services for women, practices would be wise to make use of nationally and locally available resources and campaigns.

The Look After Your Heart (LAYH) initiative was launched in April 1987 and is one of the largest and most comprehensive coronary heart disease prevention programmes in the world. It is jointly funded and managed by the Department of Health and the Health Education Authority (HEA). Death rates from coronary heart disease (CHD) in women are half those in men. There has been a promising reduction of 40 per cent among women aged 35–44 (compared with 6 per cent among women aged 55–64) between 1972 and 1987 (Coronary Prevention Group/British Heart Foundation 1988). Nevertheless, CHD accounts for 15 per cent of premature deaths among women, with threefold regional variations in mortality rates (OPCS 1989).

More importantly, the LAYH programme set out to promote healthy living and positive health, an upbeat approach which has been one of the main reasons for its growing acceptance.

The LAYH strategy has six main building blocks, which must be co-ordinated in any particular locality to be successful:

- Look After Your Employee (workplace projects)
- Look After Your Customer (commercial co-promotions, and the Heartbeat Award scheme administered by local authorities particularly in restaurants, etc.)
- Look After Your Children (schools projects)
- Look After Your Patient (primary care projects)
- Look After Your Community (community-based projects)
- Look After Yourself (LAY) (public education, mass media, publications, promotional activity).

The LAYH programme offers a number of resources to primary health care teams, including:

1. Each Regional Health Authority has a LAYH programme officer who will be able to put practitioners in touch with activities in their area (ask your FHSA for the address and telephone number).

2. No Smoking Day is held in March each year and can act as a useful focus for practice activities; similarly an alcohol-free events day is held in June each year.

3. An extensive national network of over 2000 Look After Yourself tutors has developed. Every practice should ensure that it has access to a tutor to run classes; the FHSA should be able to give information about and fund training. LAY activities usually appeal particularly to women as they focus on exercise and stress management.

4. A wide range of publications has been produced for the general public (see list at end of chapter).

5. A personal health record is being evaluated, to be owned by the patient, containing key health facts and personal health information, which may be a useful resource to offer.

6. Most FHSAs run two to three-day workshops for primary health care teams, based on a well-tested HEA model, to foster team-work and action plans for health promotion.

Other local resources

Most FHSAs have facilitators employed to provide support to practitioners in the development of protocols for health promotion programmes, and can recommend (or organize) local training for staff, methods of reaching patients, materials on which to record information, methods of audit to establish baselines and measure progress, and so on.

The local Health Promotion Unit (it may have a slightly different title) will also be able to provide advice, access to training, and information on resources.

Particularly in cities, local authorities are often very active in health promotion and may be keen to involve primary care teams. Contact the Environmental Health Department in the first instance.

ACKNOWLEDGEMENTS

With grateful thanks especially to Penny Astrop; and to all colleagues past and present, particularly those at Oxford Regional Health Authority and Oxfordshire Family Health Services Authority.

USEFUL ADDRESSES

Health Education Authority, Primary Health Care Unit, Block 10, Churchill Hospital, Old Road, Headington, Oxford OX3 7LJ. Tel: 0865 226057.

Health Education Authority, Hamilton House, Mabledon Place, London WC1H 9TX. Tel: 071 383 3833.

REFERENCES AND FURTHER READING

Charlton, A. (1990). Women and smoking. In *Promoting women's health* (ed. N. Pfeffer and A. Quick). King Edward's Hospital Fund for London.

Coronary Prevention Group/British Heart Foundation (1988). *Statistical information on coronary heart disease.* CPG/BHF, London.

Gove, W. and Hughes, M. (1981). Beliefs vs. data: more on the illness behaviour of men and women. *American Sociological Review,* **46,** 123–8.

Graham, H. (1987). The pivotal role of women in the health of the family. In *Women, health and work.* Medical Women's Federation, London.

Griffiths, J. and Adams, L. (1991). The new health promotion. In *Health through public policy* (ed. P. Draper). Green Print, Merlin Press Ltd, London.

Hart, J. T. (1990). Coronary heart disease: preventable but not prevented? *British Journal of General Practice,* **40,** 441–3.

(HPRT) Health Promotion Research Trust (1987). *Health and lifestyle survey.* Preliminary report of a nationwide survey of the physical and mental health, attitudes and lifestyle of a random sample of 9003 British adults, by R. D. Cox *et al..* HPRT.

Howie, J. G. R., Porter, A. M. D., Heaney, D. J., *et al.* (1991). Long to short consultation ratio: a proxy measure of quality of care for general practice. *British Journal of General Practice,* **41,** 48–54.

Jenkins, R. (1990). Women and mental illness. In *Promoting women's health* (ed. N. Pfeffer and A. Quick). King Edward's Hospital Fund for London.

OPCS (Office of Population Censuses and Surveys) (1989). *Mortality statistics, VS3 Deaths by cause: 1988 registrations.* OPCS, London.

Pollock, L. and West, E. (1987). Women and psychiatry today. *Senior Nurse,* **6,** 11–14.

Popay, J. and Jones, G. (1987). Women's health in households with dependent children. In *Women, health and work.* Medical Women's Federation, London.

Sanders, D. *et al.* (1989). Randomised controlled trial of anti-smoking advice by nurses in general practice. *Journal of the Royal College of General Practitioners,* **39,** 273–6.

Smith, G. D., Bartley, M., and Blane, D. (1990). The Black report on socio-economic inequalities in health 10 years on. *British Medical Journal,* **301,** 373–7.

Tannahill, A. (1985). What is health promotion? *Health Education Journal,* **44,** 167–8.

Waller, D., Agass, M., Mant, D., *et al.* (1990). Health checks in general practice: another example of inverse care? *British Medical Journal,* **300,** 1115–18.

Wells, N. (1987). The health of Britain's women. In *Women, health and work.* Medical Women's Federation, London.

Whitehead, M. (1987). *The health divide: inequalities in health in the 1980s.* Health Education Council, London.

WHO (World Health Organization) (1992). *Targets for health for all.* The health policy for Europe. Summary of the updated edition, September 1991. WHO Regional Office for Europe, Copenhagen.

Women's National Commission (1984). *Women and the health service.* Cabinet Office, London.

Women's National Commission (1988). *Stress and addiction amongst women.* Cabinet Office, London.

Recommended HEA publications for patients

Beating heart disease
Exercise: why bother?
Guide to healthy eating
Making a new start (leaflet)
LAYH: Look after yourself guide

New regulations concerning health promotion are being introduced from April 1993, which will replace remuneration for individual Health Promotion Clinics with a capitation-based allowance. There will be three levels ('bands') of allowance, depending on the previous performance of the practice and the degree of sophistication of its plans, which will be approved by the FHSA. The main focus will be on major lifestyle risk factors and coronary heart disease, to take forward the Government's strategy 'The health of the nation', published in July 1992.

Whilst the details are not clear at the time of writing, the main implications would seem to be:

- a reduction in dependence on clinics and the encouragement of a range of approaches as recommended in this chapter;
- conversely a narrow focus on major risk factors rather than the 'whole person' approach advocated here.

HMSO. (1992). *The health of the nation. A summary of the strategy for health in England*. HMSO.

17. Eating disorders

Chris Freeman and Richard Newton

INTRODUCTION

The Royal College of Physicians recently identified obesity as a major cause of health problems in the Western world (Royal College of Physicians 1983). Our society spends vast amounts of time and money in an attempt to lose weight both for health and for cosmetic reasons. Yet only 2 per cent of all dieters successfully lose weight and remain at their new thinner level. For women there is a considerable body of evidence suggesting that society's preoccupation with shape and weight and the cultural pressures placed on women to be slim are major aetiological contributions to the eating disorders anorexia nervosa and bulimia nervosa. The outcome of anorexia nervosa in GP-treated cases is unknown but the mortality rate from hospital-treated cases is comparable to the 'major' psychiatric disorders of depressive illness and schizophrenia (see Fig. 17.1).

Before discussing the specific clinical syndromes it is helpful to spend some time considering what is a normal pattern of eating and way of thinking about shape and weight. Around a third of the working population of men in the United Kingdom are overweight and a third of the working population of women are also overweight, having a Body Mass Index (BMI) of over 25. If indeed 33 per cent of the British population are out of the 'normal' weight range (BMI, weight (kg)/height^2 (m), of 20–25) then the normal weight range ceases to be normal in a statistical sense at all. It would perhaps be more reasonable to broaden the normal weight range to 20–30 on the BMI and this would then include the normal distribution of the population. The justification for maintaining the desir-

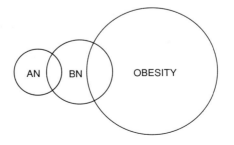

Fig. 17.1 Eating disorders: the size of the problem

able weight range at a BMI of 20–25 is that this range is associated with the lowest mortality rates on actuarial tables. However, recent reviews have raised doubts as to whether a BMI in the 25–30 range is causally related to ill health. Indeed there is some evidence to suggest that overweight women have a lower mortality rate than women in the 'normal' weight range of 20–25 (Ernsberger and Hashaw 1987). Even in the morbidly obese range (BMI >30) it seems that the distribution of excess body fat rather than its absolute quantity is the important factor. Men who tend to put on intra-abdominal adipose tissue on weight gain are putting themselves much more at risk of health problems than women who tend to lay down fat in a more even distribution over the body. And so what is thought of as a desirable weight in our society may not be based on sound medical reasons at all but on other socio-cultural factors.

In underdeveloped countries obesity is rare and seen as an important sign of beauty or power. In Tonga, for example, and in some African tribes, brides are sent to fattening houses prior to their wedding so that they will be at their most beautiful for their wedding day. In the Western world our attitudes to shape and weight have changed and continue to change with increasing influence. In general, society is prejudiced against obese people. Even at an early age pictures of fat children provoke pejorative responses from other pre-school children including 'they are cheats', 'they are sloppy', 'they are naughty', 'dirty', etc.

In the twentieth century, women are much more vulnerable to these negative attitudes than men. Susie Orbach in *Fat is a feminist issue* suggests that women who are still sexually discriminated against in a male dominated society must find it very difficult to feel that their body is the right body. Instead they try to change themselves in order to please those upon whom they are dependent or they tend to be as much as possible like those in power.

Over the last 20 years one version of the idealized body shape as evidenced by the vital statistics of the winners of the Miss American Pageant and the Playboy Centrefold has changed from a curvaceous body shape to a more tubular androgenous one that physiologically is much more difficult to attain and then maintain for women. Between 1969 and 1979 the average number of slimming articles in women's magazines increased from 1.4 per issue to 6 and the number of articles on eating disorders in the same magazines increased from 0 to 2. It was recently estimated in *Vogue* magazine that approximately 80 per cent of women felt that they were overweight and were making some efforts to slim. In a survey of young college women, 60 per cent admitted to having dieted in the last year but only 9 per cent had a BMI of over 25. Within this atmosphere of preoccupation with dieting and shape and weight it is perhaps not surprising that the average calorie intake of adults in the Western world has dropped. Conversely, however, the average BMI of women has risen slightly over the same time. To explain this discrepancy one has to look at the other side of the energy balance equation and the explanation for it may be that energy output by exercise has dropped considerably over the last 100 years with the increase in affluence and the 'conveniences' of modern life.

In addition to the social and environmental factors above, biological factors are also important in determining our weight. It seems from twin studies that body weight can be under a high degree of genetic control and this may be mediated by the 'set point' theory of weight control. The set point theory in its simplest version states that homeostatic processes tend to maintain an individual's body mass within a genetically predetermined set point or range. If someone goes on a weight reducing diet the body's metabolic rate falls to keep the body mass within its set range and if someone overeats then the metabolic rate increases to attempt to compensate.

Eating is an essential requisite of life and as such is under a high degree of central control from the eating centre of the hypothalamus. This eating centre governing hunger sensations and satiety responses is regulated by a number of feedback loops such that in a situation of under-nutrition hunger sensations and carbohydrate cravings are increased and satiety responses are diminished. Interestingly, these changes in response to starvation are much more marked in women than in men and this has aetiological implications for the development of eating disorders in women. In periods of relative over-nutrition, however, the eating centre's homeostatic regulation is less efficient, given that from an evolutionary standpoint we are adapted to surviving through periods of plenty interspersed with periods of famine.

From this brief review we can see that a vast number of factors determine both our weight and shape and also how we feel about them. What is clear from the literature, however, is that we are very unsuccessful at changing our weight via dieting. Even the most rigorously supervised and initially successful diet will lead to lasting weight reduction in only approximately 2 per cent of people. The other 98 per cent of dieters will return to at least their pre-diet and probably 'set point' weight. Indeed most dieters probably return to a weight slightly above their pre-diet weight. What we hope the rest of this chapter will do is provide some guidance on how best to recognize and help women who present in general practice with any of these three eating disorders.

ANOREXIA NERVOSA

In the introduction we have described a society preoccupied with weight, shape, dieting, and food, and within this kind of society we have to be very careful about what we define as an eating disorder that might require some psychological intervention. Although DSM IIIR, the American Psychiatric Association's classification of psychiatric disorders, contains many controversial categories, those of the eating disorders are very helpful in providing clear diagnostic criteria.

Anorexia nervosa is defined as:

1. Refusal to maintain body weight over a minimal normal weight for age and height, e.g. weight loss leading to maintenance of body weight 15 per cent below that expected or failure to make expected weight gain during a period of growth leading to body weight 15 per cent below that expected.
2. Intense fear of becoming obese even when underweight.
3. Disturbance in the way in which one's body weight, size, or shape is experienced, e.g. the individual claims to feel fat even when emaciated, or believes that one area of the body is too fat even when s/he is obviously underweight.
4. In females, the absence of at least three consecutive menstrual cycles when they would otherwise be expected to occur, i.e. primary or secondary amenorrhoea. (A woman is considered to have amenorrhoea if her periods occur only following hormone, e.g. oestrogen, administration.) It should also be noted that one can make a diagnosis of anorexia nervosa only in the absence of any other serious mental or physical illness.

Epidemiology

Anorexia nervosa is very much more common in women than in men, with a female to male ratio of at least 10:1. The peak age of onset is in adolescence between the ages of 16 and 17 and is rare in pre-pubertal girls. It is also rare for it to begin after the age of around 35 years. The disorder is increasingly recognized in all social groups and in all ethnic groups; however, it is possible to identify certain groups of young women who have a higher than expected prevalence of this disorder, e.g. ballet dancers, athletes, girls in private schools, and models. All of these at risk groups are placed under extreme pressure to maintain low body masses or low percentage body fats. The prevalence rates in these groups are around 1–2 per cent and case register estimates of the incidence of anorexia nervosa in the United Kingdom and United States range from 0.37 to 4.06 per 100 000 of the population per year (Schmukler 1985). In general practice, then, full-blown anorexia nervosa will be seen fairly rarely. However, five times as many young girls will present with sub-threshold anorexia nervosa and either themselves or their parents will request help in coping with this sub-threshold eating disorder.

Clinical features

The most obvious abnormality in someone with full-blown anorexia nervosa is that of severe weight loss. It is important to remember that all of the physical features of anorexia nervosa and most of the general psychopathology of it are consequences of starvation rather than of the anorexia nervosa itself (Keys *et al.* 1950).

The physical effects of starvation

The physical effects of starvation are largely adaptive in that these complications are secondary to the body's attempt to conserve energy for the basic activities of life. They include reduction in metabolic rate, reduced growth rate, increased cortisol secretion, loss of muscle bulk, slowing of the heart rate, fall in blood pressure, reduced renal function, shrinking and loss of function of the gastrointestinal tract, reduced wound healing, reduced temperature, loss of periods, shrinkage of the ovaries and uterus, and reduced bone mineralization. More serious short-term complications of starvation, particularly if associated with purging behaviour with laxatives or self-induced vomiting, include cardiac failure, peripheral and facial oedema, dehydration, hypoglycaemia, tetany, seizures, cardiac arrhythmias, and cardiac arrest.

Common physical symptoms complained of include: tiredness, intolerance of cold, blue extremities, dizziness, fullness after meals, swelling of face and ankles, and dry cracked skin. Common signs on examination of anorexics include lanugo hair which manifests itself as a fine growth of hair and acts as a protective heat insulating layer, loss of fatty tissue and loss of muscle bulk with emaciation of the body and face, pale skin, bradycardia, hypotension, cold, blue extremities, hypothermia, and loose folds of skin hanging from the body.

Psychological complications of starvation

Psychological complications are also usually prominent and troublesome to the sufferer. They include food preoccupation, food-related dreams, episodes of bulimia, eating rituals, other obsessional symptoms, social withdrawal, narrowing of interests, depression, lability of mood, sleep disturbance, poor concentration, and irritability.

These complications of weight loss are very important to be aware of, as often they provide a means of engaging the person in treatment when denial of actual weight loss or denial of the specific psychopathology of anorexia nervosa is prominent.

The specific psychopathology of anorexia nervosa

This is encapsulated in the first three DSM IIIR criteria outlined above. They include the markedly dysfunctional thoughts about shape and weight associated with 'an intense fear of fatness' and 'the relentless pursuit of thinness' characteristic of anorexia nervosa. This leads to control of weight and shape by:

1. Rigorous dieting or fasting with calorie counting, setting of strict calorie limits often of around 500–800 kcal per day, labelling of certain foods as forbidden and bad and therefore to be completely avoided if the person wants to have a 'good' day, rigid dietary patterns, and avoidance of many meals altogether. Often patients may resort to falsehoods and concealments to parents or friends regarding their food intake.
2. Self-induced vomiting. Often patients will induce vomiting as another method of weight control, particularly after they have exceeded their set calorie limit for that day or simply eaten what they consider to be too much at any one time.
3. Patterns of excessive exercise. Often at any available moment of the day patients suffering from anorexia nervosa will feel compelled to burn off a few extra calories by, for example, running on the spot, touching toes, aerobics, or even by rapid foot or hand tapping, etc.
4. Laxative abuse.
5. Diet pill abuse.

A number of patients with anorexia nervosa will also lose control of their food intake temporarily and have episodes of bulimia where they binge on large amounts of, usually, carbohydrate food eaten rapidly and secretively over a discrete period of time with a marked feeling of loss of control during the episode. After such a food binge most patients will then induce vomiting.

Many patients with anorexia nervosa have marked body image disturbance seeing themselves as being markedly overweight even when they are very emaciated, and this body image disturbance tends to increase with increasing weight loss. This, of course, further drives the disorder. The pursuit of thinness is not seen as unreasonable or unpleasant by the patient and indeed anorexics characteristically judge their self-control and self-esteem purely in terms of their weight. As mentioned above, denial of the problem and resistance to treatment is a common consequence of this.

Assessment and treatment

An important aim of the assessment period must be to engage the patient in treatment and to form a working relationship with him/her (see Table 17.2).

Table 17.1   *Recognizing the early signs of anorexia nervosa*

Many girls go on a diet. How can a parent or GP distinguish between 'normal adolescent dieting' and early anorexia nervosa?

1. *Denial of dieting:* Most people on a diet will admit so readily and often want to talk about dieting; about different diets that others have tried, the amount of weight loss that would be expected, how much they have cheated. The girl with anorexia nervosa will often deny being on a diet.

2. *Denial of hunger and craving:* Again, people who are dieting will admit to feeling ravenous and admit to cravings for specific foods. Many anorexics will say they are not hungry and will be very reluctant to admit to desiring particular types of high calorie food.

3. *Covering-up weight loss:* 'Normal dieters' are delighted with their weight loss, talk about the number of pounds they have lost. Anorexics will often wear clothes to hide their weight loss and in the early stages may say that they are not losing weight at all and that there is no cause for concern.

4. *Increased interest in food:* While an increased interest in food is common in most people who diet, the normal dieter will try and avoid the temptation of food. In contrast, the anorexic often takes great pleasure in preparing, handling, and cooking food for others. It seems as though this close proximity with food does not cause them distress or temptation.

5. *Needing to eat less than others:* The normal dieter does not appear to be particularly competitive with others in the family. In contrast, the anorexic always wants to have less food on her plate than other family members, particularly her sisters or mother. If she has prepared the food she will often give unrealistically large helpings to other family members.

6. *Eating slowly:* Normal dieters often eat rapidly, trying to satisfy their hunger and clearing everything from their plate. Anorexic girls will dawdle over eating, chew food for longer periods, push peas around on their plate, and always finish their meals long after others.

7. *Increasing obsessionality and perfectionism:* While these features may occur in anyone who is well into the starvation syndrome, they appear to occur early in those developing anorexia nervosa; preciseness about meal times, calorie content of food, rules about eating are mirrored by increasing obsessionality in other areas of the person's life, such as schoolwork and relationships.

Many other behavioural changes occur during early anorexia nervosa but these nearly all occur in normal dieting as well. Other features which may be significant are hoarding of food, night-time eating, becoming increasingly phobic about eating in public, increased exercise, and the use of diuretics or laxatives.

Despite the points above it is often very difficult to distinguish early anorexia nervosa from normal dieting but in at least a proportion of cases the behavioural changes around food are quite different in the two syndromes and clear inquiry about the 'nervosa' part of the syndrome such as feeling fat when getting slimmer, increased sensitivity about body shape, very low self-esteem, and negative self-worth all help make the diagnosis.

History taking should include specific questions regarding the presence of bingeing and the presence of depressive symptoms. Every opportunity should be taken to identify symptoms which are a direct consequence of the starvation syndrome and which patients themselves find distressing. This information should then be fed back to the patient. Physical examination, again with accurate feedback, should also take place, looking for any complications of starvation. In this way history taking, engagement in treatment, and education regarding anorexia nervosa occur simultaneously and the initial primary care assessment of a patient with anorexia nervosa is the most important time for this to occur. Treatment should be seen as a collaborative endeavour between the patient and the therapist. Sufferers should be encouraged to accept maximum autonomy and responsibility for themselves and in this way most patients will not require admission to hospital. However, referral to a psychiatrist with a special interest in eating disorders should probably be the norm for anybody with full-blown anorexia nervosa of any appreciable duration. Outpatient treatment of anorexia nervosa should always include full education regarding anorexia, nutritional and dietary information, and emphasis on psychological and physical symptom relief with the reversal of the starvation state rather than simply emphasizing the attainment of a particular target weight. It should include some form of psychotherapy aimed at relieving the predisposing, precipitating, and maintaining factors of this disorder for that individual.

More commonly, sub-threshold anorexia nervosa will be seen in primary care settings (see Table 17.1) and the decision regarding specialist referral may be less clear-cut. Assessment and education as outlined above should be carried out and then simple dietary changes should be suggested using the Principles Of Normal Eating which are in the appendix to this chapter as a guide. The aim is to accomplish one or two tasks from the Principles Of Normal Eating each week and so gradually over a period achieve a non-dieting approach to eating and a return to a healthy weight range. Encouragement to attend a local eating disorders self-help group is also very useful and any underlying problems may be discussed in this group setting. However, simple problem-orientated counselling can also be helpful and can be performed in the primary care setting.

Drug therapy is not helpful in the specific treatment of anorexia nervosa although concomitant depressive illness may require treatment with antidepressants. It should be remembered that low mood is one of the psychological complications of the starvation state and can be expected to reverse on achievement of a healthy weight range.

Outcome

Little is known regarding the outcome of sub-threshold anorexia nervosa although it is likely that in most patients it will resolve over a period of

Table 17.2   *The principles and management of anorexia nervosa in primary care*

1. Making the diagnosis: this is usually not difficult, and careful enquiry about the psychological aspects of the disorder will nearly always distinguish it from other causes of weight loss.

2. Do not rush into specialist referral. There are a number of steps that it is worth taking first. Anorexic adolescents are often very frightened of treatment and seeing the patient briefly over a number of weeks carrying out the steps below may in the long term be better than very early specialist referral, even when there is considerable pressure from parents.

3. Try and agree with the patient to monitor food intake at this stage without mentioning increasing intake at all. Say that it is very important to get a baseline and at present you do not want her to alter her eating habits, simply to record them as accurately as possible. Diary keeping should involve what food is eaten, where, with whom and in general what emotions and thoughts have been generated during the day. Patients should be encouraged to have a daily diary or small notebook and to carry it with them everywhere. The notebook should be regarded as a joint document between you and the patient and should be something that is brought to every consultation.

4. Try and obtain an agreement to stabilize weight so that at least the patient does not lose any more.

5. Give some simple educational information about energy balance, what happens when periods stop, and the long-term effects on bones in terms of osteoporosis. It is well worth pointing out that if the girl has not finished growing, as well as ending up slimmer she will also end up much shorter and that growth is definitely stunted by anorexia nervosa.

6. Give some simple dietary advice such as not counting calories and trying to eat small regular meals spaced out during the day rather than starving during the day and eating in the evening. Suggest that the patient uses a system of 'exchanges' similar to that used in diabetic departments, rather than counting calories.

7. With the patient's permission, give some advice to the family. Topics that may be briefly covered include 'families are not to blame for anorexia nervosa', anorexia nervosa is a psychological condition, anorexia nervosa has no single cause and is a multidetermined disorder.

8. Try and develop an atmosphere of collaboration. One of the commonest problems in the treatment of severe eating disorders is the battle that doctors get into with patients. If possible, try and create an alliance so that it becomes you and the patient fighting 'it' the anorexia.

9. Try and introduce dissonance to increase motivation: using such questions as 'How many times would I have to reassure you that you are not fat? Once? Twice? Ten times? A thousand times?' is one useful way of detaching oneself from interminable discussions about calories and body size.

Table 17.2   (*contd.*)

'Can you imagine being this way in one year, five years? ten years?'

'Can you try eating one meal—only one meal—as a non-anorexic and write down all the thoughts and feelings that this produces?'

10. In assessing change, concentrate on health rather than weight: do all you can to get away from numbers on the scales, target weight, and ideal weights and concentrate much more on pulse rate, blood pressure, body temperature, and presence or absence of periods.

   While these measures will not in themselves completely treat even a mild eating disorder they may help in forming a therapeutic alliance with the patient, a trusting relationship, and prepare the way for specialist referral if necessary.

11. When should specialist referral occur?

---

time. The longest follow-up study in full-blown anorexia nervosa has been carried out by Theander in Sweden (1985) and his work suggests a much higher mortality rate than other studies. He found a 5 per cent suicide rate at 24 years post-diagnosis and a 10 per cent mortality rate secondary to the complications of anorexia nervosa. He noted that 70 per cent of sufferers recovered by 24 years but that the likelihood of recovering from the illness after a duration of symptoms of more than 12 years was very low. The mortality rate found above is as high as that for depressive illness and that for schizophrenia.

Aetiology

Although there are many interesting theories regarding the aetiology of anorexia nervosa, few have been systematically studied. However, it is known that in twin studies one finds much higher monozygous than dizygous concordance rates and that first degree relatives of patients with anorexia nervosa have a much higher than expected incidence of both anorexia nervosa and unipolar depressive illness. It is thought that the social factors discussed at the beginning of this chapter also predispose to the development of anorexia. The importance of family factors in the aetiology of anorexia nervosa has been much debated. However, the direction of causality in terms of disturbed family dynamics has not been established. Within the individual, adolescence, low self-esteem, and the need for increasing autonomy at the time of adolescence associated with a sense of personal ineffectiveness, perfectionism, and emerging sexuality are also thought to be risk factors for the development of anorexia. In terms of maintaining factors the most important are those associated with the starvation syndrome, and those features of the specific psychopathology that produce intense denial of a problem and intense fear of weight gain. Patients suffering from anorexia nervosa can be visualized as being caught in a vicious perpetuating cycle from which they require some external help to extricate themselves.

It is important to note that in terms of outcome as many as 20 per cent of sufferers from anorexia nervosa will go on to develop full-blown DSM IIIR bulimia nervosa and that approximately half of patients who are seen with bulimia nervosa have at some point in the past met DSM IIIR criteria for anorexia nervosa. We will, therefore, now go on to discuss the clinical syndrome of bulimia nervosa.

BULIMIA NERVOSA

Bulimia nervosa is defined in DSM IIIR as:

(1) recurrent episodes of binge eating (a binge being defined as the rapid consumption of a large amount of food in a discrete period of time);

(2) a feeling of lack of control over the eating behaviour during the eating binges;

(3) regular engagement in *either* self-induced vomiting, use of laxatives or diuretics, strict dieting or fasting or vigorous exercise in order to prevent weight gain;

(4) a minimum average of two large eating episodes per week for at least three months;

(5) persistent overconcern with body shape and weight.

By convention the diagnosis is made in people within ±15 per cent of normal body weight and, therefore, someone may exhibit all of the above symptoms but if their body weight is more than 15 per cent below that expected then they would be assigned a diagnosis of anorexia nervosa. It is also important to remember that the diagnosis of bulimia should be made only in the absence of serious physical or other psychiatric illness.

Epidemiology

In surveys of college students, 20–40 per cent of students were found regularly to have loosely defined binges; and, using more stringent criteria for binge eating, perhaps 20 per cent of young women binge at least once every two months, and 4 per cent regularly induce vomiting to control weight and shape (Cooper and Fairburn 1983). The prevalence of bulimia nervosa in the general population of women under the age of 45 has remained steady over the last few years at between 1–2 per cent.

Typically, patients with bulimia nervosa are women with a female to male ratio of 100:1. They present at an average age of around 24 years although the peak age of onset of the disorder itself is around 16–17 years of age. These ages of onset and incidence may be beginning to change with increasing awareness of the disorder and increasing availability of treatment facilities leading to a younger age of onset and a shorter duration before presentation. People referred for treatment are frequently from social classes I, II, or III but population surveys reveal bulimia nervosa to occur in all social classes. It is said that bulimia is a culture-bound syndrome being rare in Third World countries and in first-generation immigrants to First World countries. Interestingly, a recent study revealed it to be more common in first-generation female Asians in Bradford than in an age-matched white population. This increased incidence appeared to occur only in families where the parents retained a very firm hold on the traditions and language of their country of origin and this finding lends some support to the strong cultural influence on the aetiology of bulimia nervosa.

Clinical features

Typically the disorder may begin during a period of dieting and indeed about 50 per cent of patients will have met the DSM IIIR criteria for anorexia nervosa sometime in the past. This is followed by profound loss of control over eating which leads to the episodes of bingeing. Patients then become involved in a cycle of dieting, bingeing, purging, and dieting that is driven by their almost continuous preoccupation with thoughts of shape, weight, and food.

A binge usually consists of fairly large amounts of carbohydrate-rich foods—bread, cakes, biscuits, and sweets—eaten very rapidly and in secret. During a binge many people feel numb and rather depersonalized although earlier on in the disorder the binge had been quite a rewarding experience and for some patients it continues to be so. The binge is associated with a profound feeling of loss of control and only stops through physical discomfort, social interruption, ending of supplies, etc. Patients then describe feeling profoundly negative about themselves and angry, disgusted, and panicky about the effects of binges on their weight. This anxiety is relieved in most patients by self-induced vomiting or less commonly by laxative abuse. The person may instead, however, decide to fast for the next day to relieve this worry and some patients compulsively exercise. After purging most patients feel depressed and describe feeling quite drowsy.

In between binges most patients are very aware of what they eat and set limits on the type and amount of food. They label diet foods as good and food that they perceive as fattening, and usually only eaten during a binge, as bad. Each element of this cycle reinforces the behaviour preceding it and each element acts as a conditioned stimulus for the following behaviour. In addition, the constant anxious preoccupation with fatness, shape, and weight leads to thoughts such as, 'I've had a sweet, that's it, my diet's blown, I may as well binge.' Therefore both cognitive and behavioural elements serve to maintain the disorder. The binges tend to be secretive and to occur when patients are on their own and are bored, anxious, lonely, or depressed. Often patients feel that bingeing is a way of coping with these feelings. The frequency of bingeing varies enormously, some people bingeing for up to two hours each day. Equally, vomiting may also vary, with many patients vomiting after non-binge meals. Often people will also have a ritual set pattern or aim of vomiting, for instance, washing their stomach out with coke or water or vomiting until only clear fluid emerges.

In addition to the abnormal eating behaviour many bulimics describe marked mood swings from around normal mood to marked depression and occasionally to quite a high mood. These mood swings often occur without any clear precipitant and reinforce the person's sense of being out of control of their own behaviour and emotions.

The picture that we are painting of a person with bulimia nervosa, therefore, is of someone who on one level is extremely distressed and unhappy about their condition, who is struggling to break out of a vicious maintaining circle, who continues to have very low self-esteem despite having a reasonably good social facade, and who is ashamed and secretive about the disorder. As well as this, patients may be intensely ambivalent about giving up their bulimia because of their continued fear of weight gain and intolerance of stress.

Physical complications of bulimia nervosa

Bulimia nervosa is also associated with a number of physical complications that all workers in this field should be aware of. Slightly more than one-third of bulimics will have either stomach or duodenal ulcers, verifiable on endoscopy, with all their associated complications. More than half complain of heartburn or dyspepsia. Up to 50 per cent will have enlarged parotid salivary glands leading to swelling of the cheeks which can aggravate bulimic patients' belief that they are overweight and need to diet. Most patients who induce vomiting erode the backs of their teeth by the action of the gastric acid and this erosion is accelerated by rigorous brushing of teeth post-emesis. It is helpful to suggest to patients the use of a fluoride-containing mouthwash after vomiting to avoid this complication. Constipation is a frequent complaint in laxative abusers on cessation of this practice. Oesophageal rupture after inducing vomiting and gastric rupture during bingeing are often fatal but fortunately extremely uncommon complications of bulimia nervosa.

Dehydration due to fluid loss in vomiting, diuretic use, or laxative abuse may lead to dizziness due to low blood pressure. Potassium loss because of vomiting can cause cardiac arrhythmias and ultimately cardiac arrest. Tetany is occasionally induced by repeated vomiting and epileptic fits are slightly more common in bulimics than in the general population. Disturbance in endocrine function may lead to irregular or absent menstrual periods, and loss of calcium from bone may lead to marked osteoporosis in later life with an increased risk of fractures.

As well as these physical complications bulimia nervosa is also associated with a high degree of psychiatric co-morbidity. We have already mentioned the marked mood swings that appear as part of the bulimia syndrome. Up to 80 per cent of patients with bulimia nervosa will, at some time in their lives, meet the DSM IIIR criteria for major depression. Perhaps up to 15 per cent will have previously received treatment for anorexia nervosa, up to 15 per cent will have taken overdoses or deliberately harmed themselves in some other way in response to environmental triggers, 5 per cent will abuse street drugs, 5 per cent will compulsively shoplift binge and non-binge items, and 3 per cent will already have run into problems with alcohol abuse.

Aetiology

Little is definitely known about the aetiology or prognosis of this condition and, therefore, much of what follows is somewhat speculative. As far as predisposing factors are concerned, however, it seems reasonably clear that there is often a family history of eating disorders, obesity, unipolar depression, or alcohol abuse. We have already mentioned the marked cultural pressures that may lead to bulimia nervosa and it also appears likely that the publicity given to bulimia nervosa in the media teaches other women how to become bulimic. Clearly a past history of anorexia nervosa also predisposes to later development of bulimia nervosa.

In terms of maintaining factors the two most important are the self-reinforcing nature of the binge–purge cycle and the continuing cultural pressures to attain an idealized weight.

In terms of outcome it seems that untreated it can be a chronic fluctuating condition that may continue well into late middle age. With treatment, perhaps two-thirds of patients will recover and perhaps one-fifth will remain severely ill. Even among the recovered group most patients continue to be disturbed by worries about food, eating, weight, and shape. It is also clear that bulimia nervosa is associated with a significant mortality rate much higher than the general population, not only due to the physical complications but also because of a marked increase in suicide among these individuals.

Assessment and treatment

Engagement and motivation to change is much easier to achieve with patients suffering from bulimia than with those suffering from anorexia nervosa and many actively seek treatment. Assessment is similar to that outlined above for anorexia nervosa but there is a particular need to look for both physical complications and psychiatric co-morbidity. Suggested treatment is along the lines outlined before, with an emphasis on specific behavioural techniques, education, and cognitive therapy. This can be done in a primary care setting either on a one-to-one basis or within a group. However, many psychiatric centres are now offering a specialist referral centre for bulimia nervosa with specialist group treatment. Again the principles of normal eating provided in the appendix can be helpful in achieving a non-dieting approach to eating and, therefore, to enable the sufferer to break out of the maintaining cycle of bingeing, vomiting, and dieting.

Antidepressant medication has consistently been shown to be effective in reducing bingeing and purging behaviour; however, it is not clear if these effects are maintained after withdrawal of the drug. In patients who have failed to respond to psychological intervention or who have concomitant depressive illness, a trial of one of the 5-HT re-uptake inhibitors should be tried in patients suffering from bulimia. Fluvoxamine in doses of up to 300 mg daily or fluoxetine at a dose of 60 mg daily can be added in as adjunctive therapy. Diary keeping is also an important part of the self-help for bulimia nervosa and patients should be encouraged not only to record every item of food that they eat in an eating diary but also to record the circumstances in which any binges took place, how they have been feeling about themselves and their shape and weight that day, and any stressful events in the patient's life that have occurred at that time. All patients should be encouraged to see treatment as an experiment in which the patient is trained to introduce certain behavioural or thinking changes. Therefore, it is possible to learn a great deal from the experiment whatever the outcome and hence one can try to avoid the idea that one outcome is a success and another is a failure. It should be remembered in those patients who are receiving a 5-HT re-uptake inhibitor as concomitant treatment for their bulimia nervosa that these drugs are not acting as antidepressants but are working as specific anti-bulimic agents by affecting serotonergic function in the eating centre of the brain located in the hypothalamic area. After an initial acute phase of treatment, which can often be fairly short (around twelve therapy sessions) some kind of long-term follow-up has consistently been shown in research to be important in the maintenance of change, and if patients are treated for their bulimia in a primary care setting formal long-term follow-up should not be neglected. Alternatively, patients may be referred to a local self-help organization for eating disorders and national

Table 17.3 *The principles of management of bulimia nervosa in primary care*

1. *Bulimia nervosa is a secret disorder:* Many women will have been to their GPs on several occasions with other complaints and been unable to confess their behaviour. They may say they were just desperate for their GP to ask them the right questions. When interviewing women with mood disorders, particularly young women, questions such as 'how has your appetite been?' or 'have you lost your appetite?' don't seem to aid disclosure. Try questions such as 'when you are down do you ever eat more than you should?' or 'when you are stressed do you ever lose control of your appetite?' or 'some people undereat in response to stress but many others overeat, how does stress affect you?' It is important to ask about the 'nervosa' symptoms of the disorder, once it has been established that binge eating is occurring. These include fear of weight gain, and extreme sensitivity about shape and weight. Other weight loss behaviours such as vomiting, and laxative and diuretic abuse should be asked about in a straightforward, matter-of-fact way, as if one expects the answer to be 'yes'.

2. *Motivation:* Increasing motivation is usually not a problem though occasionally reluctant girls are brought by their parents. It is much more difficult to achieve treatment aims that are realistic. Most sufferers want to stop their bingeing, vomiting, or purging but don't want to give up dieting and certainly don't want to put on any weight.

3. *Acknowledging the disorder:* As with many psychological disorders, the first time the story is told to a professional is very important. The bulimic patient will have fears of rejection, of being told to pull herself together, or that the GP will be repulsed by her behaviour. Reassurance that the disorder she has is common, that many women suffer from it, and that treatment is available may all help.

4. *Keeping a diary:* Introduce the idea of a diary and again stress that for the first week or two you don't want the behaviour to change. The purpose of the diary is to record her eating as accurately as possible, the number of times she binges and vomits, what factors preceded the binge, where the binge occurred, what her feelings were, and how she felt afterwards.

5. *Assess mood:* Depressive symptoms are common in bulimia nervosa. Usually they are secondary to the bulimia though sometimes it is difficult to assess which came first.

6. *Beginning to make changes:* Introduce the idea of dieting less strictly, of beginning to eat something, however small, in the morning rather than starving and of gradually moving towards three small meals including carbohydrate.

7. *Techniques to avoid bingeing:* Simple advice can be given about (a) trying to eat in company; (b) decreasing the amount of food kept in the house; (c) not shopping when hungry; (d) avoiding shops on the way home; (e) using distractions such as exercise or phoning someone.

Table 17.3   (*contd.*)

---

8. *Taking special care of risk periods:* Social events such as eating out present major stresses and rehearsing strategies for these may be important. Warn that carbohydrate craving and the likelihood of bingeing increase in the premenstrual phase.

9. *Stopping vomiting:* Usually the vomiting stops when the bingeing does, so it is not often necessary to take special steps to interrupt the vomiting. However, it is useful to encourage the idea of delaying the time between bingeing and vomiting.

10. *Advice about joining a self-help group:* For many, bulimia is a chronic relapsing disorder and self-help is an important part of treatment.

11. *Advice on practising other techniques to cope with stress:* These could be anxiety management, yoga, etc.

12. *Increasing exercise:* Simple education about energy balance (input versus output) may help.

---

contact points for these organizations can be found at the end of this chapter.

OBESITY

Definition

Quetelet's Index or the Body Mass Index of weight (kg)/height^2 (m) is now replacing the Metropolitan Life Assurance tables as an aid to defining healthy weight.

BMI   <15   Emaciated
      15–20   Underweight
      20–25   Normal or grade 0 obesity
      25–30   Overweight or grade I obesity
      30–40   Moderate or grade II obesity
      >40   Severe or grade III obesity

For the purposes of this chapter we shall consider only grade II, BMI 30–40 and grade III, BMI >40 obesity as being clinically significant. It is in this group of patients, particularly those at the top end of the grade II BMI range and within the whole of the grade II BMI range that morbidity and mortality is clearly related to obesity and where weight loss produces clear benefits.

Grade I obesity

Around a third of the population of the United Kingdom and a sixth of the population of children will have a BMI between 25 and 30. As indicated at the beginning of this chapter, the question of whether people should be described as obese if they fall within this BMI range is controversial. The major complication of being within this range is of further weight gain and a progression to grade II and then grade III obesity. Management should therefore be aimed at preventing this complication.

Outcome studies suggest that in the long term, weight gain rather than weight loss is the outcome of dieting for most people. It may be necessary for primary care workers to become advocates not of dieting but of a non-dieting approach to eating, associated with encouraging individuals to accept their body weight and shape for what they are. The 'Principles of Normal Eating' (see Appendix) can be used as an aid to promoting this non-dieting pattern which may be difficult to achieve in people who have become hooked into a pattern of preoccupation with food, shape, and weight leading to chronic mild dieting interspersed with periods of over-eating or 'comfort' eating.

It should be remembered that a proportion of people who are over-weight have all the features of bulimia nervosa save the weight control criteria and this has been recognized in the forthcoming International Classification of Diseases (ICD 10) and DSM IIIR by the inclusion of binge eating disorder categories that are not associated with a normal weight range. Acknowledgement of the binge eating problem and its treatment along similar lines to those for bulimia nervosa should be aimed for in this group of patients.

Grade II and grade III obesity

Epidemiology

Around 3 per cent of the population of the United Kingdom are moderately obese with approximately 0.3 per cent being severely obese (BMI >40). Women are more likely to be severely obese than men and in general the prevalence of obesity increases with increasing age. In developing countries obesity is common in higher socio-economic groups (SEGS) whereas in the affluent West it is more prevalent in the lower SEGS.

Aetiology

In terms of energy balance, obesity only occurs when energy input exceeds energy output for a prolonged period. The cure for obesity, therefore, is to change the equation so that energy output exceeds energy input for a similar period either by increasing metabolic rate or exercise levels or by reducing energy intake in food. However, evidence from twin studies and adoption studies suggests that weight is under a high degree of genetic control and our weight is probably maintained within a certain set range by various homeostatic mechanisms including changes in metabolic rate, hormonal responses, carbohydrate craving, and hunger and satiety responses. This genetically determined set range can be altered by various environmental influences. For example, the secretion of gastric inhibitory peptide (GIP) which stimulates insulin secretion and, therefore, fat deposition is much greater in people on high fat diets than in people taking in a similar amount of calories as carbohydrate. Weight gain in fat fed animals is, therefore, much greater than in animals fed on an equi-calorie carbohydrate diet. Obesity is also more prevalent in affluent food-rich countries than in famine-stricken food-poor countries. Palatability, availability, mood state, and cost are also important in the aetiology of obesity. It has been suggested that severe obesity can be used to avoid issues regarding sexuality or other inter- or intrapersonal problems. It is likely, then, that the aetiology of obesity involves a combination of genetic, environmental, psychological, and cultural factors. Treatment of obesity should, therefore, be similarly multifactorial.

The problems associated with obesity

Insurance company statistics suggest that mortality rates double at a BMI of 35. This mortality rate then increases exponentially with increasing BMI. In addition to the increased risk of death, however, there are a number of important medical and psychological problems associated with marked obesity.

Psychosocial problems include: low self-esteem, body image disparagement, and social disability with prejudice against the obese at work and in ordinary social intercourse with marked effects on personal and sexual relationships.

Medical problems which may reverse or be alleviated by weight loss and be exacerbated by continued obesity include: diabetes mellitus, cardiovascular disorders including hypertension and probably ischaemic heart disease, respiratory disorders, osteo-arthritis of load-bearing joints, increased operative risk, and gallstones.

Assessment of obesity

Assessment should aim at clarifying what problems the patients themselves identify, the degree of overweightness, and the presence of any complications of obesity. This should be associated with an assessment of their average dietary pattern and assessment of exercise levels, presence of binges, and the outcome of previous attempts to lose weight. Aetiological factors particularly maintaining factors of obesity should be explored and the patient helped to identify for herself the pros and cons of changing her eating habits and her weight and shape.

Management of moderate and severe obesity

Treatment of obesity should be viewed as a collaborative endeavour between patient and therapist with agreement that the patient will actively participate in all aspects of her own multicomponent treatment plan. The components of this plan will vary according to the individual and the degree of obesity. Included in it should be full education regarding the aetiology of obesity, dietary information, and the set point theory of obesity, its complications and prognosis, both treated and untreated.

Simple behavioural tasks should be introduced as soon as possible. The patient can be asked to record her food intake in a daily diary similar to the one used in treating bulimia nervosa. The Stimulus Control Techniques outlined in the 'Principles of Normal Eating' are again useful in helping people to reduce the likelihood of overeating and to learn a pattern of normal eating. Exercise should be introduced at a level sufficient for each individual. Cognitive therapy can be used to improve self-esteem and to examine the problems that arise during the course of treatment.

Most patients will also require the introduction of a weight-reducing diet sufficient to lose 0.5–1.0 kg per week. This diet may be introduced after a few weeks of assessment, during which the patient will have learnt the use of diaries and begun to experiment with the approaches to eating laid out in the 'Principles of Normal Eating'. A large number of such diet sheets leading to a daily intake of approximately 1000 kcal daily are available commercially. Research suggests that in patients with marked obesity the short-term outcome is better when patients combine a low-calorie diet with the type of behaviour changes suggested above. Very low-calorie diets consisting mostly of protein and yielding 400 kcal of energy per day have very limited value.

A number of drugs are licensed for use in the treatment of obesity. Of

Table 17.4 *The management of moderate/severe obesity in general practice*

Principles

1. Take a long-term view.
2. Try and stop further weight gain and break the diet/weight gain/diet cycle.
3. Stopping further weight gain may be a much more realistic and achievable goal than weight loss.
4. Set realistic goals for weight loss. For a 616 kg (20 stone) patient to diet down to 431 kg (14 stone) is going to take 84 continuous weeks of dieting where every week the patient has to lose 1 lb. Setting goals which have small steps is more realistic for the patient though it may take considerable effort to convince the patient of this.
5. Attend to medical complications.
6. Concentrate more on establishing different patterns of eating rather than new patterns of dieting. (Some examples are given in the 'Principles of normal eating' in the appendix at the end of this chapter.)

these, dexfenfluramine and fluoxetine are the newest and least likely to cause problems of dependence and abuse. Both these drugs lead to good short-term weight loss but on cessation of the drug weight gain occurs. However, there is some evidence that introducing them slowly as part of a more comprehensive treatment plan can lead to greater long-term weight loss.

For severe obesity, in addition to the above, surgery may need to be considered. Either a temporary intervention such as jaw wiring or permanent changes such as ileojejunal bypass surgery or gastric restriction may be considered. The results with gastric restriction surgery can be good both physically and psychologically and are maintained in the long term. However, weight loss during jaw wiring tends to be regained in the months following removal of the wire.

CONCLUSION

For people with mild eating disorders an educational approach with the use of simple behavioural and cognitive changes should be sufficient for them to attain a non-dieting, non-bingeing, non-overeating approach to food. Linked to this should be some work regarding sufferers' worries about weight and shape. Referral to a local women's self-help group can be very useful. For severe obesity, full-blown anorexia nervosa, and long-standing bulimia nervosa specialist referral should be considered.

Appendix

PRINCIPLES OF NORMAL EATING

1. *Set aside some time daily to reflect on how you are coping. Some of your strategies may not be working, try others.*

2. *Use diaries or exercise books to record your eating.*

   You may wish to do this in the form of diaries we provide or you may prefer to write down everything you eat and drink with details of times and how you were feeling while you were eating.

3. *Set yourself limited realistic goals, work from hour to hour rather than from day to day.*

   One failure does not justify a succession of failures.
   Note your successes, however modest, in your diaries.

   Every time you eat normally you are reinforcing your new good eating habits.

4. *Try to eat in company, not alone.*

5. *Do not do anything else while you eat, even if you are bingeing, except socialize.*

   For instance, do not watch TV, do not read. It is usually OK to listen to music but try to concentrate on enjoying your meal.

6. *Plan to eat three meals a day plus two snacks.*

   Try to have these meals and snacks at predetermined times. Plan your meals in detail so that you know exactly what and when you will be eating. In general you should try to keep one step ahead of the problem.

7. *Plan your days ahead.*

   Avoid both long periods of unstructured time and over-booking.

8. *Only have planned food in the house.*

   Don't stock up too far ahead. If you feel you are at risk of buying too much food, carry as little money as possible.

9. *Identify the times at which you are most likely to overeat, compulsively exercise, vomit, or binge, etc.*

   Using your recent experience and the evidence provided by your diaries, plan alternative activities that are not compatible with these activities, such as meeting a friend, exercising, or taking a bath.

10. *Whenever possible avoid areas where food is kept.*

    Try to keep out of the kitchen between meals and plan what you will do at the end of each meal. If necessary, get out of the house completely; the washing-up can wait.

11. *Don't weigh yourself more than once a week.*

    If necessary stop weighing yourself altogether. Don't try to lose weight while you are trying to learn new eating habits. Once you are eating normally you may reduce weight by cutting down the quantity you eat at each meal rather than skipping meals. Remember, gradual changes in weight are best.

12. *If you are thinking too much about your shape and weight it may be because you are anxious or depressed.*

    You tend to feel fat when things are not going well. Can you identify any current problems and do something positive to try and solve or at least minimize them?

13. *Use exercise.*

    Regular exercise increases metabolic rate and helps suppress appetite, particularly carbohydrate craving. However, avoid compulsively exercising simply in order to burn off excess calories.

14. *Take particular care in the days leading up to your period.*

For many women food cravings increase at this time.

15. *Avoid alcohol.*

It can increase cravings and reduce your control.

USEFUL TELEPHONE NUMBERS

Anorexic Aid. Tel: 0494 21431.

Anorexic Family Aid. Tel: 0603 621414.

Both organizations can provide information about self-help groups in all areas of the country.

REFERENCES AND FURTHER READING

Cooper, P. J. and Fairburn, C. G. (1983). Binge eating and self-induced vomiting in the community: a preliminary study. *British Journal of Psychiatry,* **142,** 139–44.

Ernsberger, P. and Hashaw, D. (1987). *Rethinking obesity: an alternative view of its health implications.* Human Sciences Press, New York.

Keys, A., Brozek, J., Henschel, A., *et al.* (1950). *The biology of human starvation.* University of Minneapolis Press.

Royal College of Physicians (1983). *Obesity.* A Report of the Royal College of Physicians. **17, (1),** 3–58.

Szmukler, G. (1985). The epidemiology of anorexia nervosa and bulimia. *Journal of Psychiatric Research,* **19,** 143–53.

Theander, S. (1985). Outcome and prognosis in anorexia nervosa and bulimia. *Journal of Psychiatric Research,* **19,** 493–508.

Further reading

General interest

Bruch, H. (1974). *Eating disorders: obesity, anorexia nervosa and the person within.* Routledge & Kegan Paul, London.

Duker, M. and Slade, R. (1988). *Anorexia and bulimia: how to help.* Open University Press.

Garner, D. M. and Garfinkel, P. E. (1985). *Handbook of psychotherapy for anorexia nervosa and bulimia.* Guildford Press, New York.

Gilbert, S. (1986). *The pathology of eating.* Routledge & Kegan Paul, London.

Gilbert, S. (1989). *The psychology of dieting.* Routledge & Kegan Paul, London.

Gordon, R. A. (1990). *Anorexia and bulimia: anatomy of a social epidemic.* Blackwell, Oxford.

Orbach, S. (1984). *Fat is a feminist issue,* (2nd edn). Hamlyn, London.

Anorexia nervosa

Bruch, H. (1978). *The golden cage*. Open Books, Wells.
Palmer, R. (1989). *Anorexia nervosa: a guide to sufferers and their families*. Penguin, Harmondsworth.
Slade, P. (1984). *The anorexia nervosa reference book*. Harper & Row, London.

Bulimia nervosa

French, B. (1987). *Coping with bulimia*. Thorsons, Wellingborough.
Maisner, P. and Turner, R. (1986). *The food trap*. Unwin, London.

Obesity

Ernsberger, P. and Hashaw, D. (1987). *Rethinking obesity: an alternative view of its health implications*. Human Sciences Press, New York.
Garrow, J. S. (1981). *Treat obesity seriously: a clinical manual*. Churchill Livingstone, Edinburgh.
Kano, S. (1990). *Never diet again*. Bath Press.

Assertiveness

Dickson, A. (1989). *A woman in your own right*. Quartet Books, London.

18. Drink problems

Moira Plant

INTRODUCTION

Increasingly women are presenting for help with alcohol-related problems. Research carried out in this area suggests that women are generally more likely than men to acknowledge they have problems but less likely to relate these to their alcohol consumption. This, allied to women's greater need for confidentiality, shows in their preference to attend agencies not specifically identified as alcohol services (Thom 1986). General practitioners are therefore frequently involved.

ALCOHOL CONSUMPTION LEVELS

Concern about female alcohol misuse is a reflection of a more general rise in alcohol consumption. The per capita level of alcohol consumption in the United Kingdom virtually doubled between the Second World War and 1979. Since that date per capita has been at a rather lower level. It is noted that post-war alcohol consumption has been far lower than it was during the early years of the twentieth century. This is illustrated by Fig. 18.1.

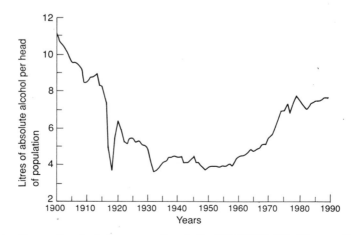

Fig. 18.1 Per capita alcohol consumption in the UK (1900–89). (Source: Thurman 1991.)

Table 18.1 *Levels of per capita alcohol consumption[1] in the European Community 1984–8*

Country	1984	1986	1988
Belgium	10.6	10.2	10.1
Denmark	10.4	10.3	10.0
France	14.1	13.5	13.3
Greece (beer and wine)	6.8	6.2	5.8
Ireland, Rep. of (incl. cider)	6.2	6.2	5.9
Italy	11.5	9.9	8.9
Luxembourg	14.9	14.1	14.2
The Netherlands	8.6	8.5	8.3
Portugal	12.4	11.0	10.0
Spain	11.2	11.5	11.3
West Germany	12.6	12.4	12.0
United Kingdom	7.1	7.2	7.4

[1] Litres of pure alcohol

Source: Brewers' Society (1990).

Overall trends in per capita alcohol consumption are important since these exert a clear influence on general levels of alcohol-related problems (Bruun *et al.* 1975; Sales *et al.* 1989). Alcohol misuse is a major national problem. Even so it is worth noting, as can be seen in Table 18.1, that per capital alcohol consumption in the UK is not exceptionally high by international standards.

Changes in drinking habits in many countries appear to be more a reflection of general national trends in per capita alcohol consumption. There is little evidence of a dramatic increase in the use of alcohol by women in comparison with their male counterparts.

The most recent figures for the UK published by the Office of Population Censuses and Surveys can be seen in Table 18.2.

The heaviest drinking women in the UK are young, unmarried career-oriented women. The proportion of females among those with some officially recorded alcohol-related problems has been increasing. Three indicators of alcohol misuse are: in-patient admissions to psychiatric hospitals for alcohol dependence and related diagnoses, liver cirrhosis mortality rates, and convictions for drunken driving and public drunkenness. In Scotland the number of women admitted to psychiatric hospitals for alcoholism and alcoholic psychosis rose from 350 in 1985 to 450 in 1989 (first admissions). The corresponding figures for men were 944 in 1985 to 975 in 1989 (first admissions). Between 1979 and 1988 there has been a 'moderate increase' in the rates of mortality from chronic liver disease and cirrhosis in women in England and Wales (Duffy 1991). Interestingly cautions and

Table 18.2   *Alcohol consumption levels for women aged 18 and over in the United Kingdom (1984–8)*

Alcohol consumption level (units per week)	1984	1986	1988
Non-drinker	13	11	12
Very low (under 1)	24	24	24
Low (1–7)	41	41	40
Moderate (8–14)	14	14	14
Fairly high (15–25)	6 ⎤	7 ⎤	7 ⎤
High (26–35)	2 ⎬9	2 ⎬10	2 ⎬10
Very high (36+)	1 ⎦	.2 ⎦	2 ⎦
Base = 100%	9399	9845	9814

Source: OPCS (1990).

convictions for drunkenness offences by women in England and Wales dropped between 1984 and 1986 (6447 and 4794 respectively), but rose again until by 1988 they had reached 6641. In Scotland, where the statistics are for those where charges have been proved, there has been a consistent decrease in numbers from 1180 in 1982 to 398 in 1988. The numbers for men show a corresponding decrease.

Female/male differences in relation to normal drinking

Past evidence suggests that women began regular drinking at an older age than men. However, more recent evidence leads to the conclusion that this gap is narrowing and that now young girls are beginning to drink at about the same age as boys (Plant *et al.* 1985). The common age of reported first drinking was 13 to 14 years.

Women are more sensitive to alcohol than are men. This may be because on average females weigh 15 per cent less than men and a smaller percentage of their body weight is in the form of water. In young women 50 per cent of their total body weight is in the form of water, in young men the corresponding level is 60 per cent, and for these two reasons alone women will show higher blood concentrations than men will after consuming the same quantity of alcohol.

Half a pint of beer, a single measure of spirits, or a single glass of wine contain roughly the same amount of alcohol: one unit. Women, more often than men, drink cocktails which may make it more difficult to calculate the amount of alcohol consumed. Such drinks often contain two or three units of alcohol in one glass. This is roughly equivalent to two or three whiskies. Other 'fashionable' drinks for women are strong lagers. These contain approximately two and a half times more alcohol than do normal beers and lagers. One pint of this type of lager has the equivalent alcohol content of approximately five single whiskies. This measurement of alcohol in units has become a very useful concept as will be seen later in this chapter.

Certain drinks pass into the bloodstream faster than others. This depends largely on beverage strength. Fortified wines such as sherry will pass into the bloodstream fastest. High alcoholic content drinks such as spirits, if taken 'neat' will cause the stomach to react by producing protective mucus to 'line' the walls and delay absorption. The pyloric sphincter will go into spasm and prevent the alcohol passing quickly into the duodenum where it is absorbed into the bloodstream. These mechanisms may give the drinker a false sense of not being affected by the alcohol until suddenly it 'hits her'.

There is also evidence to suggest that women in the childbearing age range have varying peak blood alcohol levels. Consumption of the same amount of alcohol at different times in their menstrual cycle results in changing levels, the highest being immediately premenstrually. Women on oral contraceptives metabolize alcohol more slowly, therefore it takes longer for their blood alcohol level to return to zero. This kind of information is especially important in relation to driving. A woman on oral contraceptives who has quite a lot to drink one evening may still be well over the legal limit to drive to work or drive the children to school the next morning. Other antidepressant drugs, such as benzodiazepines, when consumed at the same time as alcohol, have an additive effect.

ALCOHOL-RELATED PROBLEMS

Why do people who have been drinking in a harm-free way begin to develop problems? The reasons are many and varied. Often the explanations given appear to be no more than a desperate attempt to find some order in a frightening and uncontrollable situation. It has been suggested that men see 'triggers' for heavy drinking in work pressures while women more readily identify relationship difficulties. While this may be true, it often remains no more than a search for 'socially acceptable' answers. Some people see the problem only in terms of beverage types: 'I was fine while I stuck to the beer, it was when I started on the spirits that my problems developed'. Often this simply means that with developing tolerance the person has needed to take alcohol in a more concentrated form to maintain the necessary effect.

Some problem drinkers do not appear to realize they have a problem until some major traumatic event occurs or people begin to comment to them on the importance of alcohol in their lives. However, many will acknowledge that they themselves knew they had a drink problem long before being able to admit it to anyone else.

Physical problems

There are few organs and systems of the body which are not affected by excessive alcohol use. Many of these effects are common to both sexes.

Gastrointestinal problems

These are possibly the first to occur. Chronic gastritis, leading to gastric or duodenal ulcers, is common in heavy drinkers. One of the most common reasons for haematemesis is a tear in the gastric mucosa caused by the extreme 'retching' experienced by problem drinkers when they try to eat or even clean their teeth first thing in the morning. Difficulties with absorption of vitamins and iron often contribute to vitamin deficiencies and anaemias, particularly iron-deficiency anaemia.

Liver disease

It has been well documented that acute but heavy exposure to alcohol, for example a two- or three-day binge, can lead to fatty deposits in the liver. However, this will resolve if drinking stops and the liver is given a rest. Prolonged heavy drinking may lead to eventual scarring and cirrhosis. In the past, the accepted view was that abstinence from alcohol, even if it is too late for total return to health, will mean that there is no further physical deterioration. Recent evidence has shown that the course of alcohol-related liver disease in women differs from that in men (Hill 1984; Royal College of Physicians 1987). In women there are more frequent episodes of alcohol-related hepatitis leading more quickly to cirrhosis or cancer of the liver. Although the aetiology is unclear it has been suggested that auto-immune mechanisms play a part in the pathogenesis of alcohol-related liver disease in women. The peak age for female deaths from liver cirrhosis is 50–54 years in Scotland, slightly younger than in England and Wales (Duffy and Latcham 1986).

Cancer

In the United States a large National Cancer Survey (Williams and Horn 1977) examined the association between different types of cancer and smoking and drinking. Women seemed more prone to cancer of the lip, tongue, pharynx, and oesophagus with greater alcohol use. This survey indicated that cancer of the mouth and oesophagus were more alcohol- than tobacco-related; whereas in the case of cancer of the larynx the reverse was evident. These researchers also noted that the risk of alcohol-related cancers was greatest in parts of the body where alcohol is at its most concentrated, such as the oral cavity. Thorley has noted:

In the United States where smoking and drinking levels are similar to those in the United Kingdom, tobacco consumption causes 30 per cent of all cancer deaths but alcohol causes 3 per cent of cancer deaths and, next to tobacco, is the most significant identifiable carcinogenic factor. Tobacco and alcohol may therefore be the two factors most accessible in terms of prevention of cancer in general (Thorley 1982).

More recently media attention has been drawn to the possible causal mechanism between moderate alcohol consumption and the development of breast cancer; and a number of major studies have now been carried out. The complexities of the area are immense. Many of the studies are limited by use of inappropriate controls, such as patients suffering benign breast disease or hormone dependent cancers such as endometrial cancers. Alcohol consumption data has often not been collected in a rigorous way, but even more problematic is the collection of recent alcohol consumption data when examining a causal mechanism with a disease which could have begun up to twenty years earlier. There is enough consistency in the data to suggest an association but little evidence to prove a causal relationship (Plant 1992).

Gynaecological/obstetric problems

The occurrence of premenstrual tension in women with alcohol-related problems is greater than in the general female population and many of those suffering report self-medication with alcohol. Other studies have brought to light higher than expected rates of menstrual irregularities, hysterectomies, and infertility. Much more work needs to be done on hormone function, but the possibility of a woman with a long and troubled history of gynaecological dysfunction abusing alcohol should not be dismissed too readily (Plant, M. L. 1990).

The past few years have witnessed a resurgence of the long-established concern that maternal drinking during pregnancy may cause fetal abnormalities. The 'Fetal Alcohol Syndrome' first named by Jones and Smith (1973) has been the topic of considerable debate among researchers and clinicians in the alcohol field. The clinical features of the syndrome are illustrated by Table 18.3.

This clinical entity was initially described in relation to only eight children. The mothers of these children were all heavy alcohol abusers in Seattle. They were also in receipt of welfare payments. They were in many respects a deprived group. Their nutritional intake was poor and their intake of tobacco and other drugs was unclear. The initial naming of this syndrome was followed by a move towards the view that any amount of alcohol taken during pregnancy is harmful (Plant, M. L. 1987).

Many of the large-scale studies of this topic have been retrospective. These involved the researchers taking a group of damaged babies and then asking the infants' mothers what their alcohol consumption had been during pregnancy. The main advantage of this approach is the large number of damaged babies that can be located and included. However, the

Table 18.3

Type of abnormalities		Percentage occurrence of abnormalities
Performance	Prenatal growth deficiency	100
	Postnatal growth deficiency	100
	Developmental delay	100
	Microcephaly	91
	Short palpebral fissures	100
	Epicanthal folds	36
Craniofacies	Maxillary hypoplasia	64
	Cleft palate	18
	Micrognathia	27
Limbs	Joint anomalies	73
	Altered palmar crease pattern	73
	Cardiac anomalies	70
Other	Anomalous external genitalia	36
	Capillary hemangiomata	36
	Fine-motor dysfunction	80
		100

Source: Jones and Smith (1973).

disadvantages of this method are considerable. To take a group of women who have just experienced the trauma of delivering damaged babies and expect them to recall accurately what their alcohol consumption was 30–40 weeks earlier is a far from ideal way of gathering precise information. Another problem with some of the original studies was the lack of attention paid to 'confounding variables'. The effect of such important factors as general health, diet, social class, smoking, and other drug use was not always measured.

Current evidence in relation to this subject is fairly reassuring; but the evidence as to whether there is a dose-response relationship between alcohol consumption in pregnancy and fetal harm is conflicting. A more subtle condition known as fetal alcohol effects includes such problems as hyperactivity, poor eye–hand co-ordination, behavioural and learning difficulties. Although there is a clear association between alcohol consumption and certain fetal abnormalities, a causal relationship has not yet been fully established. Several prospective (follow-up) studies have been completed. These suggest that the overall role of alcohol in causing birth damage is relatively minor; though again it is difficult to disentangle this from other factors such as maternal age, past obstetric history, social class, diet, smoking, and illegal drug use. Given that most pregnant women are not seen even by their GPs until they are at least five or six weeks pregnant, the best advice is probably a reassuring message: 'One or two drinks once or twice a week have not been shown to be harmful. Don't drink excessively. Don't get drunk.' Many women need reassurance since some publicity and discussion of this subject may have caused unwarranted anguish and guilt.

There is some evidence that women who drink have an elevated risk of experiencing second trimester abortion (Harlap and Shiona 1980). However, there is conflicting evidence on the dosage of alcohol necessary to put the fetus at risk. This, combined with the problem of other confounding variables such as social class and use of other drugs, makes the possibility of a causal relationship far from clear. Although the likely risks of moderate drinking in pregnancy appear to have been exaggerated, there is no doubt that women should not drink excessively, use psychoactive drugs unnecessarily, or smoke during pregnancy. Alcohol and other substances pass into the breast milk. The relationship between this and more subtle cerebral harm has not yet been clarified. Again, the message must be that excessive consumption may be harmful.

It is known that men who abuse alcohol over long periods have greater than expected infertility rates with reduced sperm counts and poor sperm motility. At present there is not much comparable evidence relating to female alcohol abusers. It is, nevertheless, possible that such women may encounter enhanced difficulties in conceiving.

Psychological problems

Depression and anxiety

The association between depression and alcohol-related problems is well established. If depression is a major factor it obviously has to be treated in conjunction with the alcohol problem (see Chapter 15). The most frequently discussed antecedent of alcohol problems among women is sex-role conflict. The idea of such conflict being a contributory factor to alcohol misuse has gained some ground over the past few years.

Young women who are problem drinkers are more anxious than controls, have a lower opinion of themselves, and are more likely to reject traditional feminine roles. This is one possible explanation. However, it is equally likely that the pressures on mothers, who may be working and trying to run a home, are so great that alcohol, other drugs such as benzodiazepines, and even more commonly tobacco, may be used as a quick way to relax (Curran and Golombok 1985). The number of women in this situation is increasing. They may present at general practitioner clinics complaining of tiredness, lack of energy, and feelings of anxiety. It is worthwhile remembering that the patient may be at risk if she uses alcohol to relieve some of these symptoms. The taking of a simple drinking history is advised and is discussed below.

On the other hand, some studies of older women with a drink problem often show them presenting as 'excessively feminine' in a stereotypical way; reporting, for instance, that they wish to have lots of children and seeing their main role as care-giver and emotional support of the family.

Sexual problems

Many women with alcohol-related problems complain of sexual difficulties. Studies have found that this group suffer more frequently than the general population from vaginismus, dyspareunia, and lack of sexual responsiveness. The reasons for these difficulties are complex (see Chapter 14), but women with alcohol-related problems seem to use alcohol to 'treat' the sexual problems they experience. Many women today (possibly because of advertising images) believe that alcohol enhances sexual pleasure. They perceive alcohol as an aphrodisiac and report an increase in sexual enjoyment when drinking. However, these subjective views are at variance with the objective data on the physiological effects of alcohol on women's sexual responsiveness. Alcohol is a depressant. The subjective view may well be due, not only to a disinhibiting effect of alcohol, but to social learning. Women learn to associate drinking with sociability and sexual activity, and their expectation is that drinking will enhance sexual enjoyment.

EFFECTS ON THE FAMILY

Women play a central role in families, so it is both relevant and useful to discuss the effects of alcohol abuse here.

The stereotype of the 'lace curtain' or 'hidden housewife' drinker is in some ways misleading. Housewives are less likely to report or experience alcohol-related problems than are young, unmarried, and career-oriented women. In general, young women are more likely to experience acute problems associated with intoxication; middle-aged women are more likely to be chronic heavy drinkers.

Toddlers and younger school-age children usually spend more time with their mothers than their fathers, but existing research has paid more attention to the drinking habits of fathers than to those of mothers. The clinical literature on problem drinking mothers tends to be related to small numbers and is often psychoanalytical in perspective. However, studies have shown that in some samples of problem drinking women, the majority reported that at least one of their parents was also a problem drinker. Such females also report exceptionally high rates of affective disorders, particularly depression, among their relatives (Williams and Klerman 1984). Often evident in the children of problem drinkers are: difficulty in forming relationships, becoming easily upset, poor school performance record, primary generalized fear often arising from arguments in the home which may lead to violence, difficulty in trusting, and lack of self-confidence. These children may have little respect for authority and suffer from behavioural problems.

Conversely, in an attempt to cope with a problem drinking mother who is perceived as unreliable, inconsistent, and disorganized, the child may 'grow up too fast' and take over the running of the household and the family (Orford 1990). There is also some evidence to suggest that as young adults this group will be more likely to use alcohol unwisely, smoke, and use illicit drugs (Orford and Velleman 1990).

Available research suggests that a problem drinking father has a more damaging effect upon children than a problem drinking mother. In view of the amount of time and effort invested by mothers in their children this seems an anachronism. One of the few studies which specifically examined the children of problem drinking mothers found that regardless of social class these women showed confused, inconsistent, and ambivalent attitudes towards their offspring (Orford 1990) who themselves were distrustful, reserved, withdrawn, and dependent. As the mothers' attitudes changed after they gained sobriety, the attitudes seemed more attributable to drinking habits than to underlying chronic problems.

Recently a great deal of media attention has been given to the issue of child abuse. There is little research evidence on the possible association with alcohol. Children of problem drinking women are more likely to experience neglect than violence. However, given the sometimes chaotic lifestyle of some of these women, the children may not be protected as well as they might be in fraught situations such as parental arguments or paternal abuse. This may be an important clinical issue.

There is always a risk that the husband who continues to drink may undermine the treatment plan of his wife. Many studies report a high rate of separation or divorce in alcohol-abusing women. Some have suggested that husbands of problem drinking women are less likely to remain in the relationship than are wives of problem drinking men (Vannicelli 1984).

ALCOHOL AND 'RISKY SEX'

Alcohol has long been associated with sexual behaviour for a wide variety of physical, psychological, and social reasons (MacAndrew and Edgerton 1969; Soloman and Andrews 1973; Plant, M. A. 1990); and the AIDS epidemic has greatly increased the risks. In consequence, researchers have recently examined the possible association between alcohol consumption and 'high risk' or unprotected sexual contacts. Recent interest in this topic owes much to the work of Stall (1987) and his co-workers. These researchers reported that among gay men in the USA, alcohol and drug use were associated with marked increases in high risk sexual activities. Several subsequent British and American studies have confirmed these findings (Strunin and Hingson 1987; Temple and Leigh 1990). It is also evident that prolonged heavy or dependent drinking may weaken the human immune system. This may make people more susceptible to HIV infection if they are exposed to the virus (Plant, M. A. 1990).

A Scottish study by Robertson and Plant (1988) examined contraceptive use among young people who had married while teenagers. These individuals were asked whether their first sexual encounters had involved contraceptive use and whether they had been immediately preceded by drinking. Females who had consumed alcohol were much less likely than other females to have used contraceptives, 24 per cent compared with 68 per cent. A more recent Scottish study by Bagnall *et al.* (1990) concluded that young adults who frequently combined sexual activity and alcohol consumption were seven times more likely than other young people to engage in risky sex. Alcohol frequently leads to 'disinhibition' (Room and Collins 1983), when people behave (or believe that they behave) in a less careful or restrained way than would otherwise be the case. In fact sexual activity is influenced by many factors.

POLY DRUG MISUSE

This topic is important enough to warrant attention, even in a chapter on alcohol. Studies show that many women, particularly those between 45 and 49 years of age, are prescribed anxiolytic or antidepressant medication. Women in general have also not been as successful as men in cutting down smoking, and are more likely than men to self-medicate with over-the-counter products.

Available evidence should alert professionals to the very real risk of women abusing a number of substances. It is suggested that there may be 'hydraulic' or substitution effect in relation to patterns of psychoactive drug use. When the availability of one substance is reduced by choice, or by other factors such as price, this may be compensated for by increased recourse to another substance, legal or illegal. Care should therefore be taken both when initially prescribing and when discontinuing anxiolytic or antidepressant medication. As noted earlier, taking a simple drinking history would be advisable in these circumstances.

TAKING A DRINKING HISTORY

A useful way for practitioners to avoid the discomfort of approaching a suspected problem drinker for information on alcohol consumption is to incorporate a drinking history into all routine health checks.

One of the simplest and quickest ways is to take a week's drinking diary. The patient is asked what she had to drink on each of the past seven days, starting with the previous day and working back. The information elicited should include all alcohol consumed throughout the day, lunch-time drinks, early-evening, and so on; the beverage type, whether beer, spirits, or wine; and the quantity. Over the past few years it has become fashionable for females to drink strong lagers, so information on beverage type is important. Other important information to collect includes: times and places the drinking occurred, the people in whose company the patient was drinking, and how the patient felt at the time of the drinking episode. The doctor should check if last week's drinking was typical and, if not, how it varied from the normal week.

For most people their drinking will not be a cause for concern. However, there are now well-established guidelines agreed upon by the Royal Colleges of General Practitioners (1987), Physicians (1987), and Psychiatrists (1986) showing safe/risky levels of consumption. These can be seen in Table 18.4.

These figures can be compared with the total weekly consumption noted from the diary and the information should then be fed back. If the doctor is concerned about either the levels or patterns of the woman's consumption, this also should be relayed to the patient.

It should be noted that the weekly 'low risk' levels suggested above should be spread out over the week, for example, 12 units taken as two units over six days has a very different effect from 12 units taken on one occasion. For this reason it may be helpful to ask the patient for such details as places and people involved in the patient's heaviest drinking times so that she can identify 'at risk' times. There are a couple of publications now available by Robertson and Heather which provide easily understood information on this: *So you want to cut down your drinking?* (1984) and *Let's drink to your health* (1986). These both contain well-presented information plus a diary which can be used to monitor alcohol consumption levels.

Some women may feel they would like to reduce their consumption even though their drinking is not problematic. In this case it may help

Table 18.4   *Sensible drinking levels for women*

Level of risk	Weekly consumption
Low	below 14 units
Intermediate	15–21 units
High	over 22 units

Source: Health Education Authority (1990).

to have some hints available. The following are just a few of the simple steps:

1. Don't drink daily; make two or three days in the week drink-free.
2. Find other ways of relaxing and improving your self-image, e.g. join a keep-fit group. This will not only help to fill in your time, it will also give you support and company other than your heavy-drinking friends.
3. Find ways of coping with emotional problems which are safer than drinking.
4. Don't use alcohol every night to aid sleep. Try some of the many relaxation techniques now available.
5. Don't drink on an empty stomach.
6. Make every second drink non-alcoholic.
7. Sip the drink, don't gulp.
8. Put the glass down between sips. This increases the length of time it takes to finish a drink.

MANAGEMENT

As with so many problems, social or medical, the earlier the difficulty is detected the sooner help can be initiated and the more hopeful the prognosis becomes.

A number of concerns are of particular relevance to the interaction between female problem drinkers and their doctors. Alcohol misuse has an implicit moral component. It is an assumption, and a dubious one, that female patients will be treated better by female professionals than they would be by males. The reality is often different, perhaps partly because women doctors are largely trained by men. Furthermore, regardless of professional group or gender, a person with alcohol-related problems is often seen as not worthy of attention. Alcohol problems are frequently viewed as self-inflicted, and treatment, when given, is often grudged. In a strange sense women professionals often regard female problem drinkers as 'letting the side down'. Comments such as 'it's always worse in a woman' are not uncommon from both the patients themselves and the professionals. It is often difficult to accept that the professionals' own biases or standards of behaviour can 'get in the way of therapy'. Women problem drinkers do not need judgements or criticisms. They may judge and revile themselves more readily than anyone else.

It is important early on in therapeutic relationships of this kind to try to develop a collaborative approach and encourage the woman to take responsibility for her own future treatment. Women in general, and problem drinkers in particular, often feel very guilty about taking time for themselves. They need to be shown how vitally important it is to have their needs met in healthier, more constructive, and safer ways than drinking excessively. Feelings of lack of competence, confidence, and power make the initial act of seeking professional help extremely difficult; so because of the shame of self-disclosure some women with alcohol problems go through the trauma of withdrawal without any help. The following is an extract from a letter sent to a colleague:

I cannot put my address because I feel my patient husband has put up with enough . . . I reached the bottom, my work was suffering, my health, suicide never out of my mind. I had two choices, suicide or stand up and be counted . . . One Sunday night I found myself out of my secret stock. I was like a demented animal. My understanding husband went to the off-sales and bought me the whisky. This was the best thing that could have happened. The owner remarked: 'She's sent you tonight.' I never thought he knew. My husband told me this on his return with great sorrow on his face. I felt anger, despair, and above all shame. I vowed I would stop. The next six months were a nightmare. I had the shakes, nausea, strange feelings I am unable to describe, horrible dreams, terror, and anguish. Sometimes I felt this indeed was death as I paced the floor night after night. Never once did I ask for help, too ashamed to ask a doctor or Alcoholics Anonymous.

Most of the early research into the management of alcohol problems related to patients in specialized treatment units. The resulting bias in the literature has led to a commonplace assumption that all people with alcohol-related problems have to be admitted to hospital and given high doses of drugs to help them through the withdrawal phase. The above extract from the letter goes against many of the widely-held beliefs about alcohol misuse. These include the view that people with alcohol-related problems need to be hospitalized and to have careful observation by qualified personnel to survive withdrawal from alcohol. Certainly there are times when this is necessary, for example, when there is a physical component to the alcohol problem. However, it is evident that many people undergo successful withdrawal from alcohol without any medical intervention. The sad fact is that not only do people who go to specialist agencies self-select, but so too do people who go to their general practitioners.

It is clear from research carried out both in the UK and elsewhere that, as noted earlier, women are less likely to go to specialist alcohol agencies and more likely to visit other sources of help, such as marriage guidance councils, women's support groups, and GPs. The risk is that some such agencies may be unable or indeed unwilling to recognize the woman's alcohol problem. This may be due to lack of training. Many professionals also admit that they do not feel confident or qualified to treat people with alcohol-related problems. They do not know how to approach patients and so they avoid the issue altogether. The other comment often made by professionals is, 'What's the use, she'll only give up when she wants to.'

This is to some extent true. However, people can be helped to come to a decision about their drinking by having help to clarify just how far the problem has developed and whether alcohol has taken over from all their former interests. It is also of great importance that people have appropriate information at hand if and when they decide to seek help. The most useful aid for GPs, recently updated, is the DRAMS Scheme which is available from the Health Education Board for Scotland (see also Wallace and Haines 1985; Anderson *et al.* 1987).

If the patient is unsure of whether drinking is causing a problem in her life, the doctor can suggest that she keeps a diary of her drinking for the next two weeks, or until her next appointment. It should be stressed that this record must be honest. Reassuring the patient that she need not show the diary to anybody may help to make it more accurate. This is not an exercise to bring back to the 'teacher', but a form of self-assessment to aid in recognition of possible problems. At the second appointment any such problems can be discussed.

The doctor may wish at this point to assess alcohol-related physical harm, partly because this information needs to be gained, but also because doctors in general often feel comfortable in this role and patients quickly become aware of the doctor's feelings. Although blood tests are sometimes used as an aid in identifying a drink problem, their accuracy is questionable and they should not be seen as a very accurate measure of harm. However, results of these tests when discussed with the patient make it more difficult for her to avoid the issue of alcohol-related physical harm.

Enquiry should then be made about relationships, work, financial problems, etc. These need not be discussed in detail during this first interview; it simply states to the patient that the doctor takes what she is saying seriously and feels it is important enough not to be dismissed lightly. It is an opportunity for the woman to 'stop running' and stand still long enough to take stock of her life. Information should also be taken to assess the possibility (noted above) of a primary depression; and of the use or misuse of substances such as tobacco, and other legal or illicit drugs.

If this is the first meeting between patient and GP specifically about a drink problem it may not be the time to make great plans. Perhaps the most important part of this session is the feeling the patient develops of being taken seriously, and the emerging feeling of trust of the GP. However, the patient should get a clear message from the doctor stating the part drink has played in the difficulties that have been described.

Treatment

It may be that a simple clear statement that drinking has played a large part in the woman's problems and that she should reduce her alcohol consumption to within the one to 14 units a week band will be enough to ensure an improvement in the situation. The practitioner may wish to help further and as noted earlier a package has been designed, and recently extensively updated (Health Education Board for Scotland), for this purpose. If, however, patient and doctor agree that abstinence is necessary, at least in the short term, then thought must be given to methods of managing withdrawal. Clearly if the patient is very ill and in need of in-patient care then it is important to explain the reasons for this and to contact the nearest appropriate clinic. Whether this is a ward in a local general or psychiatric hospital or a specialized unit will depend on which facilities are available locally.

A few psychiatric community nurse teams are now providing a home detoxification service. This is run in conjunction with the patient's general practitioner who assesses the physical condition of the patient and agrees on a regime of an appropriate drug to cover withdrawal. The nurses thereafter monitor the patient's condition over the first five- to six-day period. This particular treatment will be more appropriate for some problem drinkers than others. Moreover this type of home detoxification is only possible if there is a dependable supportive relative or close friend willing to be involved. Patients with marked physical harm due to their drinking may be more safely detoxified in a hospital setting.

If the GP feels strongly that admission is necessary then it may be helpful to meet with the patient and her partner (if any) to explain the importance of the move. However, it must be kept in mind that for women with families this may not be an acceptable or indeed a viable proposition. The next step therefore is to assess and bring in the local support systems, e.g. the patient's family, the district nurse, health visitor, community psychiatric nurse, Alcoholics Anonymous, or the local council on alcoholism. The patient will then be given medication if the doctor thinks this is necessary. No one has ever proved that going through withdrawal without the aid of medication if it is needed makes the problem drinker either a better person or less likely to drink excessively thereafter. There are a number of preparations on the market to aid with this process. The one used by many specialist agencies is a regime of chlordiazepoxide which covers six days.

Day 1   20 mg q.i.d.
Day 2   10 mg q.i.d.
Day 3   10 mg q.i.d.
Day 4   10 mg t.i.d. (8 a.m., 6 p.m., 10 p.m.)
Day 5   10 mg b.d.
Day 6   10 mg nocte

A vitamin supplement is also helpful on an outpatient basis. A one-off dose of intravenous high potency Parentrovite with a daily follow-through of 250 mg thiamin orally has been found to be advantageous. During the period of withdrawal the patient will need support and encouragement.

Some practitioners will at this stage offer the patient disulfiram treatment. This drug is not a cure but it can enable the patient to start reorganizing her life in a less self-destructive pattern during a period of enforced sobriety. It can be particularly useful for women who drink impulsively as it can give them some time to think before they drink. The disulfiram is taken daily and the patient is made aware of the risks of drinking alcohol while on this drug. Further information can be obtained from routine drug sources.

These drugs are only an aid to recovery. The main changes have to be a continuing process of self-awareness, regaining confidence, and control over self. For women in particular continuing contact with other female problem drinkers either at a local agency or simply with other females at a woman's self-awareness group is often extremely helpful. The main problem with alcohol agencies such as Alcoholics Anonymous is that many of them often have only a minority of female clients or members. It is for this reason that follow-up in a women's group is often more useful and supportive.

Follow-up

As noted above, the use of blood tests is of limited initial value. However, repeating tests to show how the body is recovering may encourage the patient to persevere when the going becomes difficult. It should be noted that women in the childbearing years may continue to have liver problems even after cessation of heavy drinking. In these cases, continuing abnormal liver function tests should not be automatically taken as an indication of heavy drinking without further proof.

There will be times when the agreed goals set by patient and practitioner are not met, e.g. the patient has a drink. This is not uncommon and should be seen rather as a learning situation which, when discussed and any reasons clarified and understood, will add strength to future efforts. The major risk during these periods of relapse is the patient feeling that she has let her GP down and feeling too guilty or ashamed to return. It is for this reason that the steady building up of a relationship, with the personal responsibility clearly based in the patient and the support role based in the practitioner, is of such great importance.

The practitioner's role

As noted above, the role of the practitioner is one of support. He or she is ideally seen by the patient as someone who can be trusted, someone who will listen to what the patient is thinking and feeling, and yet remain non-judgemental; someone who will not turn away from her even if she has relapsed.

Occasionally difficulties can arise if the practitioner feels, for instance, that there may be some risk to the children of a problem drinking mother. The steps in this case are the same as for any 'at risk' children. It must be stressed that the trust which can be developed between problem drinker and practitioner necessitates complete honesty about the doctor's concerns regarding the children.

It becomes clear that there are many facets to the problem drinker. It should be acknowledged that working with such people may be an emotionally draining, stressful experience. It is important for professionals in this situation to allow themselves the use of support systems, be they other general practitioners in a group practice or other professionals such as specialist alcohol workers. It is never helpful for colleagues to adopt an 'I told you so' attitude if a patient relapses. An acknowledgement of how it feels is much more helpful.

ABSTINENCE OR CONTROLLED DRINKING

The long and interesting debate on whether abstinence or controlled drinking is the better treatment is beyond the scope of this chapter. Interested readers are referred to the Heather and Robertson (1983) review of the subject. It is enough to say here that controlled drinking is a viable option for some people with alcohol-related problems. As noted above, owing to the fact that much of the initial research into treatment was conducted in specialist units there was little or no attention paid to the possibility of some people returning to moderate, harm-free, or controlled drinking. Since research has widened its scope people have become more aware of this as a useful option.

CONCLUSION

This chapter has attempted to clarify some of the issues particularly relevant to women with alcohol problems. Information on how to take a simple drinking history as part of a routine examination is recommended for this group of patients who have particular difficulty in acknowledging drinking problems.

ACKNOWLEDGEMENT

This chapter is based upon a review funded by the Scotch Whisky Association.

USEFUL ADDRESSES

Alcohol Concern, 305 Gray's Inn Road, London WC1X 8QF.

Scottish Council on Alcoholism, 147 Blythswood Street, Glasgow G2 4EN.

REFERENCES AND FURTHER READING

Anderson, P., Wallace, P., and Jones, H. (1987). Cut Down on Your Drinking (kit).

Bagnall, G., Plant, M. A., and Warwick, W. (1990). Alcohol, drugs and AIDS-related risks: results from a prospective study. *AIDS Care*, **2**, 309–17.

Breeze, E. (1985). *Women and drinking*, Office of Population Censuses and Surveys. HMSO, London.

Brewers' Society (1990). *UK statistical handbook*. Brewers' Society, London.

Bruun, K., Edwards, G., Lumio, M., *et al.* (1975). *Alcohol control policies in public health perspective*, Vol. 25. Finnish Foundation for Alcohol Studies, Helsinki.

Camberwell Council on Alcohol (ed.) (1980). *Women and alcohol*. Tavistock, London.

Curran, V. and Golombok, S. (1985). *Bottling it up*. Faber & Faber, London.

Dight, S. (1976). *Scottish alcohol habits*. HMSO, London.

Duffy, J. C. and Latcham, R. W. (1986). Liver cirrhosis mortality in England and Wales compared to Scotland: an age-period-cohort analysis 1941–1981. *The Journal of the Royal Statistical Society*, **149**, (1), 45–59.

Duffy, J. C. (1991). *Trends in alcohol consumption patterns 1978–1989*. NTC Publications, England.

El-Guebaly, N. (1979). On being the offspring of an alcoholic: an update. *Clinical and Experimental Research*, **3**, 1480.

Grant, M. (1984). *Same again*. Pelican, Harmondsworth.

Harlap, S. and Shiona, P. H. (1980). Alcohol, smoking and the incidence of spontaneous abortions in the first and second trimester. *Lancet*, **2**, 173–6.

Health Education Authority (1990). *A women's guide to sensible drinking*. HEA, London.

Heather, N. and Robertson, I. (1983). *Controlled drinking*. Methuen, London.

Heather, N. and Robertson, I. (1989). *Problem drinking* (2nd edn). Oxford University Press.

Hill, S. Y. (1984). Vulnerability to the biomedical consequences of alcoholism and alcohol-related problems. In *Alcohol problems in women* (ed. S. C. Wilsnack and L. J. Beckman), pp. 121–54. Guildford Press, New York.

Jones, K. L. and Smith, D. W. (1973). Recognition of the fetal alcohol syndrome in early infancy. *Lancet*, **2**, 999–1001.

Kalant, O. J. (1980). *Alcohol and drug problems in women: research advances in alcohol and drug problems*, Vol. 5. Plenum Press, London.

Kline, J., Shrout, P., Stein, Z., *et al.* (1980). Drinking during pregnancy and spontaneous abortion. *Lancet*, July 26, 176–80.

MacAndrew, C. and Edgerton, R. R. (1969). *Drunken comportment: a social explanation*. Aldine, Chicago.

Orford, J. (1990). Alcohol and the family: an international review of the literature with implications for research and practice. In *Research advances in alcohol and drug problems*, Vol. 10, (ed. L. T. Kozlowski, H. M. Annis, H. D. Cappell *et al.*). Plenum, New York.

Orford, J. and Velleman, R. (1990). Offspring of parents with drinking problems: drinking and drug-taking as young adults. *British Journal of Addiction*, **85**, 779–94.

Plant, M. A. (ed.) (1982). *Drinking and problem drinking*. Junction/Fourth Estate, London.

Plant, M. A. (1990). Alcohol, sex and AIDS. *Alcohol and Alcoholism*, **29**, 293–301.

Plant, M. A., Peck, D. F., and Stuart, R. (1984). The correlates of serious alcohol-related consequences and illicit drug use amongst a cohort of Scottish teenagers. *British Journal of Addiction*, **79**,(2), 197–200.

Plant, M. A., Peck, D. F., and Samuel, E. (1985). *Alcohol, drugs and school-leavers*. Tavistock, London.

Plant, M. L. (1987). *Women, drinking and pregnancy*. Tavistock, London.

Plant, M. L. (1990). *Women and alcohol: a review of international literature on the use of alcohol by females*. World Health Organization, Geneva.

Plant, M. L. (1992). Alcohol and breast cancer: a review. *International Journal of the Addictions*, **27**, (2) 107–28.

Robertson, I. and Heather, N. (1984). *So you want to cut down your drinking?* Scottish Health Education Group, Edinburgh.

Robertson, I. and Heather, N. (1986). *Let's drink to your health: a self-help guide to sensible drinking*. British Psychological Society, Leicester.

Robertson, J. A. and Plant, M. A. (1988). Alcohol, sex and risks of HIV infection. *Drug and Alcohol Dependence*, **22**, 75–8.

Room, R. and Collins. G. (ed.) (1983). *Alcohol and disinhibition: nature and meaning of the link*, Research Monograph No. 12. National Institue on Alcohol Abuse and Alcoholism, Rockville, Maryland.

Royal College of General Practitioners (1987). *Alcohol: a Balanced View*. Royal College of General Practitioners, London.

Royal College of Physicians (1987). *A great and growing evil: the medical consequences of alcohol abuse*. Tavistock, London.

Royal College of Psychiatrists (1986). *Alcohol: our favourite drug*. Tavistock, London.

Sales, J., Duffy, J., Plant, M. A., *et al.* (1989). Alcohol consumption, cigarette sales and mortality in the United Kingdom: an analysis of the period 1970–1985. *Drug and Alcohol Dependence*, **24**, 155–60.

Health Education Board for Scotland (1990). *The DRAMS Scheme: helping problem drinkers*. Health Education Board for Scotland, Edinburgh.

Soloman, D. and Andrews, G. (ed.) (1973). *Drugs and sexuality*. Panther, St. Albans.

Stall, R. (1987). The prevention of HIV infection associated with drug and alcohol use during sexual activity. In *AIDS and substance abuse* (ed. L. Siegel), pp. 73–88. Harrington Park Press, New York.

Strunin, L. and Hingson, R. (1987). Acquired immune deficiency syndrome and adolescents: knowledge, beliefs, attitudes and behaviors. *Pediatrics*, **79**, 825–8.

Temple, M. and Leigh, B. (1990). *Alcohol and sexual behaviour in discrete events. I. Characteristics of sexual encounters involving and not involving alcohol.* Paper presented at Alcohol Epidemiology Symposium, Kettil Bruun Society, Budapest, Hungary.

Thom, B. (1986). Sex differences in help-seeking for alcohol problems. 1. Barriers to help-seeking. *British Journal of Addiction,* **81,** 777–88.

Thorley, A. (1982). The effects of alcohol. In *Drinking and problem drinking,* p. 47. Junction Fourth Estate, London.

Vannicelli, M. (1984). Treatment outcome of alcoholic women: the state of the art in relation to sex bias and expectancy effects. In *Alcohol problems in women* (ed. S. C. Wilsnack and L. J. Beckman). Guildford Press, New York.

Wallace, P. and Haines, A. (1985). Use of a questionnaire in general practice to increase the recognition of problem drinkers. *British Medical Journal,* **290,** 1949–53.

Williams, C. N. and Klerman, L. V. (1984). Female alcohol abuse: its effects on the family. In *Alcohol problems and women* (ed. S. C. Wilsnack and L. J. Beckman), pp. 280–312. Guildford Press, New York.

Williams, R. R. and Horn, J. W. (1977). Association of cancer sites with tobacco and alcohol consumption and socioeconomic status of patients: interview study from the Third National Cancer Survey. *Journal of the National Cancer Institute,* **58,** 525–47.

Wilsnack, S. C. and Beckman, L. J. (1984). *Alcohol problems in women.* Guildford Press, New York.

19. Women and smoking

Patti White

For many years the urgency of the epidemic of smoking-related diseases among men overshadowed women's smoking and its health consequences. In the late 1970s there was a dawning realization that there were nearly as many women smoking as men, and smoking diseases—traditionally thought of as men's diseases—were killing women in epidemic proportions. Girls had started to smoke more too and the tobacco industry, ever alert to the opportunities of winning new customers, increasingly targeted the female market. It soon became apparent how very little was known about women's smoking habits and the factors that influenced women to become and continue to be smokers. Now more information is available on this critical subject, but much remains to be done to understand and to help women smokers.

TRENDS IN WOMEN'S SMOKING

In the early decades of this century, smoking was almost exclusively a male habit, but gradually it became more socially acceptable for women to smoke. Greater numbers of British women began to take up the habit about the time of the Second World War, but even in 1948 about 7 in 10 men smoked cigarettes compared to 4 in 10 women (Wald and Kiryluk 1988).

Now the proportions of men and women who smoke cigarettes are nearly the same. Since 1972, questions about smoking have been asked biennially in the General Household Survey. The most striking aspect of smoking prevalence over this period is the narrowing of the gap between the proportions of men and women who smoke cigarettes (see Fig. 19.1). The prevalence of cigarette smoking has declined more steeply among men, falling from 52 per cent in 1972 to 31 per cent in 1990. Among women, 42 per cent were cigarette smokers in 1972 compared with 29 per cent in 1990 (OPCS 1991).

Since 1972, smoking prevalence for both sexes has been higher in Scotland than in Great Britain as a whole but whereas men's smoking fell between 1972 and 1988, prevalence among women actually rose between 1984 (35 per cent) and 1988 (37 per cent). In 1988, smoking prevalence among women in Great Britain as a whole was 30 per cent (ASH Scotland and EB for Scotland 1991).

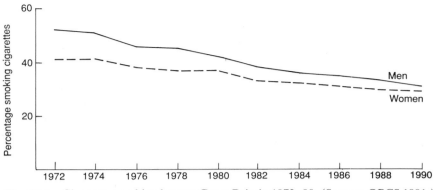

Fig. 19.1 Cigarette smoking by sex: Great Britain 1972–90. (Source: OPCS 1991.)

The comparatively more rapid decline in men's cigarette smoking has fostered a commonly held belief that women are not as good as men at giving up smoking. But the difference in men's and women's so-called 'quit rate' diminishes when all tobacco use is taken into account. When women stop smoking cigarettes they rarely switch to cigars or a pipe as men sometimes do. There is evidence that former cigarette smokers continue to inhale when they switch to other forms of smoking. It has been argued that these smokers have probably not realized a significant health benefit from giving up cigarettes and should not be classified as non-smokers (Jarvis 1984).

Younger smokers

Smoking among younger people continues to be one of the most worrying aspects of current cigarette-smoking patterns. Between 1988 and 1990 smoking prevalence increased among women aged 16–24 years, although it fell among older women. In 1990, smoking prevalence was higher among women in the 16–19 age group (32 per cent) than among men (28 per cent) of the same age (OPCS 1991).

The 1990 OPCS survey of smoking among secondary school children showed that 10 per cent of 11- to 15-year-olds in England and Wales were regular smokers, as were 12 per cent of those in Scotland. Smoking prevalence rises with age: in 1990 about a quarter of British 15-year-olds were regular smokers. Over a quarter of these regular smokers were already reporting consumption of 10 or more cigarettes a day (Lader and Matheson 1991).

Ethnicity

It is difficult to get a clear picture of smoking trends in black and minority ethnic groups in Great Britain because data on smoking status usually relies on a record of the individual's country of birth. While this gives information on immigrants, it misses out the British-born members of these groups. However, there are some indications of smoking prevalence among different ethnic groups.

Unlike the situation in North America and elsewhere, cigarette smoking seems to be more prevalent in the white population of Britain than in other ethnic groups. An analysis of General Household Survey data for 1978 and 1980 showed that heavy smoking was lower than the national average for those born in the West Indies and lower still for those born on the Indian subcontinent (Balarajan and Yuen 1986).

Studies of smoking habits of pregnant women have also found that white women are more likely to smoke, and to smoke more heavily, than Asian or Afro-Caribbean women. One antenatal clinic study found about a third of pregnant women of European origin were smokers compared with about a quarter of Afro-Caribbean women and about a tenth of Oriental and Asian women (Waterson and Murray-Lyon 1989).

Although cigarette smoking may be rare among Asian women, chewing 'pan', a mixture of betel nut, lime, and tobacco, is not uncommon; use of tobacco in this way is associated with an increased risk of oral cancer.

Smoking is likely to become more of a problem among minority ethnic groups as their British-born children become assimilated into the cultural norms of their peers. Research commissioned by the Health Education Authority found similar smoking rates among 16–19-year-old Afro-Caribbean and white youngsters living in England. However, fewer Asian youths smoked (HEA/MORI unpublished).

SMOKING AND DISEASE

It is by now almost a cliché that smoking is the leading preventable cause of premature death in the UK. In 1988, the total of smoking-attributable deaths was estimated to be 111 000—or about one death every five minutes (HEA 1991). Nearly 8 in 10 smoking-attributable deaths are due to coronary heart disease, lung cancer, and chronic obstructive lung disease, although tobacco use is associated with an impressive range of diseases (Table 19.1).

Because men started smoking cigarettes about a generation before women did, it was not at first apparent that women were liable to smoking-related diseases. But in reality, in addition to the smoking-related diseases that men are subjected to, women experience some that are specific to their gender.

Cancer

Lung cancer
In 1988, over 8400 women in the UK died prematurely due to smoking-attributable lung cancer (HEA 1991). Female lung cancer rates have

Table 19.1   *Smoking-related diseases*

Cardiovascular diseases:
  Coronary heart disease
  Cerebrovascular disease
  Atherosclerotic aortic aneurysm
  Atherosclerotic peripheral vascular disease

Cancer:
  Lung, laryngeal, oral, oesophageal, bladder, liver, pancreatic, renal, gastric, cervical; leukaemia

Diseases of the respiratory system:
  Chronic bronchitis
  Emphysema

Peptic ulcer disease

Complications of pregnancy

Source: US DHHS (1989).

increased by about two and a half times in the last 20 years, reflecting the great surge in women's smoking during the Second World War and after.

Breast cancer kills more British women than does lung cancer, but the relative importance of these diseases is changing. The UK is exhibiting what appears to be a trend common to Western countries: lung cancer is overtaking cancer of the breast as the leading cause of cancer mortality among women. In the US, this was the case by the mid-1980s and it has been predicted that the UK will follow suit early in the next century. In Scotland and some parts of England more women are already dying of lung cancer than of breast cancer.

Lung cancer risk increases with the number of cigarettes smoked per day, the duration of smoking, and the tar level of the cigarette smoked. A smoker of 1–14 cigarettes a day has an eight times greater risk of lung cancer than does a non-smoker. For those who smoke more than 25 a day, the risk rises to 25-fold. However, stopping smoking reduces the risk of lung cancer compared to smokers. The risk of lung cancer in ex-smokers is about 30 to 50 per cent less than that of continuing smokers (US DHHS 1990).

Other cancers

A number of studies have suggested that women who smoke are at increased risk of developing cervical neoplasia or invasive cancer. One study (La Vecchia *et al.* 1986) found the risk of developing cervical neoplasia to be 1.8 times higher and that of developing cervical cancer 1.7 times higher among current smokers than among those who had never smoked. The risk increased with the number of cigarettes smoked and was apparently greater for women who started smoking at younger ages. Ex-smokers have a substantially lower risk of cervical cancer than do continuing smokers, even in the first few years after cessation (US DHHS 1990).

Cancer of the endometrium is one of the few diseases for which there is evidence of lower risk among smokers. The risk of endometrial cancer among current smokers is approximately 30 per cent lower than that among non-smokers. The reasons for this lower risk are not well understood, but it may be due to the effects of smoking on oestrogen production.

Cardiovascular disease

The UK death rates from coronary heart disease (CHD) are among the highest in the world. Cigarette smokers have about twice the risk of dying from CHD compared with lifetime non-smokers. The relative importance of smoking as a risk factor is even more pronounced in younger women. It has been estimated that cigarette smoking may account for as much as two-thirds of the incidence of myocardial infarction in women under 50 (Rosenberg *et al.* 1985).

It is estimated that stopping smoking halves the excess risk of CHD caused by smoking after one year of abstinence. After 15 years, risk of CHD is similar to that of people who have never smoked. For people with diagnosed CHD, stopping smoking significantly reduces the risk of having another heart attack (US DHHS 1990).

For young women who use oral contraceptives, smoking increases the risk of a heart attack, stroke, or other cardiovascular disease tenfold. The risk is even higher for women over the age of 45.

Cigarette smoking is a major independent risk factor for the development of peripheral vascular disease in women. Female smokers also experience an increased risk of subarachnoid haemorrhage but stopping smoking reduces the risk.

Chronic obstructive pulmonary disease

About three-quarters of all deaths from chronic obstructive pulmonary disease (COPD) in the UK are attributable to smoking. The association of smoking and chronic bronchitis observed in men has been confirmed in women (Doll *et al.* 1980). For women who reported smoking 15 or more cigarettes a day, the mortality rate due to chronic bronchitis and emphysema was more than five times as great as in non-smokers. Deaths from these diseases were more than doubled in smokers compared to non-smokers and were twice as high in current heavy smokers (25 or more cigarettes a day) as in light smokers (15 or fewer cigarettes a day).

Smoking and reproduction

Pregnancy

The effects of maternal smoking on the fetus have been documented since the late 1950s. Children born to mothers who smoke during pregnancy are, on average, 200 g lighter than children born to comparable women who do not smoke. The relationship of smoking and low birthweight persists after adjustment for other factors such as race, parity, maternal size, and socio-economic status. The more cigarettes a woman smokes during pregnancy, the greater the probable reduction in birthweight.

However, giving up smoking is of considerable benefit. Women who quit smoking before becoming pregnant have infants of the same weight as those born to women who have never smoked. Pregnant smokers who quit any time up to the 30th week of pregnancy deliver infants with higher birthweight than do those who continue to smoke throughout pregnancy (US DHHS 1990).

On average, smokers have more complications of pregnancy and labour which can include placenta previa, abruptio placenta, bleeding during pregnancy, and premature rupture of the membranes. Several studies have demonstrated an association between maternal smoking and spontaneous abortion.

Other reproductive conditions

Women who smoke are more likely to have problems with fertility and take longer to conceive, but quitting smoking appears to return fertility to that of lifetime non-smokers. Several reports also show an increased risk of ectopic pregnancy in smokers. It has been suggested that current smokers may have a twofold increased risk of ectopic pregnancy compared with never-smokers (US DHHS 1990). Recent research has shown an association between smoking and abnormal menstrual patterns such as prolonged, heavy, painful, or irregular periods. Women smokers are also liable to experience the menopause about two years earlier than non-smokers. A dose-response effect has been found with heavier smokers having an even earlier menopause than lighter smokers. Osteoporosis is also more common in smokers than in non-smokers.

WHY DO GIRLS AND WOMEN SMOKE?

Starting to smoke

The great majority of adult smokers started smoking as children and adolescents. Children's attitudes and beliefs are reflections of the environment in which they live and boys and girls share many of the same pressures to smoke. Siblings' and parents' smoking and that of friends are important influences on young smokers, although girls may be slightly more influenced by parents' smoking and less by their peer group.

Children's smoking is also influenced by all the factors that affect adult smoking but some have a more marked effect on children. In recent years there has been extensive research which demonstrates the influence of tobacco advertising and promotion on children. Although tobacco advertising has been banned from British television for more than a quarter of a century, nearly two-thirds of children claim to have seen such advertising. This is almost certainly because of extensive tobacco sponsorship of sporting events on television (HEA 1990).

Cigarettes are heavily advertised in the media that are seen almost exclusively by women and girls—women's magazines. Although a direct appeal to femininity (or masculinity) is forbidden by rules governing tobacco advertising which are agreed between the tobacco industry and the government, brands aimed at women are frequently associated with the words 'slim', 'thin', or 'light', reinforcing the belief that smoking will make you thin. Even though the government has taken some steps to restrict cigarette advertising in magazines with a large proportion of young female readers, a collective readership of seven million young women aged 16–25 is still exposed to tobacco advertising from this source (ASH 1990).

For many young people the immediate, positive aspects of smoking outweigh the seemingly remote possibilities of disease, disability, and premature death. Beliefs about the perceived 'benefits' of smoking, such as calming the nerves, promoting relaxation, aiding concentration, and so on, are more important to girls than to boys. Girls are also more likely to believe that smoking will help them control their weight. One study of teenagers' smoking habits found that the main anxiety about stopping smoking among 16-year-old girls was the fear of putting on weight. The belief that smoking controlled weight was closely related to girls' smoking (Charlton 1984).

What keeps women smoking?

Girls carry many of their reasons for smoking with them into adulthood. Social influences, such as smoking by other family members and friends, smoking in the work-place, and tobacco advertising directed at women, help to maintain the smoking habit.

Both men and women at the lower end of the socio-economic scale smoke more than their middle-class counterparts. Smoking is also related to education, with those with fewer educational qualifications being the most likely to smoke (see Fig. 19.2).

Nicotine is, of course, a powerful psycho-active drug and for many smokers a dependence on nicotine can make giving up smoking very difficult.

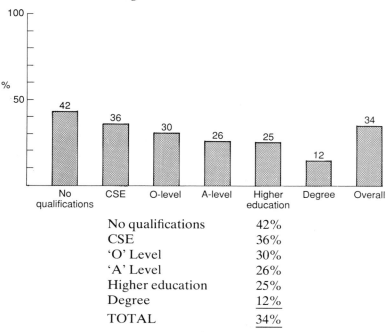

No qualifications	42%	
CSE	36%	
'O' Level	30%	
'A' Level	26%	
Higher education	25%	
Degree	12%	
TOTAL	34%	

Fig. 19.2 Cigarette smoking by highest educational qualification attained by women aged 16–19 years not in full-time education, Great Britain, 1988. (Source: OPCS 1989.)

Even teenage smokers can become dependent on nicotine surprisingly quickly. Although the number of cigarettes they smoke daily is small compared to adults, girls show the same withdrawal symptoms as adult smokers.

There are also strong psychological factors that influence women's smoking. It has been argued (Jacobson 1986) that women are more psychologically dependent on cigarettes than are men because women use cigarettes as a release from stress and as a method of suppressing the anger that a sexist society finds unacceptable in a woman.

The role of stress and the use of smoking as a 'coping mechanism' has been the subject of spirited discussion in the last decade. One difficulty is determining what women mean by 'stress'. By all measures, women's lives are more stressed than are men's. In general, women have more responsibilities than men do, and although this greater burden makes women's lives more stressed, they cope with it. One major study of smoking attitudes and behaviours confirmed that women experience more stress but that this is not an obstacle to stopping smoking (Marsh and Matheson 1983).

Those women who are most likely to say that smoking is a vital ingredient in their ability to cope are those who are living on low incomes, often in poor housing and with pre-school children. For women struggling to care for a family on a small budget, cigarettes are often the only thing they spend money on for themselves. Unlike clothes, magazines, or make-up, cigarettes are seen by some women as a necessary luxury that helps them deal with 'nerves', anger, fatigue, and even hunger (Graham 1987). Cigarettes occupy a very important place in these women's lives. Even women who are not living in conditions of deprivation can use cigarettes as a treat for themselves, perhaps to take an 'adult' break from the kids, or to share with a friend over a cup of coffee. The kind of emotional investment women make in smoking can both postpone the decision to try to give up and trigger a relapse into smoking.

HELPING SMOKERS TO STOP

How do smokers quit?

Stopping smoking is not an event when a smoker is 'cured' of her habit, but a dynamic process involving changing beliefs and behaviour. It has been convincingly argued that smokers weigh up their beliefs about the comparative costs and benefits of smoking and, even if their beliefs are wrong, try to act on them. Thus, for some smokers, the perceived benefits of smoking—such as a way to help them 'cope' or control weight, or as a source of pleasure and relaxation—may seem of greater benefit than the expense of their habit or a 'remote' possibility of disease (Marsh and Matheson 1983).

The process of moving from being a 'contented' smoker to one who thinks about trying to give up and eventually makes an attempt to do so is influenced by a variety of factors. Some of these factors are internal, such as physical dependence on nicotine; others are external, such as anxiety about the health consequences, the price of cigarettes, or the recommendation to quit from a GP.

The process of stopping smoking has been described as a revolving door (Fig. 19.3) from which a smoker may eventually exit. It is possible to encourage and help smokers at different points throughout this process. For example, health education may move a 'contented' smoker to think about stopping. A suggestion to stop, from a doctor or other respected person, might give a smoker the determination to make a serious attempt at quitting.

Research indicates that at any one attempt, most smokers will relapse. It is common for smokers to go through a cycle of deciding to stop, making an

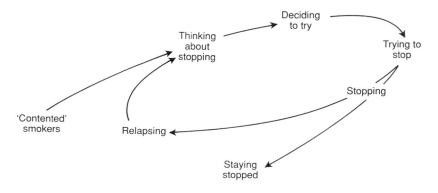

Fig. 19.3   Stopping smoking as a process. (Source: Raw 1988.)

attempt to do so, and relapsing several times before achieving long-term abstinence.

While some smokers may find the high prospects of such 'failure' discouraging and may be daunted by the length of time it may take them finally to give up smoking, there is potentially much to find encouraging in this understanding of the process of smoking cessation. On this view, what may be immediately a failed attempt to achieve one's goal may well be a stage in the progress towards success.

General practitioners' advice

Research from the UK, Australia, and the US indicates that general practitioners can encourage and help smoking patients to quit through routine use of brief smoking cessation techniques. Now, with a growing number of health promotion clinics in general practice and the need to offer routine health checks, the role of the GP in smoking cessation will increase.

A GP can achieve a small but marked reduction in the proportion of smoking patients just by offering simple cessation advice (Russell *et al.* 1979). The addition of an offer of nicotine chewing gum doubles the success rate (Russell *et al.* 1983). Using other minimal intervention techniques, such as measuring expired-air carbon monoxide levels, increases the success rate, especially among social classes IV and V (Jamrozik *et al.* 1984).

As a matter of routine, a brief smoking history should be obtained from each patient and her current smoking habits—smoking status and amount smoked—recorded. Every opportunity should be sought to inform those who smoke of the dangers of smoking and especially the benefits of stopping. Advice can be supported with simple literature and, where appropriate, the offer of nicotine gum and/or patches.

Several different national agencies provide a range of materials to help smokers, including the cessation leaflets available from the national health education agencies. Most local health promotion units will also be able to provide supporting materials, publications as well as videos, and will often be able to lend local practices a carbon monoxide monitor. (These monitors, now very easy to use and compact in size, are available in the UK at a modest cost.) Many health promotion units also organize local events and publicity around No Smoking Day, an event that is increasingly important in motivating smokers and providing a focus for setting a date to try to give up.

Other support for smokers

Nicotine replacement

Nicotine replacement is the only cessation treatment that has received extensive clinical evaluation. While the gum has been with us for years, two new forms of nicotine delivery, a kind of nose spray and a transdermal patch, are being tested in the UK. Nicotine chewing gum (Nicorette) seems to be most suitable for heavier smokers and those who, although motivated, may have already made several attempts to give up. The gum is available in two strengths, 2 mg or 4 mg of nicotine per piece. The 4-mg is available on prescription but the 2-mg strength can now be purchased over the counter.

The gum does not feel or taste like normal chewing gum and it is important that it is used according to the instructions. Nicotine chewing gum has been shown to be most effective when used as part of a stop-smoking programme. It is not, however, recommended for pregnant women or nursing mothers.

Support groups

The cost effectiveness of smokers' support groups has sometimes been questioned. The criticism is that such intensive support can only be offered to a comparatively small number of smokers and thus these groups are not cost effective when compared with more minimal techniques, such as GPs' advice, that reach a much larger number of smokers. This argument overlooks the greater health risks for heavier, addicted smokers and a very real need for help among a minority of smokers.

Although an estimated 90 per cent of ex-smokers give up without formal support, the remaining 10 per cent may need more help. People who go to the trouble of attending groups tend to be heavier, more dependent smokers (Raw and Heller 1984). Heavier smokers are more at risk of smoking-related diseases and are therefore an important target for help. An effective smokers' support group is the most efficient way to provide help for this group of smokers. Quitline is a service of the charity QUIT which offers telephone advice to smokers but also keeps a list of local smokers' support groups and counselling services.

Over the counter aids

There are many products on the market designed to help smokers quit. These include tablets, herbal and dummy cigarettes, filters, tapes and videos, books, hypnosis, and acupuncture. Clearly, none of these offers a sure-fire route to success. What is needed for a successful attempt at quitting is determination and self-confidence. These aids can be a useful support to those who are trying to quit, but none has been shown to be more effective than the others.

Many of these products are available in pharmacies and health food stores. Tablets and lozenges, some containing small amounts of nicotine and others using lobelia, a plant of the same family as tobacco, are said to decrease the craving for nicotine. There are also astringent products, usually containing silver acetate, that leave an unpleasant taste in the mouth after a cigarette is smoked.

Some smokers try filters or low tar cigarettes to cut down on nicotine as a prelude to giving up altogether. Unfortunately, this is usually self-defeating as smokers tend to compensate for the loss of nicotine by inhaling more deeply or taking more puffs from each cigarette. Generally, cutting down is more difficult than stopping 'cold turkey'. Other smokers switch to herbal cigarettes in an attempt to give up nicotine before breaking the other habits associated with smoking. Herbal cigarettes are themselves dangerous to health as they contain tar and carbon monoxide.

Many would-be ex-smokers are interested in acupuncture and hypnosis, perhaps because they view these treatments as a form of 'cure'. Smokers sometimes find them useful. The only drawback is the cost.

Smoking cessation and weight gain

It has long been received knowledge that only about a third of smokers gain weight after stopping smoking, while a third maintain weight, and the other third lose weight. But a 1990 review of the evidence by the US Surgeon General involving 15 studies and more than 20 000 persons confirmed what ex-smokers had claimed all along: a majority of ex-smokers, about 8 people in 10, put on weight after quitting. However, the average weight gain was small. It was found that on average continuing smokers gained about 0.8 lb while ex-smokers gained about 5 lb. Thus, smoking cessation produced an approximate 4 lb greater weight than continuing smoking.

Individual weight gains were quite variable, but the risk of large weight gain after quitting smoking was found to be very low: less than 4 per cent of ex-smokers gained more than 20 lb (DHHS 1990).

Greater food consumption and decreases in resting energy expenditure are thought to be largely responsible for weight gain after giving up smoking. Most short-term evaluations of eating changes that take place after smoking cessation have found that food consumption, particularly of sweet foods and simple carbohydrates, increases after stopping smoking. Advice about diet and exercise should be helpful to patients in avoiding or at least minimizing weight gain after quitting.

Several studies have indicated that smokers who use nicotine chewing gum as an aid to stopping smoking gain less weight than those who give up unaided. However, the use of nicotine gum seems to delay rather than prevent weight gain.

CONCLUSION

The picture of smoking among British women is not all gloomy. As a whole, smoking prevalence has been falling gradually among British women for nearly twenty years. However, there is no room for complacency since smoking is particularly high in some populations, including Scottish women and women in lower socio-economic groups. Especially worrying is the large number of young women starting to smoke.

Many of the adverse consequences of smoking can be avoided if smokers quit. This is often true even when symptoms of smoking-related disease have already manifested themselves. General practitioners have a unique opportunity to improve women's health by advising and encouraging their patients to give up smoking.

USEFUL ADDRESSES

ASH (Action on Smoking and Health), 109 Gloucester Place, London W1N 3PH. Tel: 071 935 3519. (Fact sheets, a selection of leaflets, posters, signs, stickers, fortnightly Information Bulletin and quarterly Newsletter. Library and information service. Resource list available.)

ASH Scotland, 8 Fredrick Street, Edinburgh EH2 2HB. Tel: 031 225 4725.

HEA Helios Project, Bristol Polytechnic, Redland Hill, Bristol BS6 6UZ. Tel: 0272 238317. (HELIOS stands for Health Education Local Initiatives on Smoking. The project supports health education officers and others with help and advice in smoking prevention work.)

National Smoking Cessation Resource Centre, QUIT Ltd, 102 Gloucester Place, London W1H 3DA. Tel: 071 487 2858. (Keeps a list of all the smoking cessation support groups and group leaders in the country, Leaflets, books, videos, newsletter available. Send for the Resource List.)

QUITLINE: 071 487 3000. (Telephone counselling service for people trying to stop smoking. Weekdays 9.30 am to 5.30 pm, individual counselling; a recorded message at other times.)

Smokestop, Department of Psychology, The University, Southampton S00 5NH. Tel: 0703 583741. (Training courses for smoking cessation self-help group leaders held regularly in Southampton.)

REFERENCES AND FURTHER READING

ASH (Action on Smoking and Health) Women and Smoking Working Group (1990). *Smoke still gets in her eyes.* ASH, London.
ASH (Action on Smoking and Health) Scotland and Health Education Board for Scotland (1991). *The smoking epidemic: counting the cost in Scotland.* ASH/HEB Scotland, Edinburgh.
Balarajan, R. and Yuen, P. (1986). British smoking and drinking habits: variation by country of birth. *Community Medicine,* **8,** 237–9.
Charlton, A. (1984). Smoking and weight control in teenagers. *Public Health,* **98,** 277–81.
Doll, R., Gray, R., Hafner, B., *et al.* (1980). Mortality in relation to smoking: 20 years' observations on female British doctors. *British Medical Journal,* **280,** 967–71.
Graham, H. (1987). Women's smoking and family health. *Social Science and Medicine,* **25,** 47–56.
HEA (Health Education Authority) (1990). *Beating the ban.* Health Education Authority, London.
HEA (Health Education Authority) (1991). *The smoking epidemic.* Health Education Authority, London.
HEA (Health Education Authority)/MORI (1990). *Young adults' health and lifestyles: smoking* (unpublished).
Jacobson, B. (1986). *Beating the ladykillers.* Pluto Press, London.
Jamrozik, K., Vessey, M., Fowler, G., *et al.* (1984). Controlled trial of three different antismoking interventions in general practice. *British Medical Journal,* **288,** 1499–503.
Jarvis, M. (1984). Gender and smoking: do women really find it harder to give up? *British Journal of Addiction,* **79,** 57–61.
Lader, D. and Matheson, J. (1991). *Smoking among secondary school children in 1990.* HMSO, London.
La Vecchia, C. *et al.* (1986). Cigarette smoking and the risk of cervical neoplasia. *American Journal of Epidemiology,* **123,** 22–9.
Marsh, M. and Matheson, J. (1983). *Smoking attitudes and behaviour.* HMSO, London.
OPCS (Office of Population Censuses and Surveys) (1989). *General household survey 1988.* HMSO, London.
OPCS (Office of Population Censuses and Surveys) (1991). *General household survey: cigarette smoking 1972 to 1990.* OPCS Monitor, SS91/3.
Raw, M. (1988). *Help your patient stop.* British Medical Association/Imperial Cancer Research Fund/World Health Organization/International Union Against Cancer, London.

Raw, M. and Heller, J. (1984). *Helping people stop smoking.* Health Education Council, London.

Rosenberg, L. *et al.* (1985). Myocardial infarction and cigarette smoking in women younger than 50 years of age. *Journal of the American Medical Association,* **253,** 2965–9.

Russell, M., Wilson, C., Taylor, C., *et al.* (1979). Effect of general practitioners' advice against smoking. *British Medical Journal,* **2,** 231–5.

Russell, M., Merriman, R., Stapleton, J., *et al.* (1983). Effect of nicotine chewing gum as an adjunct to general practitioners' advice against smoking. *British Medical Journal,* **287,** 1782–5.

US DHHS (Department of Health and Human Services) (1990). *The health benefits of smoking cessation: a report of the Surgeon General.* Public Health Service Centers for Disease Control, Atlanta.

Wald, N. and Kiryluk, S. (ed.) (1988). *UK smoking statistics.* Oxford University Press.

Waterson, E. and Murray-Lyon, I. (1989). Alcohol, smoking and pregnancy: some observations on ethnic minorities in the United Kingom. *British Journal of Addiction,* **84,** 323–5.

Index